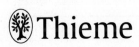

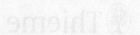

Pocket Atlas of Nutrition

Hans Konrad Biesalski, M.D.

Professor
Institute of Biological Chemistry and Nutrition Sciences
University of Hohenheim
Stuttgart, Germany

Peter Grimm, Ph.D.

Institute of Biological Chemistry and Nutrition Sciences
University of Hohenheim
Stuttgart, Germany

With the cooperation of Susanne Nowitzki-Grimm, Ph.D.

Translated and adapted for the American market by Sigrid Junkermann, M.S., B.A., Adj. Asst. Prof. of Biology and Nutrition, F.I.T., SUNY

177 color plates

Thieme
Stuttgart · New York

Library of Congress Cataloging-in-Publication Data

Biesalski, Hans Konrad
[Taschenatlas der Ernährung. English]
Pocket atlas of nutrition/
Hans Konrad Biesalski, Peter Grimm;
with the co-operation of Susanne Nowitzki-Grimm; translation and adaption to the
American market by Sigrid Junkermann. –
Rev. translation of 3rd German ed.
p.; cm.
Includes bibliographical references and index.
ISBN 3-13-135481-X (alk. paper) –
ISBN 1-58890-238-2 (alk. paper)
1. Nutrition–Handbooks, manuals, etc.
2. Nutrition–Atlases.
[DNLM: 1. Nutrition–Handbooks.]
I. Grimm, Peter, M.D. II. Title.
QP141.B5413 2005
613–dc22
2004028350

1st German edition 1999
2nd German edition 2002
1st French edition 2001

This book is an authorized and
completely revised translation based
on the 3rd German edition published and
copyrighted 2004 by Georg Thieme Verlag,
Stuttgart, Germany. Title of the German
edition: Taschenatlas der Ernährung

Translator: Sigrid Junkermann, New York

Color plates: Karin Baum, Mannheim

© 2005 Georg Thieme Verlag,
Rüdigerstrasse 14, 70469 Stuttgart,
Germany
http://www.thieme.de
Thieme New York, 333 Seventh Avenue,
New York, NY 10001 USA
http://www.thieme.com

Cover design: Cyclus, Stuttgart
Typesetting by Satzpunkt Ewert, Bayreuth
Printed in Germany by Appl, Wemding

ISBN 3-13-135481-X (GTV)
ISBN 1-58890-238-2 (TNY)   1 2 3 4 5

Important note: Medicine is an ever-changing science undergoing continual development. Research and clinical experience are continually expanding our knowledge, in particular our knowledge of proper treatment and drug therapy. Insofar as this book mentions any dosage or application, readers may rest assured that the authors, editors, and publishers have made every effort to ensure that such references are in accordance with **the state of knowledge at the time of production of the book.**
Nevertheless, this does not involve, imply, or express any guarantee or responsibility on the part of the publishers in respect to any dosage instructions and forms of applications stated in the book. **Every user is requested to examine carefully** the manufacturers' leaflets accompanying each drug and to check, if necessary in consultation with a physician or specialist, whether the dosage schedules mentioned therein or the contraindications stated by the manufacturers differ from the statements made in the present book. Such examination is particularly important with drugs that are either rarely used or have been newly released on the market. Every dosage schedule or every form of application used is entirely at the user's own risk and responsibility. The authors and publishers request every user to report to the publishers any discrepancies or inaccuracies noticed. If errors in this work are found after publication, errata will be posted at www.thieme.com on the product description page.

Foreword

The important role of nutrition in promoting health and preventing disease is well established. Although scientific understanding of the roles of various nutrients in human health has progressed rapidly over the past century, nutritional deficiencies remain a threat to the lives and health of millions of people throughout the world, particularly children. At the other end of the nutritional spectrum, a global epidemic of obesity is also threatening the lives and health of millions. Despite appearances, overweight and obesity are often associated with poor nutrition. Although poor nutritional status has long been associated with increased risk of infectious disease, a large body of evidence now supports the association of poor nutrition with increased risk of noninfectious chronic diseases.

Obesity is associated with an increased risk of several cancers, including colon cancer and postmenopausal breast cancer. It has been estimated that diet modification could potentially prevent as many as one third of cancers worldwide. Epidemiologists at Harvard have estimated that as much as 70% of stroke and colon cancer, 80% of coronary heart disease and 90% of type 2 diabetes could be prevented by a healthy diet, regular physical activity, and avoidance of smoking. After reviewing the large body of evidence linking diet and chronic disease risk, a number of expert panels have made surprisingly similar recommendations for a healthy diet:

- Achieve and maintain a healthy body weight
- Increase consumption of fruits, vegetables, legumes, and nuts
- Replace saturated and *trans* fats with unsaturated fats
- Replace refined grains with whole grains
- Limit sugar and salt intake
- Drink alcohol in moderation (if at all)

Although basic to health, the study of nutrition is complex and integrates knowledge from disciplines as varied as physiology, molecular biology, chemistry, psychology, sociology, economics and public policy. In this edition of the *Pocket Atlas of Nutrition*, Professors Biesalski and Grimm are providing health and nutrition professionals, students and motivated consumers with a useful nutrition resource that is broad in its scope yet concise in its delivery. The first section of the book provides the reader with an important foundation in nutrition science, including essential topics such as body composition, energy requirements, appetite regulation, and the physiology of nutrient digestion and absorption. Subsequent chapters on macronutrients (carbohydrates, proteins and fats) and micronutrients (vitamins and minerals) discuss relevant clinical issues, as well as current intake recommendations. A section on nutrition in specific life situations addresses important nutritional issues specific to the elderly, pregnant and lactating women, young children, and athletes, while a section on nutritional medicine provides additional information on the role of nutrition in chronic disease prevention and treatment. Throughout the book detailed figures clarify and expand on information discussed in the text.

Unlike some nutrition texts, the *Pocket Atlas of Nutrition* does not shy away from controversy. In addition to presenting the often-criticized U.S. Department of Agriculture Food Guide pyramid, the authors also discuss the merits of the Healthy-Eating Pyramid created by the Harvard School of Public Health and a pyramid based on the Mediterranean diet. Discussions of food quality, food additives and food safety that cover controversial topics from the genetic modification of foods to bovine spongiform encephalopathy (BSE) will be of interest to consumers and clinicians alike.

Despite the fact that there is general agreement among scientists regarding the basic components of a healthy diet, the proportion of the population that actually follows these guidelines is relatively small. Although consumers are interested in the relationship between diet and health, many are confused about what they should eat and whether they should take supplements.

Contributing to this confusion are seemingly contradictory nutritional sound bites supplied by the news media and well-funded marketing campaigns from food, dietary supplement, and weight loss industries. Now, more than ever, there is a need for nutrition and health professionals who understand and communicate consistent and accurate information regarding healthy diets and lifestyles. The *Pocket Atlas of Nutrition* will be a useful study guide and an excellent reference for those who want to learn more about the science of nutrition.

Jane Higdon, Ph.D.
Linus Pauling Institute
Oregon State University
Corvallis, Oregon

Preface

After 30 years of advice to eat low fat, the United States, followed closely by many other, mostly but not exclusively, industrialized nations, is witnessing an unprecedented epidemic increase in obesity and diabetes, to name just two. The cost of these developments to the individual and to society is enormous, and the projected cost for the future staggering. It is evident that the increase in obesity and diabetes is strongly related to faulty nutrition. Proper nutrition is probably the most effective and cost-effective prevention for these and many other diseases, including most cancers.

It should be clear to anyone by now that proper nutrition involves much more than having three meals a day. The written media abound with nutritional advice and information. Many books promote often extremely controversial guidelines for weight loss and better health. Frequently, articles and books are based on unproven assumptions, anecdotal evidence, or single scientific studies that seem to point in one or the other direction. The reader who tries to make sense of it all tends to be utterly confused.

Yet, even though nutritional science is relatively young, it is a hard science and many aspects have been thoroughly researched. Our knowledge of other aspects, such as the functions and effects of many secondary phytochemicals, or the multiple interactions between many body chemicals during nutrition-related metabolism, is evolving continually. Nutritional science is an interdisciplinary endeavor based on chemistry, biology, physiology, and anatomy, which are often hard to understand and even harder to present in a condensed, easy to assimilate fashion.

So where can the interested layperson turn for information? Where do professionals dealing with nutritional questions, physicians, nurses, pharmacists, teachers, etc.—who often have little or no nutritional training—turn for easily accessible, reliable, up-to-date, and comprehensive information? Where can dietitians and nutritionists quickly look up scientifically sound and up-to-date information about a particular nutritional topic?

This is where the *Pocket Atlas of Nutrition* comes in. It provides well-presented basic knowledge and presents the state of the art of nutritional science today. Of course, it cannot provide the in-depth approach of textbooks of nutrition, nutritional medicine, and related fields. We are hoping, though, that the compact presentation of knowledge typical of Thieme's Pocket Atlas series will provide the reader with quick insights and a relatively easy to obtain overview. If the book raises in the reader a skeptical attitude toward quickly drawn conclusions, that was our intent.

Recent advances in molecular biology have allowed nutritional science to advance rapidly, and the information resulting from this research is increasingly complex. Yet, even most recent research findings have been included in these chapters, sometimes still marked as open questions.

Nutritional science remains a work in progress. In tune with the latest concerns about public health, this edition includes several new chapters on preventive nutrition and more emphasis has been placed on nutritional medicine.

Hans Konrad Biesalski
Peter Grimm
Sigrid Junkermann (Translator)

As the translator and as a teacher of biology and nutrition, I found it an exciting endeavor to render this German book in English and adapt it to the American market. It made me research a number of topics, compare European with American conditions, deepen aspects of my knowledge, confirm and revise others, and overall gain a deeper insight into the state of the art and the present direction of nutritional science. I also wish to express my gratitude to Angelika Findgott of Thieme International for having found me and given me the opportunity to do this work, for being a great editor, collegial, wonderful, and fun to work with.

Sigrid Junkermann

The authors are glad to have secured the collaboration of Ms. Sigrid Junkermann for this English edition. She has not only produced an accurate translation of fine literary quality but has also, through her familiarity with American conditions and guidelines and her tireless commitment and dedication to the quality of the book, succeeded in adapting this edition optimally to the standard practice and terminology of English-speaking health care professionals.

We are grateful to the readers for suggestions and criticism, as well as for comments relating to the content.

H.K.B., P.G.

Contents

Introduction

Introduction 2
Preventive Nutrition:
A Science in Flux 4
Preventive Nutrition:
The Mediterranean Diet 6
The RDA and DRI 8
Assessing Current Status 10

Body Composition
Variable: Body Composition 12
Water in Body and Foods 14
Anthropometrics 16
Experimental Methods 18
Nutrient Compartmentalization:
Cellular Distribution 20
Nutrient Compartmentalization:
Distribution to the Organs–
Homeostasis 22

Energy Metabolism
The Biochemistry of Energy
Transfer 24

How Food Energy is Used 26
Individual Energy Requirements . . . 28
Energy Requirements 30
Tissue-Specific Energy Metabolism . 32
Control of Energy Metabolism 34

Food Intake
Regulation of Food Intake: Hunger
and Satiety 36
Leptin 38
Stomach Function 40

Nutrient Uptake
Anatomy and Histology 42
Cellular Mechanisms 44
The Colon: Active and Passive
Functions 46
Enterohepatic Circulation 48
Regulation of Digestion 50
Principles of Digestion 52

The Nutrients

Carbohydrates
Structure and Properties 56
Digestion and Absorption 58
Metabolism: Distribution and
Regulation 60
Metabolism: Glucose Storage 62
Glucose Homeostasis: Insulin and
Glucagon 64
Metabolic Homeostasis:
Blood Glucose Aspects 66
Glucose Tolerance 68
Fructose and Galactose 70
Sugar Alcohols: Metabolism 72
Sugar Alcohols: Occurrence 74
Glycoproteins 76
Fiber: Structure 78

Fiber: Effects 80
Occurrence and Requirements 82

Lipids
Classification 84
Fatty Acids 86
Lipid Digestion 88
Absorption 90
Transport 92
LDL-Receptor-Mediated
Metabolism 94
HDL Metabolism 96
Postprandial Lipid Distribution 98
Lipoprotein Lipase 100
Fatty Acids: Metabolism 102
Cholesterol: Biosynthesis 104

X   Contents

Cholesterol: Homeostasis 106
Regulatory Functions:
Membrane Structure 108
Regulatory Functions:
Eicosanoids 110
Regulatory Functions:
Influence of Nutrition 112
Occurrence and Requirements 114

Proteins
Proteins as a Source of Nitrogen ...116
Classification:
From Chain to 3-D Structure 118
Essential Building Blocks:
The Amino Acids 120
Digestion and Absorption 122
Metabolism 124
Amino Acid Homeostasis 126
Regulatory Functions:
Endothelial Functions 128
The Blood-Brain Barrier 130
Protein Quality 132
Occurrence and Requirements 134

Fat-Soluble Vitamins
Vitamin A: Chemistry 136
Vitamin A: Uptake and
Metabolism 138
Vitamin A: Functions 140
Vitamin A: Regulation of Gene
Expression 142
Vitamin A: Occurrence and
Requirements 144
β-carotenes: Chemistry and
Metabolism 146
β-carotenes: Functions,
Occurrence, and Requirements 148
Vitamin D: Chemistry and
Metabolism 150
Vitamin D: Functions 152
Vitamin D: Occurrence and
Requirements 154
Vitamin E: Chemistry and
Metabolism 156
Vitamin E: Functions, Occurrence,
and Requirements 158

Vitamin K: Chemistry, Metabolism,
and Functions 160
Vitamin K: Occurrence and
Requirements 162

Water-Soluble Vitamins
Ascorbic Acid: Chemistry,
Metabolism, and Functions 164
Ascorbic Acid:
Occurrence and Requirements 166
Thiamin: Chemistry, Metabolism,
and Functions 168
Thiamin: Occurrence and
Requirements 170
Riboflavin: Chemistry, Metabolism,
and Functions 172
Riboflavin: Occurrence and
Requirements 174
Niacin: Chemistry, Metabolism,
and Functions 176
Niacin: Occurrence of
Requirements 178
Pantothenic Acid: Chemistry,
Metabolism, and Functions 180
Pantothenic Acid:
Occurrence and Requirements 182
Biotin: Chemistry, Metabolism,
and Functions 184
Biotin: Occurrence and
Requirements 186
Pyridoxine: Chemistry, Metabolism,
and Functions 188
Pyridoxine: Occurrence and
Requirements 190
Cobalamin: Chemistry,
Metabolism, and Functions 192
Cobalamin: Occurrence and
Requirements 194
Folic Acid: Chemistry, Metabolism,
and Function 196
Folic Acid: Occurrence and
Requirements 198

Vitamin interactions
B Vitamin Interactions 200
Free Radicals: Formation and
Effects 202

Free Radicals: Endogenous
Systems 204
Free Radicals: Exogenous
Systems 206
Vitamin-Like Substances:
Choline and Inositol 208
Vitamin-Like Substances:
Nonvitamins 210

Minerals and Trace Elements
Calcium: Metabolism and
Functions 212
Calcium Homeostasis 214
Calcium: Occurrence and
Requirements 216
Phosphorus 218
Magnesium 220
Sulfur 222
Sodium Chloride 224
Potassium 226
Iron: Metabolism 228
Iron: Functions 230
Iron: Occurrence and
Requirements 232
Iodine: Metabolism 234
Iodine: Function and Deficiency ... 236
Iodine: Occurrence and
Requirements 238
Fluorine 240
Selenium: Metabolism and
Functions 242
Selenium: Occurrence and
Requirements 244
Zinc: Metabolism and Functions .. 246
Zinc: Occurrence and
Requirements 248
Copper: Metabolism and
Functions I 250
Copper: Functions II, Occurrence,
and Requirements 252

Manganese 254
Molybdenum 256
Chromium 258
Vanadium 260
Tin and Nickel 262
Cobalt, Boron, and Lithium 264
Silicon, Arsenic, and Lead 266

Other Nutrients, Additives, and Contaminants
Secondary Phytochemicals:
An Overview..................... 268
Secondary Phytochemicals: Effects
and Activity 270

Nonnutritive Nutrients
Alcohol: Metabolism 272
Alcohol and Health 274
Alcohol and Nutrition 276
Herbs and Spices 278
Additives: An Overview 280
Sweeteners 282
Contaminants I: Nitrate/Nitrite ... 284
Contaminants II:
Residues and Pollutants 286
Pre- and Probiotics 288
Functional Foods and
Nutraceuticals 290

Food Quality
Quality Defined 292
New Methods for Quality
Optimization I: Preservation 294
New Methods for Quality
Optimization II: Genetic
Modification 296
Nutrient Content, Processing, and
Storage 298
Hygiene 300

Applied and Medical Nutrition

Nutritional Guidelines
Nutrition for Healthy People I 304
Nutrition for Healthy People II 306

Vegetarianism 308
Separation Nutrition 310
Outsider Diets 312

Nutrition in Specific Life Stages
Pregnancy 314
Lactation 316
From Neonate to Adolescent 318
Seniors 320
Athletes 322
Ergogenic Aids 324

Selected Issues in Food Safety
Drugs and Diet I 326
Drugs and Diet II 328
Prion Diseases 330
Prion Diseases in the U.S. 332
Creutzfeldt-Jakob Disease
(CJD and vCJD) 334

Medical Nutrition
Eating Disorders 336

Underweight 338
Obesity 340
Diabetes Mellitus: Pathogenesis ... 342
Pathologies Associated with
Diabetes Mellitus 342
Molecular Mechanisms 342
Pathologies of Fat Metabolism:
Hyperlipoproteinemia 344
Therapy 344
Metabolic Syndrome:
Insulin Resistance Syndrome 346
Osteoporosis 348
Age-Related Macular
Degeneration (AMD) 350
Cancer 352
Chronic Inflammatory Bowel
Disease (CIBD) 354

Appendix

Table of Measures 358
General References 359
Selected Websites 359

Figure Sources 360
Index 361

Abbreviations

11-β-OHSD	11-β-hydroxysteroid dehydrogenase	Arg	Arginine
5HT	5-hydroxytryptamine	As	Arsenic
5-methyl-THF or H_3C-PteGLU	5-methyl-tetrahydrofolic acid	As_2O_3	Arsenic trioxide
		Asp	Aspartic acid
AA	Amino acids	ATP	Adenosine triphosphate
AAS	Amino acid score	AUC	Area under the curve
ACAT	Acyl-CoA cholesterol acyl-transferase	B	Boron
		BCCA	Branched chain amino acids
Acetyl-CoA	Acetyl coenzyme A		
ADH	Antidiuretic hormone	BIA	Bioelectrical impedance
ADH	Alcohol dehydrogenase		
		BMI	Body mass index
ADI	Acceptable Daily Intake	BMR	Basal metabolic rate
		BN	Bulimia nervosa
ADP	Adenosine diphosphate	BRFSS	Behavioral Risk Factor Surveillance System (CDC)
AGE	Advanced glycylation end products	BSE	Bovine spongiform encephalopathy
AHEI	Harvard School of Public Health Alternative Healthy Eating Index	BV	Biological value
		Ca	Calcium
		CaBP	Calcium-binding protein
AI	Adequate Intake	CAD	Coronary artery disease
ALDH	Aldehyde dehydrogenase		
		CCK	Cholecystokinin
AMD	Age-related macular degeneration	CCO	Cytochrome C oxidase
		CDC	Centers for Disease Control
AMDR	Acceptable Macronutrient Distribution Range	CE	Cholesterol esters
		CETP	Cholesterol ester transfer protein
AMP	Adenosine monophosphate	CH_3-Pte	Methyl tetrahydrofolic acid
AMR	Advanced meat recovery	CIBD	Chronic inflammatory bowel disease
AN	Anorexia nervosa		
ANF	Atrial natriuretic factor	CJD	Creutzfeldt-Jakob disease
APHIS	Animal and Plant Health Inspection Service	CLA	Conjugated linoleic acid
		CM	Chylomicrons
ARAT	Acyl-CoA-retinol acyl-transferase	Co	Cobalt
		CoA	Coenzyme A
AREDS	Age-related eye disease study	Cp	Ceruloplasmin

Cr	Chromium	FDC	Follicular dendritic cell
CRALBP	Cellular retinal-binding protein	FD&C	Federal Food, Drug, and Cosmetic (Act)
CRBP	Cellular retinol-binding protein	Fe	Iron
CRF	Corticotropin releasing factor	FEMA	Federal Emergency Management Agency
CRIP	Cysteine-rich intestinal protein	FFA	Free fatty acids
Cu	Copper	FMN	Flavin mono-nucleotide
CuSOD	CuZn-Superoxide dismutase	G6P	Glucose-6-phosphate
CVD	Cardiovascular disease	GAG	Glycosaminoglycan
		Gal	Galactose
CWD	Chronic wasting disease	GI	Glycemic index
		GL	Glycemic load
Cys	Cysteine	GLC	Glucose
DBP	Vitamin D-binding protein	GlcNAc	N-acetyl-glucosamine
		Gln	Glutamine
DFE	Dietary folate equivalents	GLP-1	Glucagon-like peptide 1
		GLU	Glutamate
DLW	Doubly labeled water technique	GLU	Glucoronic acid
		Gly	Glycine
DM	Diabetes mellitus	GM	Genetic modification
DRI	Dietary Reference Intakes	GMP	Good manufacturing practices
DT	Delirium tremens	GR	Glutathione reductase
EAR	Estimated Average Requirement	GRAS	Generally Recognized As Safe
ECW	Extracellular water	GSH-Px	Glutathione per-oxidase
EDRF	Endothelium-derived relaxing factor	GST	Glutathione-S-trans-ferase
EER	Estimated energy requirement	GTF	Glucose tolerance factor
ER	Endoplasmic reticulum	H_2S	Hydrogen sulfide
		H_3BO_3	Boric acid
F	Fluorine	H_3C-Pte-GLU	Methyl-tetrahydro-folate
F^-	Fluoride		
FA	Fatty acids	H_4-Pte-GLU	Tetrahydrofolic acid
FABP	Fatty acid binding protein	Hb	Hemoglobin
		HCA	Hydroxy citrate
FAD	Flavin adenine dinu-cleotide	HDL	High-density lipo-proteins
FAE	Fetal alcohol effects	HEI	USDA Healthy Eating Index
FAS	Fetal alcohol syndrome		
FC	Free cholesterol	HFCS	High fructose corn syrup

His	Histidine	Mn	Manganese
HMB	Hydroxymethyl butyrate	MnSOD	Manganese-SOD
		Mo	Molybdenum
HMG	Hydroxymethylglutaryl	MoO_4^{2-}	Molybdate
HUS	Hemolytic uremic syndrome	MSG	Monosodium glutamate
		NA	Nicotinic acid
I	Iodine	NAD^+	Nicotinamide adenine dinucleotide
I^-	Iodide		
ICW	Intracellular water	NADP	Nicotinamide adenine dinucleotide phosphate
IDDM	Insulin-dependent diabetes mellitus		
IDL	Intermediate-density lipoproteins	NADPH	Dihydro-nicotinamide adenine dinucleotide phosphate
IF	Intrinsic factor	NE	Nicotinamide
IgG	Immunoglobulin G	Neo-DHC	Neohesperidine DHC
IM	Intramuscular	N-HDL	Nascent high-density lipoproteins
IP	Inositol phosphate		
IPP	Isopentenyl diphosphate	Ni	Nickel
IRS	Insulin receptor substrate	NIDDM	Non-insulin dependent diabetes mellitus
IU	International units	NMN	Nicotinic acid mononucleotide
IUPAC	International chemical nomenclature		
		NO	Nitrogen monoxide
		NO_3^-	Nitrate
K	Potassium	NO-R	S-Nitrosocysteine
kcal	Kilocalories	NOS	NO synthase
LCAT	Lecithin cholesterol acyl-transferase	NPU	Net protein utilization
		NPY	Neuropeptide Y
LDL	Low-density lipoproteins	nvCJD	new variant Creutzfeldt-Jakob disease
Li	Lithium		
LNAA	Long-chain neutral amino acids	OP	Organophosphate
		P	Phosphate
LPL	Lipoprotein lipase	PAF	Platelet activation factor
Lys	Lysine		
MAO	Monoamine oxidases	PAH	Phenylalanine hydroxylase
MCL	Maximum contaminant level		
		PAI	Plasminogen activator inhibitor
MCT	Medium-chain triglycerides		
		PAL	Physical activity level
MEOS	Microsomal ethanol oxidation system	Pb	Lead
		PDCAAS	Protein digestibility-corrected amino acid scores
Met	Methionine		
MGP	Matrix Gla-proteins	PEM	Protein energy malnutrition
MJ	Mega joule		

PER	Protein efficiency ratio
PG	Polygalacturonase
Phe	Phenylalanine
PI	Phosphatidyl inositol
PKC	Protein kinase C
PKU	Phenylketonuria
PL	Phospholipids
PL	Pyridoxal
PM	Pyridoxamine
PMN	Polymorphonuclear leukocytes
PP	Pellagra preventive
PPS	Pentose phosphate shunt
Prot-SH	Sulfur-containing proteins
PRPP	Phospho ribosyl-1-diphosphate
PRPP	5-Phosphoribosyl-1-diphosphate
Pte	Pteridine
PTP	Phospholipid transfer protein
PUFA	Polyunsaturated fatty acids
R	Retinol
RA	Retinoic acid
RAR	Retinoic acid receptors
rBGH	Recombinant human growth hormone
RBP	Retinol-binding protein
RDA	Recommended Dietary Allowances (U.S.)
RDA	Recommended Daily Amounts (UK)
RDI	Reference Daily Intake (U.S.)
RDI	Recommended Daily Intakes (Australia)
RE	Retinol Equivalents
RE	Esterified Retinol
RE	Retinyl ester
REM	Remnants
RFBPs	Riboflavin-binding proteins
RfD	Reference dose
RME	Receptor-mediated endocytosis
RNI	Reference Nutrient Intake (UK)
ROS	Reactive oxygen species
RPE	Retinal pigment epithelium
R-PteGLU$_n$	Non-methylated pteroyl polyglutamate
SAD	Seasonal affective disorder
SD	Standard deviations
Se	Selenium
SeO$_3^{2}$	Selenite
SeO$_4^{2-}$	Selenate
Ser	Serine
Si	Silicon
Sia	Sialic acid
SiO$_2$	Silicon oxide
SiO$_4^{4-}$	Silicate
Sn	Tin
SO$_2$	Sulfur dioxide
SO$_3^{2-}$	Sulfite
SO$_4^{2-}$	Sulfate
SOD	Superoxide dismutase
SR material	Specified risk material
SRM	Specified risk material
TBG	Thyroxine-binding globulin
TDP	Thiamin diphosphate
TEF	Thermic effect of food
TfR	Transferrin receptors
TG	Triglycerides
TG	Triacyl glycerole
THFA	Tetrahydrofolate
Thr	Threonine
TSE	Transmissible spongiform encephalopathy
TTP	Thiamin triphosphate
TTR	Transthyretin
UCP1	Uncoupling protein 1
UDP-	Uridine phosphate
UL	Tolerable Upper Intake Level

USP	United States Pharmacopeia	VO_4^{3-}	Vanadate
UWL	Unstirred water layer	X5P	Xylulose-5-phosphate
V	Vanadium	XO	Xanthine oxidase
vCJD	Variant Creutzfeldt-Jakob disease	YOPI	Young, old, pregnant, and immunocompromised
VLDL	Very low density lipoproteins	Zn	Zinc
VO^{2+}	Vanadyl	αTE	α-Tocopherol equivalents

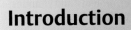
Introduction

Introduction

Human foods are made up of essentially six basic component types (five groups of nutrients and water), each of which has different functions in the body (**A**). Carbohydrates and lipids represent our main energy sources. Proteins, vitamins, minerals, and trace elements are essential for growth and development of tissues. Water, proteins, and vitamins are needed for metabolism as well as for its regulatory functions. While energy nutrients (carbohydrates, lipids, proteins) are partially interchangeable in terms of their use, vitamins, minerals, and trace elements always play very specific roles. Consequently, a lack of any of these components results in nutrient-specific—albeit not always symptomatic—**deficiencies**. The commonality of all nutrient deficiencies is that they interfere primarily with growth. Consequently, growth rates can be used to demonstrate the value of balanced nutrition. Here is an example: in 1880, only 5 % of male college students were over 1.80 m (6 ft) tall, by 1955 that percentage had reached 30 %. Improved availability of nutrients since the beginning of the twentieth century has greatly increased **life expectancy**. Even though theoretical "availability" is more than sufficient in industrialized countries today, major improvements may still be possible through adjustments of **nutrient ratios**. According to present knowledge, a nutrition that prevents disease can be described in the following simplified manner: lipids <35 % (i. e., less than 35 % of total calories consumed), and predominantly from plant sources; proteins ~15 %, also predominantly from plant sources; and carbohydrates >55 %, with a high fiber content. This means a reduction in foods from animal sources and consumption of a varied array of plant foods with a high proportion of fruits and vegetables, all minimally processed.

Such general recommendations are not sufficient, though, since there is great diversity among people (**B**). Nutrition professionals (nutritional scientists, home economists, dietitians, physicians, etc.) need detailed information about individual nutrients to do justice to all the complexity. For this reason, many countries have developed recommendations intended to represent basic guidelines for **desirable nutrient intakes**. In the U.S., these recommendations are issued by the Food and Nutrition Board under the National Research Council. The most recent ones, the **Dietary Reference Intakes** (**DRI**), were established in conjunction with the Canadian Health authorities.

As **nutritional science** evolves, these recommendations are revised periodically, and new findings challenge old ideas all the time. On the other hand, external factors are changing as well. Over the past decades, many occupations have progressively evolved towards lower levels of physical activity, and, in many cases, increasing income levels. These factors have a major impact on food choices and nutrient requirements.

A. Basic Components of Foods

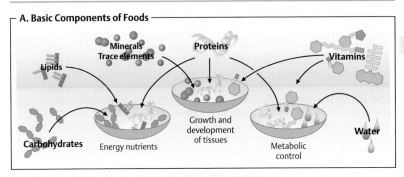

Lipids

Minerals
Trace elements

Proteins

Vitamins

Carbohydrates

Energy nutrients

Growth and
development
of tissues

Metabolic
control

Water

B. Factors with Short or Long-Term Impact on Food Choices

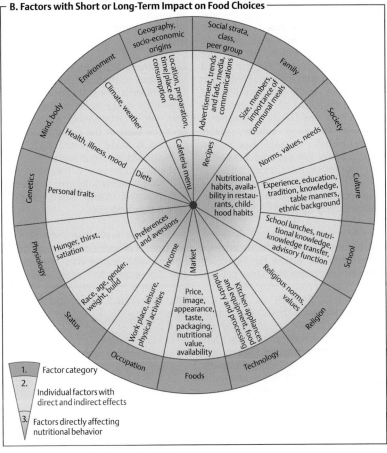

Geography,
socio-economic
origins

Social strata,
class,
peer group

Environment

Family

Location,
preparation,
time/place of
consumption

Advertisement, trends
and fads, media,
communications

Size, members,
importance of
communal meals

Climate, weather

Society

Mind, body

Cafeteria menu

Health, illness, mood

Recipes

Norms, values, needs

Genetics

Personal traits

Diets

Nutritional
habits, availa-
bility in restau-
rants, child-
hood habits

Experience, education,
tradition, knowledge,
table manners,
ethnic background

Culture

Preferences
and aversions

Hunger, thirst,
satiation

School lunches, nutri-
tional knowledge,
knowledge transfer,
advisory function

School

physiology

Income

Market

Race, age, gender,
weight, build

Religious norms,
values

Religion

Status

Work place, leisure,
physical activities

Price,
image,
appearance,
taste,
packaging,
nutritional
value,
availability

Kitchen appliances,
food industry
and equipment, processing

Occupation

Foods

Technology

1. Factor category

2. Individual factors with
direct and indirect effects

3. Factors directly affecting
nutritional behavior

Preventive Nutrition:
A Science in Flux

Controversy is an integral part of nutritional science. Like many other aspects, preventive nutrition is a controversial issue. During the past decades, reducing fat intake while increasing carbohydrate intake was recommended across the world. These recommendations were based on the observation that, in the Western industrial nations, high fat intakes seemed to correlate with a high incidence of coronary artery disease. Even though many details about the effects of various fatty acids had been known since the sixties, the message was simplified to state "Fats are bad." It was assumed that a general reduction in fat intake would automatically lead to a reduced load of saturated fatty acids. Thus, low-fat diets became a standard. The food industry gladly picked up on this message, especially in the U.S. where low-fat products have a high market-share. Admonitions that called this fat-free strategy arbitrary were published repeatedly, but remained largely unheard.

As early as three decades ago, some scientists proposed that a high carbohydrate intake—or rather the intake of high-glycemic index foods (see p. 68)—might lie at the root of many degenerative diseases. As early as 1972, the American physician Dr. R.C. Atkins proposed a nutritional revolution by recommending consumption of more fats and fewer carbohydrates. The recent publication of a new food pyramid by Harvard scientists (**A**) gives new support to his thesis.

While whole grain products should be part of every meal, all foods with a high glycemic index, like white bread, baked potatoes, polished rice, pasta, and sweets have been banned into the pyramid's upper levels. Their approach differentiates between refined and whole, simple and complex carbohydrates, taking into account their glycemic index and glycemic load. Additionally, strict distinctions are drawn between various types of fatty acids: vegetable oils are placed at the base, milk products, butter, and red meat moved up. Micronutrient intakes appear to be suboptimal regardless of such "healthy" nutrition; hence, multivitamin and mineral supplements are recommended.

Government authorities have not yet subscribed to these opinions (**B**). Their recommendations still consider a high overall fat intake to be the main problem, while carbohydrate foods represent the basis of the pyramid. No distinction is made between foods with high and low glycemic loads.
It remains to be seen whether the official recommendations on preventive nutrition will change based on these recent developments.

To emphasize preventive and therapeutic aspects of nutrition, they are highlighted with orange bars next to the text. The orange bars mark those passages that pertain to prevention or therapy, and clinical or nutritional medicine.

A. Harvard Food Pyramid

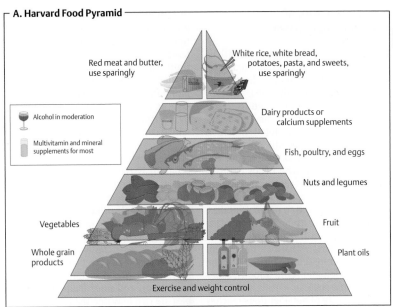

Red meat and butter, use sparingly

White rice, white bread, potatoes, pasta, and sweets, use sparingly

Alcohol in moderation

Multivitamin and mineral supplements for most

Dairy products or calcium supplements

Fish, poultry, and eggs

Nuts and legumes

Vegetables

Fruit

Whole grain products

Plant oils

Exercise and weight control

B. USDA Food Pyramid

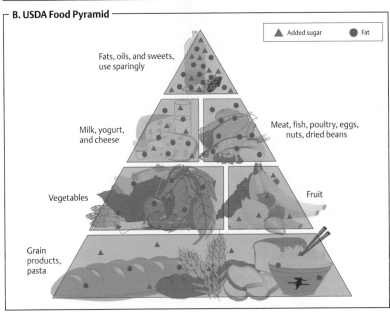

▲ Added sugar   ● Fat

Fats, oils, and sweets, use sparingly

Milk, yogurt, and cheese

Meat, fish, poultry, eggs, nuts, dried beans

Vegetables

Fruit

Grain products, pasta

Preventive Nutrition: The Mediterranean Diet

Nutrition in accordance with the official guidelines could be considered as preventive, in spite of recent discussions about antioxidant vitamins, for instance. Nutrient data derived from scientific research provide an important foundation for institutional nutrition plans (e.g., hospitals, nursing homes); however, they are too abstract for the general consumer, who needs easy-to-apply nutritional recommendations. Translated into practical recommendations and compared to present intakes, a preventive nutrition should increase the consumption of whole grains, fruits, and vegetables, enhance the use of plant over animal fats, and reduce the intake of fried and refined foods, especially simple sugars.

The popularity of outsider diets teaches that recommendations are more successful and attractive if combined with a "lifestyle" image, as may be provided, for instance, by the "**Mediterranean Diet**" (A).

Mediterranean food consumption patterns with their high proportion of various vegetables, grains, plant oils (olive oil, in particular), fish, small amounts of animal fats and meat, largely coincide with present-day ideas about a preventive diet. As early as in the 1950s, the "Seven Countries Study" found that, compared to Northern Europe and the U.S., Mediterranean countries had very low levels of heart disease.

Persons whose data were collected in the 1950s and 1960s are still followed within the framework of this study. They show that in the Mediterranean, too, the amounts of saturated fatty acids consumed increase with increasing wealth, lessening the preventive properties of the diet. In principle, the traditional Mediterranean is largely transferable to Western industrialized nations, since a great variety of foods is available. The high level intake of monounsaturated (olive oil) and n-3-fatty acids (fish) can be achieved in part by consuming rapeseed (canola) oil, which contains both components.

The National "5 A Day for Better Health" program is the National Cancer Institute's attempt to convince people to adopt a healthier nutrition. It propagates the simple principle of eating fruit or vegetables five times a day. Since these are recommended to be eaten "in addition," restrictions—which people tend to dislike or reject—are not necessary. Also, the principle is easy to remember; and since fruit and vegetables are rich in water, the resulting satiety automatically leads to lower intakes of other foods. Alternatively (max. twice/day), fruit or vegetables juices may be taken instead. Whether the "5 A Day" campaign will achieve the desired reduction in nutrition-related diseases remains to be seen within the coming years and decades.

A. The Mediterranean Diet

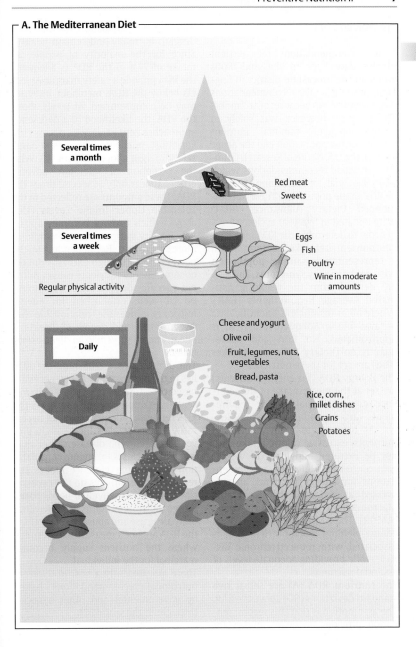

Several times a month

Red meat
Sweets

Several times a week

Eggs
Fish
Poultry
Wine in moderate amounts

Regular physical activity

Daily

Cheese and yogurt
Olive oil
Fruit, legumes, nuts, vegetables
Bread, pasta

Rice, corn, millet dishes
Grains
Potatoes

The RDA and DRI

Early recommendations for nutrient intakes date back to the mid-1800s when, in the Lancashire district in England, nutrient intake recommendations were established because of a famine. The purpose, however, was solely to ensure adequate minimal nutrient intakes for the population and the army. In 1941, the U.S. National Research Council first issued recommendations which had the goal of achieving "perfect health" in the population. These **Recommended Dietary Allowances** (RDA) were updated in five-year cycles.

In order to determine the RDA for a specific nutrient, its intake is determined in a **representative sample population with no deficiency symptoms**. The RDA are derived from the resulting **Estimated Average Requirements (EAR)**. Where no or insufficient scientific data are available, an **Adequate Intake (AI)** is approximated. No RDA and consequently no **Dietary Reference Intakes** (DRI) are set for these nutrients.

The **Energy RDA** (for energy nutrients) are set at the mean intake of the reference groups. Actual energy requirements vary depending on activity levels. As opposed to many nonenergy nutrients, excessive caloric intake cannot be excreted and leads to weight gain. Since the **DRI** (2002), recommendations for energy nutrients are expressed as a range, the **Acceptable Macronutrient Distribution Range** (AMDR). The AMDR is the range of an energy-yielding macronutrient that is associated with reduced chronic disease while providing adequate levels of essential nutrients.

The **Nutrient RDA (A)** are set at two standard deviations (SD) above the EAR. The assumption is that this recommendation provides adequate intakes for 97.5 % of the population, so that they develop normally and remain healthy. Since for the majority of people, an intake of 77 % of the RDA is adequate, the RDA provide a safety margin. At levels below the RDA, metabolic integrity may be compromised. At levels above the RDA, the likelihood of a deficiency approaches zero.

For most nutrients, there is a large safety margin above the RDA (**B**). With the exception of selenium, adverse effects appear only at several times the RDA. These amounts are reflected in the **Tolerable Upper Intake Levels** (UL), above which toxicity becomes apparent. Toxicity symptoms may be mild or more severe (e. g., B_6), depending on the nutrient. Even though excessive intake of some energy nutrients causes nutrient-specific degenerative symptoms, no UL were established for energy nutrients, since the relationship between intake and degree of disease is linear, and no threshold could be established.

The difficulty in establishing the RDA lies in the fact that they are by necessity based on estimates derived from representative samples of the population. The RDA represent adequate, but not necessarily optimal intakes. Increasingly, prevention of chronic disease rather than just deficiencies is taken into consideration when setting reference intakes. The representative samples do not necessarily account for individual needs based on age, nutritional status, genetic variability, drug use and abuse, etc. Therefore, the RDA are not a measure to determine where the nutrient supply becomes marginal for the individual.

There are presently a host of different nutritional recommendations issued by governmental and other agencies throughout the world (**C**).

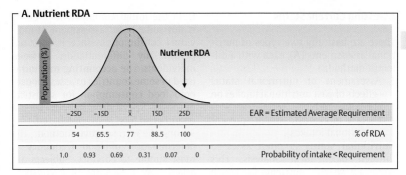

A. Nutrient RDA

- **Nutrient RDA**

	−2SD	−1SD	x̄	1SD	2SD	EAR = Estimated Average Requirement
	54	65.5	77	88.5	100	% of RDA
1.0	0.93	0.69	0.31	0.07	0	Probability of intake < Requirement

B. DRI

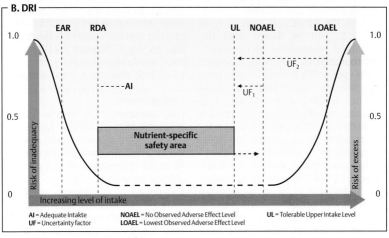

EAR   RDA   UL   NOAEL   LOAEL

UF_2

- - - - AI UF_1

Nutrient-specific safety area

Risk of inadequacy

Increasing level of intake

Risk of excess

AI = Adequate Intakte
UF = Uncertainty factor
NOAEL = No Observed Adverse Effect Level
LOAEL = Lowest Observed Adverse Effect Level
UL = Tolerable Upper Intake Level

C. Nutritional Recommendations

RDA	**R**ecommended **D**ietary **A**llowances	US	(1943)
RDA	**R**ecommended **D**aily **A**mounts	UK	(1979)
RNI	**R**ecommended **N**utrient **I**ntakes	Canada	(1983)
RDI	**R**ecommended **D**aily **I**ntakes	Australia	(1986)
EAR	**E**stimated **A**verage **R**equirement	UK	(1991)
		US	(1994)
RNI	**R**eference **N**utrient **I**ntake	UK	(1991)
	Food Guide Pyramid	US	(1992)
HEI	USDA **H**ealthy **E**ating **I**ndex	US	(1994)
UL	Tolerable **U**pper Intake **L**evels	US	(1994)
DRI	**D**ietary **R**eference **I**ntakes	US and Canada	(1997)
AI	**A**dequate **I**ntake	US	(1997)
AHEI	Harvard School of Public Health **A**lternative **H**ealthy **E**ating **I**ndex	US	(2002)
AMDR	**A**cceptable **M**acronutrient **D**istribution **R**ange	US	(2002)
EER	**E**stimated **E**nergy **R**equirement	US	(2002)

Assessing Current Status

There are basically two types of nutritional assessments (**A**), each with a different method:

1. Assessment of nutritional status (effects of past nutritional intakes on the body) and
2. Dietary intake assessment (present nutritional intakes).

Nutritional status is often assessed through biochemical analysis. This works for specific nutrients for which there is a measurable indicator. Conclusions on the nutritional availability of iron, e.g., can be drawn from the amount of hemoglobin in the blood. **Anthropometrics**, i.e., body measurements (see p. 16), provide a more general measure. Besides height and body weight, determination of skin fold thickness has been gaining increasing importance. Anthropometric measurements represent cumulative results of many different factors and do not differentiate among the various nutrients. Clinical symptoms caused by nutritional deficiencies tend to become apparent very late. A long-term low iron supply, e.g., will eventually result in clinical symptoms like pallor and reduced performance levels—symptoms that could have been averted through early intervention.

Direct **dietary intake assessment** can be ongoing (prospective) or retrospective. With the **weighing method**, all foods consumed are actually weighed, whereas the **protocol method** uses amount estimates. The **inventory method** assesses the food consumption of an entire household by registering use of food items, as well as leftovers and waste. For example, a large amount of food is made available to a family and after a week the remainder subtracted from the initial amount. This method is not suitable for assessment of individual consumption since it does not permit any differentiation between individuals. The **accounting method** is used in some countries to assess household food consumption for statistical purposes. Selected households keep a record of all food items purchased.

Among the retrospective methods, the determination of **food frequency** is most simple to conduct. Subjects are asked how frequently they consume specific food groups. A **diet history** is more informative since additional factors like nutrition-related behaviors are also recorded. **24-hour recall** presupposes good memory in the participants, as all food items consumed within 24 hours have to be recalled—including their amounts.

Food consumption can also be assessed indirectly through official agricultural statistics. This, however, does not permit differentiation among different segments of the population and does not account for waste.

The results of all methods presented naturally contain errors. In a study conducted with 140 participants (**B**), a 24-hour recall was compared with the "actual" observed food consumption. During the recall, all types of foods were regularly omitted or listed erroneously. Cooked vegetables were omitted in more than 50% of all cases, whereas sugar was listed erroneously in nearly 30% of all cases.

A. Methods for Nutritional Assessment

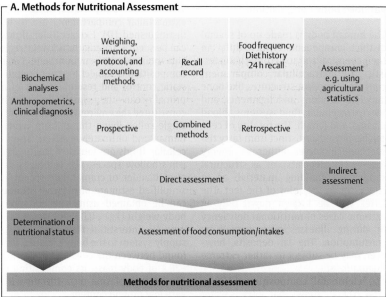

Biochemical analyses Anthropometrics, clinical diagnosis	Weighing, inventory, protocol, and accounting methods	Recall record	Food frequency Diet history 24 h recall	Assessment e.g. using agricultural statistics
	Prospective	Combined methods	Retrospective	
	Direct assessment			Indirect assessment
Determination of nutritional status	Assessment of food consumption/intakes			

Methods for nutritional assessment

B. Foods Listed in Food Intake Assessment

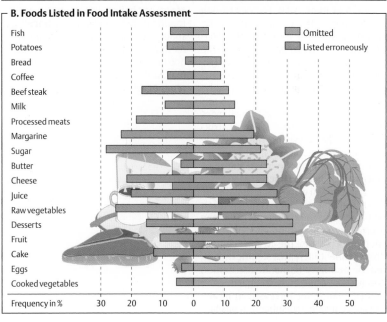

Omitted
Listed erroneously

Fish
Potatoes
Bread
Coffee
Beef steak
Milk
Processed meats
Margarine
Sugar
Butter
Cheese
Juice
Raw vegetables
Desserts
Fruit
Cake
Eggs
Cooked vegetables

Frequency in %   30   20   10   0   10   20   30   40   50

Variable: Body Composition

The human body is made up of several distinct components, which differ in their chemical and structural characteristics. The **extracellular compartment** consists of support structures like bone lamellae, tendons and ligaments, and the extracellular fluid systems, blood plasma, and lymph. The **totality of cells** can be viewed as distinct from **fatty tissue**, which serves either as energy reserve (fat deposits), or as structural support or building material, as in cheeks or in the soles of the feet. The latter will be broken down only in extreme cases of nutritional deficiency or during illnesses accompanied by consumption. The fat deposits, however, may be subject to rather extreme fluctuations.

The **"elemental" composition** of a 70 kg (154 lb) male shows that ~60 % is water and 16 % or more is fat. Besides carbon (C), hydrogen (H), and oxygen (O), the chemical elements nitrogen (N), calcium (Ca), and phosphorus (P) are the most abundant in terms of mass (**A**). Most other naturally occurring elements can also be found in the human body; however, their significance is often unknown. Chemical composition changes with age. These changes are most striking during the first year of life (**B**). While the water content drops rapidly, fat content, protein in muscle mass, and minerals, mostly in bone, increase.

The reduction in water content with age is accompanied by **redistribution** between body compartments (**C**). In the central nervous system, skin, and subcutaneous tissue, the water content drops while it increases significantly only in muscle and fatty tissue. Redistribution also occurs within body compartments; intracellular water increases in all organs except skin and subcutaneous fat.

Within **total body water,** intra- and extracellular compartments are to be distinguished (**D**). **Extracellular fluids** can be seen as a mediator between cells and their external environment. Their composition is subject to strict homeostatic control and resembles that of a primal ocean—the primal ocean which constituted the environment of ancient, single-celled living things from which humankind ultimately evolved. **Transcellular fluids** are found in the organism's hollow spaces, like the digestive tract, bladder, or cranial fluid spaces. A simplified estimate of **plasma volume** can be obtained using the equation: body weight (kg) × 0.035 = plasma volume [l]. **Interstitial fluid** serves as a supply system to the body's tissues. It is found between the cells and makes up ~20 % of body mass. Its composition is similar to a plasma ultra-filtrate with very low protein content.

More than half of the total body water is found inside the cells. The **intracellular space** is the site of cellular metabolism. As opposed to other fluid spaces, it is not homogeneous and its composition may differ greatly between different types of cells.

A. Body Composition

		Fetus (gest. week 20–25)	Premature birth	Neonate	Child (age 4–5)	Adult male
Body weight	(kg)	0.30	1.50	3.50	14.00	70.00
Fat	(g/kg)	5.00	35.00	160.00	160.00	160.00
Water	(g/kg)	880.00	830.00	700.00	630.00	600.00
Composition of lean body mass:						
Water	(g/kg)	880.00	850.00	820.00	695.00	720.00
Total N	(g/kg)	15.00	19.00	23.00	38.20	34.00
Na	(g/kg)	2.30	2.30	1.88	1.84	1.84
K	(g/kg)	1.68	1.95	2.07	2.54	2.70
Cl	(g/kg)	2.69	–	1.94	1.77	1.56
Ca	(g/kg)	4.20	7.00	9.60	21.10	22.40
Mg	(g/kg)	0.18	0.24	0.26	0.36	0.50
P	(g/kg)	3.00	3.80	5.60	10.50	12.00
Fe	(mg/kg)	58.00	74.00	94.00	64.20	74.00
Cu	(mg/kg)	3.00	4.00	5.00	3.30	2.00
Zn	(mg/kg)	20.00	20.00	20.00	22.30	30.00

B. Age-Dependent Changes in Body Composition

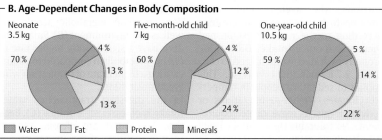

Neonate 3.5 kg — 70 %, 4 %, 13 %, 13 %

Five-month-old child 7 kg — 60 %, 4 %, 12 %, 24 %

One-year-old child 10.5 kg — 59 %, 5 %, 14 %, 22 %

☐ Water ☐ Fat ☐ Protein ☐ Minerals

C. Age-Dependent Changes in Body Water Content

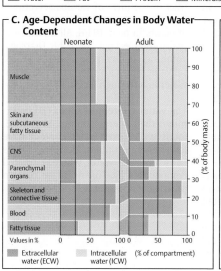

Neonate   Adult

Muscle
Skin and subcutaneous fatty tissue
CNS
Parenchymal organs
Skeleton and connective tissue
Blood
Fatty tissue

Values in %   0   50   100 0   50   100

(% of body mass)

☐ Extracellular water (ECW)   ☐ Intracellular water (ICW)   (% of compartment)

D. The Body's Fluid Spaces

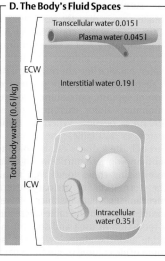

Total body water (0.6 l/kg)

Transcellular water 0.015 l
Plasma water 0.045 l
ECW
Interstitial water 0.19 l
ICW
Intracellular water 0.35 l

Water in Body and Foods

Homeostasis of the **water balance** (A) ensures stability of the water content. This stable balance is achieved through various hormonal feedback mechanisms in conjunction with osmoreceptors. The total average daily water intake results from a combination of drinking, intake of water contained in solid foods, and **oxidation water**. The latter is an end-product of the oxidative metabolism of energy nutrients. The oxidation of 1 g carbohydrate yields 0.6 ml of water; of 1 g protein, 0.42 ml; and of 1 g fat 1.07 ml. Based on a mixed nutrition, the average daily total amounts to 300 ml of oxidation water.

According to the recently established **Dietary Reference Intake** (DRI), to be properly hydrated, women need to consume 2.7 l, men 3.7 l water/d. This applies to sedentary people in temperate climates. Higher temperatures or activity levels increase these requirements. No **Tolerable Upper Intake Level** (UL) has been established for water. In the average person, ~80% of water intake comes directly from fluids and ~20% from water contained in foods. Approximately 1.5 l is excreted through the urine. The kidneys can influence water balance by altering the rate of **reabsorption**. To ensure proper excretion of sodium, potassium, and urea, a minimum fluid excretion of 300–500 ml is needed. When no drinking water is available, the water loss through the kidneys can be minimized with appropriate nutrition. This means minimizing those foods that result in the formation of **urinary excreted metabolites**. For instance, lowering intake of protein and table salt results in a reduction of urea and sodium in the urine and, therefore, lowers the minimum urine volume required. In particu-lar situations, e. g., for a prematurely born baby with kidney insufficiency, this mechanism becomes important. **Water loss** via skin and lungs amounts to 0.9 l/d. Increased respiratory frequency, as occurs in higher elevations, dry and warm surroundings, as well as during physical activity, can greatly increase these losses; 0.5 l/h may be lost via the skin alone in extreme situations. Concurrent loss of sodium takes place, decreasing, however, with regular training. If water loss exceeds 3 l/d, sodium loss needs to be replenished, as does water.

Human **fluid requirement** is, therefore, dependent on metabolic activity, as well as the environment (**B**). Small children have a significantly higher rate of energy metabolism compared to adults, causing a higher rate of respiration with greater water loss.

In the digestive tract, actual water intake is of lesser significance (**C**). Each day, ~8 l of fluids are released into the tract in the form of various secretions. Together with the fluids we drink, this amounts to over 10 l/d, all of which is reabsorbed except for 0.2 l. Diarrhea, vomiting, or increased secretions of saliva or bile acids can greatly increase water loss through feces.

The **water content of foods** (D) determines their energy content. In general, foods with lower water content have lower energy content. Many vegetables consist of >90% water, whereas isolated components like oil or sugar contain practically no water.

A. Water Balance

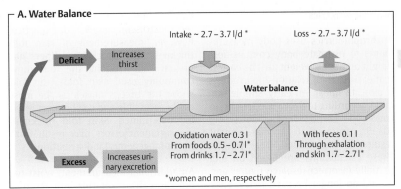

Intake ~ 2.7 – 3.7 l/d *

Loss ~ 2.7 – 3.7 l/d *

Deficit → Increases thirst

Water balance

Excess → Increases urinary excretion

Oxidation water 0.3 l
From foods 0.5 – 0.7 l*
From drinks 1.7 – 2.7 l*

With feces 0.1 l
Through exhalation and skin 1.7 – 2.7 l*

*women and men, respectively

B. Fluid Requirements

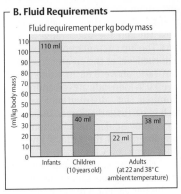

Fluid requirement per kg body mass

(ml/kg body mass)

Infants 110 ml
Children (10 years old) 40 ml
Adults (at 22 and 38°C ambient temperature) 22 ml, 38 ml

C. Water Exchange in the Intestinal Tract

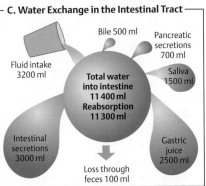

Fluid intake 3200 ml

Bile 500 ml

Pancreatic secretions 700 ml

Saliva 1500 ml

Total water into intestine 11 400 ml Reabsorption 11 300 ml

Intestinal secretions 3000 ml

Gastric juice 2500 ml

Loss through feces 100 ml

D. Water Content of Foods

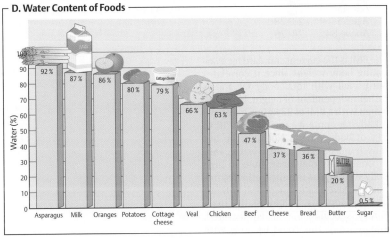

Water (%)

Asparagus 92 %
Milk 87 %
Oranges 86 %
Potatoes 80 %
Cottage cheese 79 %
Veal 66 %
Chicken 63 %
Beef 47 %
Cheese 37 %
Bread 36 %
Butter 20 %
Sugar 0.5 %

Anthropometrics

Anthropometrics uses body measurements to estimate body composition. Height and body weight are the easiest to measure. Their relationship in adults is close to linear. An early, simple formula, according to **Broca** was height (in cm) −100 = normal weight. Subtracting 10–15% from that normal weight resulted in the so-called "ideal" weight. These calculations are based on old, partially incorrect research figures and should no longer be used today. They suggest a very low weight as "ideal = healthy." The "health value" of such a lowest possible body weight is no longer accepted today.

The **Body Mass Index** (BMI) provides a more accurate anthropometric measurement (**A**). It is calculated from body weight (kg) divided by the square of height (m^2); hence the BMI unit is kg/m^2. The desirable BMI is also age-dependent:

Age 19–24:	19–24
Age 25–34:	20–25
Age 35–44:	21–26
Age 45–54:	22–27
Age 55–64:	23–28
Above 64:	24–29

The BMI is the current standard for evaluating body weight since it correlates fairly well with total body fat and is rather independent of height. However, a man with a BMI of 27 kg/m^2 may have a body fat content ranging from 10 to 31% of body weight. Not only fat, but muscle mass, extracellular water, and/or bone mass may contribute to high body weight. For instance, athletes frequently have a rather high BMI without large fat deposits. To address this inaccuracy, subcutaneous fat is measured. Theoretically, this could be done with an ultrasound device or through infrared spectroscopy. In everyday practice, however, measurement of skin fold thickness with **precision calipers** has proven valid. Among the four most commonly used skin folds, the fold above the triceps muscle is the most easily accessible and can be most reliably determined. **Skin fold thickness** measurement errors may result from nonhomogeneous fat distribution.

An additional measurement, **waist-to-hip ratio** (**B**), takes this into account. Waist circumference is measured while standing, between the lower edge of the lowest rib and the upper edge of the pelvis. The hip circumference is measured at the level of the greater trochanters. A ratio above 0.88 in women and above 1.0 in men indicates an android or abdominal fat distribution pattern, which is particularly closely associated with cardiovascular complications and other illnesses. If the ratio is low, the gynoid type prevails, with a lesser health risk. The waist-to-hip ratio is a particularly valuable tool for determining whether weight reduction is necessary in case of moderate overweight.

A. Body Mass Index (BMI) for Age Group 19 – 34

Height in meters

Weight (kg)	1.48		1.52		1.56		1.60		1.64		1.68		1.72		1.76		1.80		1.84		1.88		1.92		1.96		2.00
120	55	53	52	51	49	48	47	46	45	44	43	42	41	40	39	38	37	36	35	35	34	33	33	32	31	31	30
118	54	52	51	50	48	47	46	45	44	43	42	41	40	39	38	37	36	36	35	34	33	33	32	31	31	30	30
116	53	52	50	49	48	46	45	44	43	42	41	40	39	38	37	37	36	35	34	34	33	32	31	31	30	30	29
114	52	51	49	48	47	46	45	43	42	41	40	39	39	38	37	36	35	35	34	33	32	32	31	30	30	29	29
112	51	50	48	47	46	45	44	43	42	41	40	39	38	37	36	35	35	34	33	32	32	31	30	30	29	29	28
110	50	49	48	46	45	44	43	42	41	40	39	38	37	36	36	35	34	33	32	32	31	30	30	29	29	28	28
108	49	48	47	46	44	43	42	41	40	39	38	37	37	36	35	34	33	33	32	31	30	30	29	29	28	28	27
106	48	47	46	45	44	42	41	40	39	38	38	37	36	35	34	33	33	32	31	31	30	29	29	28	28	27	27
104	47	46	45	44	43	42	41	40	39	38	37	36	35	34	34	33	32	32	31	30	30	29	28	28	27	27	26
102	47	45	44	43	42	41	40	39	38	37	36	35	34	34	33	32	32	31	30	30	29	28	28	27	27	26	26
100	46	44	43	42	41	40	39	38	37	36	35	35	34	33	32	32	31	30	30	29	28	28	27	27	26	26	25
98	45	44	43	42	41	40	39	38	37	36	35	34	33	32	32	31	30	30	29	28	28	27	27	26	26	25	25
96	44	43	42	40	39	38	38	37	36	35	34	33	33	32	31	30	30	29	28	28	27	27	26	26	25	24	24
94	43	42	41	40	39	38	37	36	35	34	33	33	32	32	31	30	30	29	28	28	27	26	26	25	25	24	24
92	42	41	40	39	38	37	36	35	34	34	33	32	32	31	30	30	29	28	28	27	26	26	25	25	24	23	23
90	41	40	39	38	37	36	35	34	34	33	32	32	31	30	29	29	28	28	27	26	26	25	25	24	24	23	23
88	40	39	38	37	36	35	34	34	33	32	31	30	30	29	28	28	27	27	26	25	25	24	24	23	23	22	22
86	39	38	37	36	35	34	34	33	32	31	30	30	29	28	28	27	27	26	25	25	24	24	23	23	22	22	21
84	38	37	36	35	34	33	32	31	30	30	29	28	28	27	27	26	25	25	24	24	23	23	22	22	21	21	21
82	37	36	35	35	34	33	32	31	30	30	29	28	28	27	26	26	25	25	24	24	23	23	22	22	21	21	20
80	37	35	35	34	33	32	31	31	30	29	28	28	27	26	26	25	25	24	24	23	23	22	22	21	21	20	20
78	36	35	34	33	32	31	30	30	29	28	28	27	26	26	25	25	24	24	23	23	22	22	21	21	20	20	20
76	35	34	33	32	32	31	30	29	28	28	27	27	26	26	25	24	24	23	23	22	22	21	21	20	20	20	19
74	34	33	32	31	30	30	29	28	28	27	26	26	25	24	24	23	23	22	22	21	21	20	20	20	19	19	19
72	33	32	31	30	30	29	28	27	27	26	25	25	24	24	23	23	22	22	21	21	20	20	19	19	18	18	18
70	32	31	30	30	29	28	27	27	26	25	25	24	24	23	23	22	22	21	21	20	20	19	19	18	18	18	18
68	31	30	29	29	28	27	27	26	25	25	24	24	23	22	22	21	21	20	20	19	19	18	18	18	17	17	17
66	30	29	29	28	27	26	26	25	24	24	23	23	22	22	21	20	20	19	19	19	18	18	17	17	17	16	16
64	29	28	28	27	26	26	25	24	24	23	23	22	22	21	21	20	20	19	19	18	18	18	17	17	16	16	16
62	28	28	27	26	25	25	24	23	23	22	22	21	21	20	20	19	19	18	18	18	17	17	16	16	16	15	15
60	27	27	26	25	25	24	23	23	22	22	21	21	20	19	19	18	18	18	17	17	16	16	16	15	15	15	15
58	26	26	25	24	24	23	23	22	21	21	20	20	19	19	18	18	17	17	16	16	16	15	15	15	15	14	14
56	26	25	24	24	23	22	22	21	21	20	19	19	18	18	18	17	17	16	16	16	15	15	15	14	14	14	14
54	25	24	23	23	22	22	21	21	20	20	19	18	18	18	17	17	16	16	15	15	15	14	14	14	14	13	13
52	24	23	23	22	21	21	20	20	19	19	18	18	17	17	16	16	16	15	15	14	14	14	13	13	13	13	13
50	23	22	22	21	21	20	20	19	19	18	18	17	17	16	16	15	15	15	14	14	14	13	13	13	13	12	12
48	22	21	21	20	20	19	19	18	18	17	17	16	16	15	15	15	14	14	14	14	13	13	13	12	12	12	12

Morbid obesity | Obesity | Overweight | Normal weight | Underweight

B. Waist-To-Hip Ratios in Women

Waist circumference in centimeters

Hip circumference in centimeters	50	55	60	65	70	75	80	85	90	95	100	105	110	115	120	125	130	135	140	145	150
50	1.00	1.10	1.20	1.30	1.40	1.50	1.60	1.70	1.80	1.90	2.00	2.10	2.20	2.30	2.40	2.50	2.60	2.70	2.80	2.90	3.00
55	0.91	1.00	1.09	1.18	1.27	1.36	1.45	1.55	1.64	1.73	1.82	1.91	2.00	2.09	2.18	2.27	2.36	2.45	2.55	2.64	2.73
60	0.83	0.92	1.00	1.08	1.17	1.25	1.33	1.42	1.50	1.58	1.67	1.75	1.83	1.92	2.00	2.08	2.17	2.25	2.33	2.42	2.50
65	0.77	0.85	0.92	1.00	1.08	1.15	1.23	1.31	1.38	1.46	1.54	1.62	1.69	1.77	1.85	1.92	2.00	2.08	2.15	2.23	2.31
70	0.71	0.79	0.86	0.93	1.00	1.07	1.14	1.21	1.29	1.36	1.43	1.50	1.57	1.64	1.71	1.79	1.86	1.93	2.00	2.07	2.14
75	0.67	0.73	0.80	0.87	0.93	1.00	1.07	1.13	1.20	1.27	1.33	1.40	1.47	1.53	1.60	1.67	1.73	1.80	1.87	1.93	2.00
80	0.63	0.69	0.75	0.81	0.88	0.94	1.00	1.06	1.13	1.19	1.25	1.31	1.38	1.44	1.50	1.56	1.63	1.69	1.75	1.81	1.88
85	0.59	0.65	0.71	0.76	0.82	0.88	0.94	1.00	1.06	1.12	1.18	1.24	1.29	1.35	1.41	1.47	1.53	1.59	1.65	1.71	1.76
90	0.56	0.61	0.67	0.72	0.78	0.83	0.89	0.94	1.00	1.06	1.11	1.17	1.22	1.28	1.33	1.39	1.44	1.50	1.56	1.61	1.67
95	0.53	0.58	0.63	0.68	0.74	0.79	0.84	0.89	0.95	1.00	1.05	1.11	1.16	1.21	1.26	1.32	1.37	1.42	1.47	1.53	1.58
100	0.50	0.55	0.60	0.65	0.70	0.75	0.80	0.85	0.90	0.95	1.00	1.05	1.10	1.15	1.20	1.25	1.30	1.35	1.40	1.45	1.50
105	0.48	0.52	0.57	0.62	0.67	0.71	0.76	0.81	0.86	0.90	0.95	1.00	1.05	1.10	1.14	1.19	1.24	1.29	1.33	1.38	1.43
110	0.45	0.50	0.55	0.59	0.64	0.68	0.73	0.77	0.82	0.86	0.91	0.95	1.00	1.05	1.09	1.14	1.18	1.23	1.27	1.32	1.36
115	0.43	0.48	0.52	0.57	0.61	0.65	0.70	0.74	0.78	0.83	0.87	0.91	0.96	1.00	1.04	1.09	1.13	1.17	1.22	1.26	1.30
120	0.42	0.46	0.50	0.54	0.58	0.63	0.67	0.71	0.75	0.79	0.83	0.88	0.92	0.96	1.00	1.04	1.08	1.13	1.17	1.21	1.25
125	0.40	0.44	0.48	0.52	0.56	0.60	0.64	0.68	0.72	0.76	0.80	0.84	0.88	0.92	0.96	1.00	1.04	1.08	1.12	1.16	1.20
130	0.38	0.42	0.46	0.50	0.54	0.58	0.62	0.65	0.69	0.73	0.77	0.81	0.85	0.88	0.92	0.96	1.00	1.04	1.08	1.12	1.15
135	0.37	0.41	0.44	0.48	0.52	0.56	0.59	0.63	0.67	0.70	0.74	0.78	0.81	0.85	0.89	0.93	0.96	1.00	1.04	1.07	1.11
140	0.36	0.39	0.43	0.46	0.50	0.54	0.57	0.61	0.64	0.68	0.71	0.75	0.79	0.82	0.86	0.89	0.93	0.96	1.00	1.04	1.07
145	0.34	0.38	0.41	0.45	0.48	0.52	0.55	0.59	0.62	0.66	0.69	0.72	0.76	0.79	0.83	0.86	0.90	0.93	0.97	1.00	1.03
150	0.33	0.37	0.40	0.43	0.47	0.50	0.53	0.57	0.60	0.63	0.67	0.70	0.73	0.77	0.80	0.83	0.87	0.90	0.93	0.97	1.00

Gynoid < 0.80 | Intermediate 0.80 – 0.88 | Android > 0.88

Experimental Methods

Bioelectrical impedance (BIA) is based on differences in conductivity between bodily tissues (**A**). Water-containing tissues have low impedance since they are highly conductive because of the presence of electrolytes. Fatty tissues have greater resistance, and cell membranes function as electrical condensers. Since electricity of different frequencies flows preferentially in different compartments, the measurement of impedance, combined with phase displacement, permits conclusions about the three compartments: fatty tissues, lean body mass, and water. BIA is considered to produce reliable and well-reproducible values for healthy people. The simplicity of the method's use is advantageous: the four stick-on electrodes don't bother the patient. However, changes in plasma electrolytes, use of diuretics, or dextrose infusions can greatly disturb the results.

Measurements of **conductivity**, like the BIA, are based on the different conductivities of different tissues. Since the person to be measured has to be placed inside a magnetic coil, the method is not practical as a routine.

Body composition can also be determined through various **isotope dilution methods** (**B**). These are used to determine just one compartment—total body water. The method is based on the assumption that fatty tissue is water-free and hence cannot take up any electrolytes. By additionally defining that lean body mass has a constant 73.2% degree of hydration, all three compartments can be determined through appropriate calculations. The most commonly used isotopes are deuterium oxide (^2H_2O), tritium-labeled water (^3H_2O), and the potassium isotopes ^{42}K and ^{43}K. The respective isotope is injected, losses are measured in urine, blood levels are measured after an equilibration phase, and the resulting dilution factor is used to determine total body water. Measurements of total body potassium using the ^{40}K method differ somewhat. The isotope occurs naturally at a level of 0.0118 % of body potassium and can be determined using a whole body counter. An assumption is made that potassium is found in lean body mass at a fixed concentration of 8 mmol/kg. Just as with the injected isotopes, this makes it possible to calculate all three compartments. Isotope measurements are also subject to errors. The assumptions mentioned do not apply to pathological conditions like sepsis, stress, malnutrition, or obesity.

Underwater weighing (**C**) is considered the standard for determining body fat. The subject has to be submerged under water. The displaced water in the vessel corresponds to the body volume. If the body weight is known, the density (D) (in g/cm^3) can be calculated. Since body water has a constant density of 1.0 g/cm^3, and the density of lean body mass and fat are also near constant, D can be used to estimate the respective proportions of the three compartments. Any change in density is interpreted primarily as a change in body fat content.

A. Impedance Measurement of a Body Section with Tetrapolar Electrodes

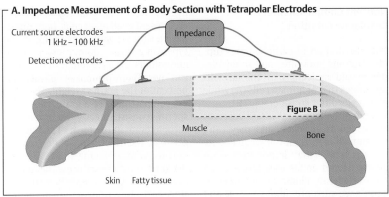

Current source electrodes
1 kHz – 100 kHz

Detection electrodes

Impedance

Figure B

Muscle

Bone

Skin   Fatty tissue

B. Isotope Dilution Methods

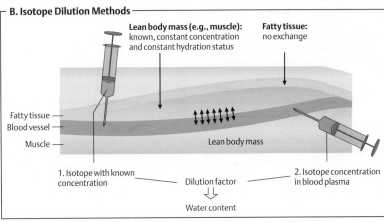

Lean body mass (e.g., muscle):
known, constant concentration
and constant hydration status

Fatty tissue:
no exchange

Fatty tissue
Blood vessel
Muscle

Lean body mass

1. Isotope with known
concentration

Dilution factor

2. Isotope concentration
in blood plasma

Water content

C. Underwater weighing

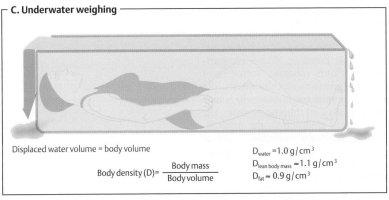

Displaced water volume = body volume

$$\text{Body density (D)} = \frac{\text{Body mass}}{\text{Body volume}}$$

$D_{water} = 1.0 \ g/cm^3$
$D_{lean\ body\ mass} \approx 1.1 \ g/cm^3$
$D_{fat} \approx 0.9 \ g/cm^3$

Nutrient Compartmentalization: Cellular Distribution

The distribution of carbohydrates, lipids, proteins, vitamins, and other elements and molecules in animal cells resembles that of human cells (**A**) while plant cells differ considerably (**B**).

In animal cells, carbohydrate reserves are stored as glycogen, and they can't store much of it. Their role as an energy reserve is of lesser importance since energy stored as fat uses space much more efficiently. Plants, except in seeds, don't have such problems of space and efficiency. They can, therefore, afford the uneconomic luxury of storing energy as large amounts of starch. Plant cell walls usually consist of polysaccharides, indigestible to humans, which are also called fiber or roughage.

Lipids are always found in fat droplets made of triglycerides or vitamin A esters. They are also found in all biological membranes, which consist mostly of phospho- and sphingolipids. Human and animal cell membranes also contain cholesterol. Plant cell membranes do not.

Proteins are found in all cells and throughout all compartments, as well as all extracellular fluids. This reflects their importance in the structure and function of all living things.

Most **vitamins, minerals, and trace elements** are associated with proteins and hence also found in all cell compartments. Plants contain intracellular organelles known as chloroplasts, not found in animal and human cells, which are the sites of photosynthesis. The structure of chlorophyll—the light absorbing molecule—resembles that of hemoglobin; however, whereas hemoglobin contains iron, chlorophyll has a magnesium ion in its center.

Even though nearly all nutrient types are present in all plant cells, their distribution varies greatly, depending on cell types. In a cereal grain, most vitamins and minerals (**C**) are found in the aleuron layer. This layer makes up just a few percent of the grain's weight. The largest compartment of a grain, the endosperm, consists nearly exclusively of carbohydrate in the form of starch. The germ, on the other hand, is rich in vitamin B_1, vitamin E, and lipids. Usually, the germ is removed during the milling process to increase the shelf life of flour since hydrolysis or oxidation of the lipids contained in it would affect taste over time.

The aleuron layer and the germ are theoretically the nutritionally most valuable components of a cereal grain. In reality, though, most people prefer the vitamin- and mineral-deficient white flour.

Animal cells have similarly diverse **distribution patterns**. Muscle cells contain a high percentage of protein, whereas liver cells are rich in vitamins A, D, B_{12}, and folate. Fatty tissues consist mostly of lipids, with which vitamin E and carotenoids are associated.

A. Animal Cell

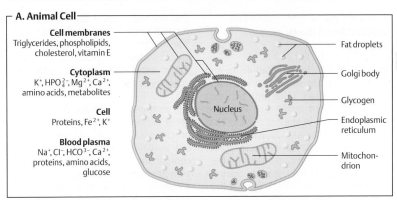

Cell membranes
Triglycerides, phospholipids,
cholesterol, vitamin E

Cytoplasm
K^+, HPO_4^{2-}, Mg^{2+}, Ca^{2+},
amino acids, metabolites

Cell
Proteins, Fe^{2+}, K^+

Blood plasma
Na^+, Cl^-, HCO_3^-, Ca^{2+},
proteins, amino acids,
glucose

Fat droplets

Golgi body

Glycogen

Endoplasmic
reticulum

Mitochon-
drion

Nucleus

B. Plant Cell

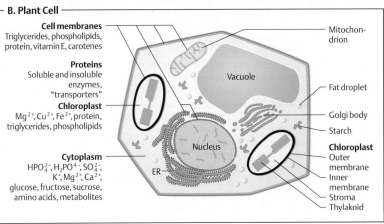

Cell membranes
Triglycerides, phospholipids,
protein, vitamin E, carotenes

Proteins
Soluble and insoluble
enzymes,
"transporters"

Chloroplast
Mg^{2+}, Cu^{2+}, Fe^{2+}, protein,
triglycerides, phospholipids

Cytoplasm
HPO_4^{2-}, $H_2PO_4^-$, SO_4^{2-},
K^+, Mg^{2+}, Ca^{2+},
glucose, fructose, sucrose,
amino acids, metabolites

Mitochon-
drion

Vacuole

Fat droplet

Golgi body

Starch

Chloroplast
Outer
membrane
Inner
membrane
Stroma
Thylakoid

Nucleus

ER

C. Structure of a Grain

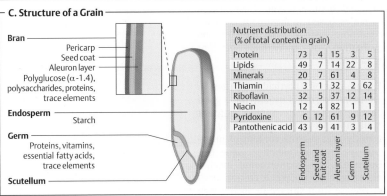

Bran
Pericarp
Seed coat
Aleuron layer
Polyglucose (α-1.4),
polysaccharides, proteins,
trace elements

Endosperm
Starch

Germ
Proteins, vitamins,
essential fatty acids,
trace elements

Scutellum

Nutrient distribution
(% of total content in grain)

	Endosperm	Seed and fruit coat	Aleuron layer	Germ	Scutellum
Protein	73	4	15	3	5
Lipids	49	7	14	22	8
Minerals	20	7	61	4	8
Thiamin	3	1	32	2	62
Riboflavin	32	5	37	12	14
Niacin	12	4	82	1	1
Pyridoxine	6	12	61	9	12
Pantothenic acid	43	9	41	3	4

Nutrient Compartmentalization: Distribution to the Organs— Homeostasis

Nutrient intake, loss, metabolism, and requirements are subject to considerable changes over time and between individuals. Even intake can never be constant. This is in spite of the fact that most foods are always available nowadays, due to extensive world trade. Other factors like age, gender, or a person's state of health, lead to varying nutrient needs, different metabolization, and storage capacities.

The fact that none of the measurable parameters have a "normal" value is a result of the important impact of **genetic variability**: Instead, there is just a more or less narrow normal range. One of the causes is a certain variability of the amino acid sequence of proteins. For instance, there are several forms of hemoglobin, which differ in their oxygen-binding capacity. Under normal conditions this does not necessarily affect their physiological function. But in some cases (sickle-cell anemia, thalassemia) it does. A similar situation can be assumed to exist with regard to enzymes and transport proteins involved in nutrient metabolism. These variables, based on mostly intracellular conditions, need to be factored into the evaluation of individual nutrient requirements.

The amount of a particular nutrient in the blood plasma is usually not a good parameter for determining nutrient availability. Nevertheless, the body frequently uses plasma content of nutrients as internal reference value (**A**). Hormonal and nonhormonal mechanisms regulate uptake, excretion, and/ or release from storage in such a way that the registered value in the plasma is equal to the internal reference value. The function of this **homeostasis** is to ensure adequate nutrient supply to those tissues that need them most urgently at a given time.

The example of **vitamin A** shows that these homeostatic mechanisms often preclude a simple assessment of nutrient availability from easily accessible compartments like blood (**B**). With a sufficient vitamin A supply, the vitamin A content of the liver—its main storage organ—is 300–1000 µg vitamin A/g. Serum content ranges between 50 and 90 µg/dl (with individual variations). Even if no more vitamin A is consumed, the blood level is maintained for 12–15 months during which the liver contents continue to decrease. A marginal deficiency in the serum is detectable only during the last stage, just before complete exhaustion of liver storage.

Additionally, the wide range of normal values makes it hard to interpret serum values. Consequently, a serum value within normal range is of no diagnostic value and cannot be used to infer the vitamin A status of the entire organism.

A. Homeostasis: Comparing Internal Reference and Actual Values

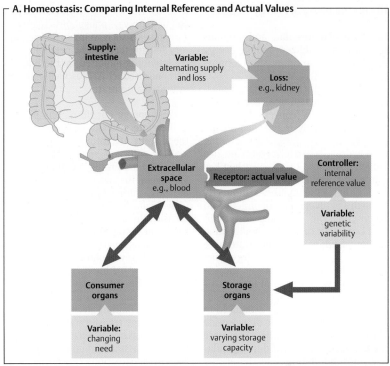

Supply: intestine

Variable: alternating supply and loss

Loss: e.g., kidney

Extracellular space e.g., blood

Receptor: actual value

Controller: internal reference value

Variable: genetic variability

Consumer organs

Variable: changing need

Storage organs

Variable: varying storage capacity

B. Retinol Homeostasis

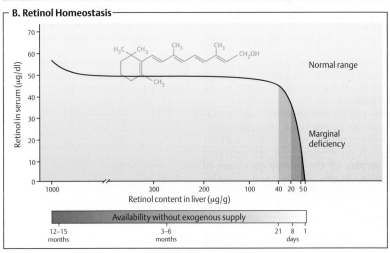

Retinol in serum (µg/dl)

Retinol content in liver (µg/g)

Normal range

Marginal deficiency

Availability without exogenous supply

12–15 months

3–6 months

21 8 1 days

The Biochemistry of Energy Transfer

The carbohydrates, fat, and proteins consumed are oxidized, and the energy that is released in the process is transferred to ATP (**A**).

The key substance for this energy transfer is **acetyl-coenzyme A** (acetyl-CoA). Carbohydrates are converted to pyruvate during **glycolysis** and then further to acetyl-CoA. The fatty acids resulting from hydrolysis of triglycerides are also broken down into this two-carbon key compound. Amino acids from proteins are either metabolized indirectly through a pyruvate stage or directly into acetyl-CoA. The resulting acetyl-CoA pool can either be used to build amino and fatty acids or enter the **citrate cycle** where it is oxidized for energy gain. During this process, carbon dioxide (CO_2) forms when carbon atoms get oxidized; the coenzyme nicotinamide adenine dinucleotide (NAD^+) is reduced to NADH and flavine adenine dinucleotide (FAD) is reduced to $FADH_2$. These are subsequently reoxidized during **oxidative phosphorylation,** and the energy released in the process is stored as ATP energy. Organisms need a sophisticated respiratory apparatus for this purpose alone: oxygen has to be made available in order to oxidize NADH, and the CO_2 resulting from oxidation of energy nutrients' carbon atoms needs to be eliminated.

The energy metabolism's major metabolic pathways share mutually interactive control mechanisms without which an efficient and self-regulated interplay of the energy pathways of carbohydrates, lipids, and proteins would be impossible. Energy use functions as an important control value, overall. Many enzymatic pathways of the energy metabolism are inhibited when a cell receives more energy than it needs. The second enzyme of the glycolytic pathway, phosphofructokinase-1, represents such an important regulatory enzyme for an early metabolic step. Its activity is inhibited by the energy-rich end product ATP, as well as by an intermediate, citrate.

A rapid energy transformation process is, therefore, necessitates the removal of the forming ATP through energy use, as well as sufficient supply of substrate and oxygen. **Aerobic metabolism** prevails when the two latter requirements are met. During physical activity it is unavoidable for the oxygen supply to be occasionally insufficient for the necessary energy transformation. This leads to incomplete performance of the last step, oxidative phosphorylation. Its substrate NADH builds up and in turn inhibits the citrate cycle upstream, leading in turn to a build-up of pyruvate, which inhibits glycolysis. Thus, the entire energy transformation is halted. The body has one alternative allowing it to extract a small amount of energy— even in this situation—converting pyruvate into lactate. While this is a dead-end pathway, it removes pyruvate so that glycolysis can again produce at least a small amount of ATP. This **anaerobic metabolism** enables sudden, maximal muscle performance without any required preparatory steps.

A. Transfer of Nutrient Energy to High-Energy Compounds

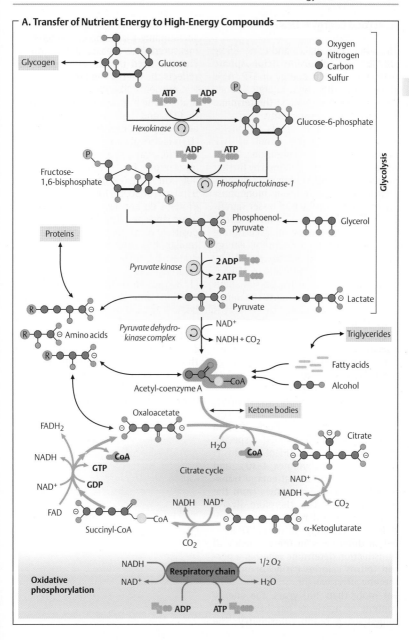

How Food Energy Is Used

The adult body makes and uses ~85 kg (187 lb) of **adenosine triphosphate** (**ATP**) per day. The energy in ATP (**A**) is stored in the high-energy bonds between the phosphates; the terminal bond has the highest energy.

Hydrolysis of these bonds (**B**) yields ~8 kcal (33.47 kJ) per 1 mol of ATP under physiological conditions. Additional energy can be obtained by further breakdown of ADP (adenosine diphosphate) to AMP (adenosine monophosphate)—this reaction is of lesser significance, though. In a reversal of the above hydrolysis, the energy released during the metabolic breakdown of energy nutrients is used to synthesize ATP by attaching a phosphate group to ADP.

Even though in a healthy person about 95 % of the energy nutrients consumed are absorbed, only part of that energy is converted into ATP energy (**C**).

Fifty percent of the **metabolizable energy** (also called physiological calorific content) of the metabolized energy nutrients is immediately converted to heat energy. A few percent are used for digestion, modification, distribution, and storage of energy nutrients. This postprandial **thermic effect of food** (**TEF**) used to be called "specific dynamic action." The TEF of proteins is 14–20 %, of carbohydrates 4–10 %, and of fats 2–4 %. The actual energy transduced to ATP energy comes from the remaining ~40 %. One, therefore, always consumes considerably more energy than will ultimately end up as ATP. Individual differences in the efficiency of transduction determine whether a person "burns calories easily" or not and thereby affect weight.

For more than 100 years, the energy content of nutrients has been determined using **bomb calorimetry**. The temperature changes in the medium surrounding the bomb calorimeter are measured. The measured heat difference is called the **calorific value** and reflects the energy content.

For nutrients like lipids and carbohydrates, which are completely oxidized to CO_2 and H_2O in metabolism, the **actual** (physiological) **calorific value** (**D**) is identical to the bomb calorimetric calorific value, assuming complete absorption. For carbohydrates, it is 400 kcal (1680 kJ)/100 g, for lipids 930 kcal (3890 kJ)/100 g.

Proteins do not have a uniform caloric value since proteins differ in their composition of amino acids. On average, though, it is similar to that of carbohydrates: for instance, the physiological calorific value of casein is 4.25 kcal (17.8 kJ)/g. Nitrogen (N) contained in proteins cannot be fully oxidized by the body. It is used to make urea, which is excreted by the kidneys. Since the N in urea is not oxidized, some of the energy consumed with proteins is always lost through the urine. Therefore, for proteins, the actual, physiological calorific value is always lower than the calorific value determined by bomb calorimetry.

A. Adenosine triphosphate

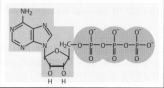

B. ATP hydrolysis

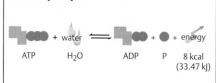

ATP + H₂O ⇌ ADP + P + energy 8 kcal (33.47 kJ)

C. Food Energy

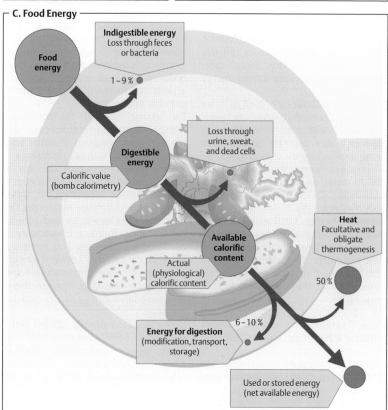

Food energy

Indigestible energy
Loss through feces or bacteria
1–9 %

Digestible energy

Calorific value (bomb calorimetry)

Loss through urine, sweat, and dead cells

Available calorific content

Actual (physiological) calorific content

Heat
Facultative and obligate thermogenesis
50 %

Energy for digestion
(modification, transport, storage)
6–10 %

Used or stored energy
(net available energy)

D. Use of Nutrients for Making ATP

Nutrient	ATP formed/ 100 g nutrient	Physiological calorific value/100 g nutrient	Required nutrient energy/1 mol ATP
Carbohydrates (starch)	23.5 mol	410 kcal (1720 kJ)	17.4 kcal (73.2 kJ)
Fat (tristearate)	51.4 mol	930 kcal (3890 kJ)	18.1 kcal (75.7 kJ)
Protein (casein)	20.4 mol	425 kcal (1780 kJ)	20.8 kcal (87.3 kJ)

Energy Requirements

Human energy requirements can be divided into three essential components (**A**): basal metabolism, energy required for physical activity, and energy used for food-induced thermogenesis. There are a number of additional minor factors, often neglected because of their lesser share in the basal metabolism, like increase in metabolic rate due to body, organ, or muscle growth. Mental activity, though perceived as work, does not impact energy metabolism.

The **basal metabolic rate** (BMR) is by no means constant, but varies between individuals and over time. Sleeping induces a 10 % decrease compared to being awake. Intense cold causes a 2–5 % increase. Temperatures above 30° C (86° F) cause an increase of 0.5 % per additional °C. Women, having more body fat, generally have a lower BMR compared to men. Until ages 4–5, basal metabolism increases significantly in relation to body weight, then decreases slowly until age 20–25. With increasing age, a decrease in metabolically active tissue (mainly muscle tissue) further reduces BMR. Individual variations in the significance of thermogenesis versus ATP synthesis account for people's different levels of metabolic efficiency.

Energy consumption does correlate with body weight (**B**), but depends predominantly on lean body mass. Since increasing body weight usually goes along with an increase in metabolically inactive fatty tissue, body mass increases usually do not result in large increases in energy consumption.

Most people greatly overestimate energy use through **physical activity** (**C**). Nowadays, high-energy-use activities are, for the most part, restricted to professional or semi-professional athletes.

Energy consumption is determined by the number of muscle fibers used and the intensity of their use. This type of activity always requires increased oxygen consumption resulting in an increase in respiratory rate and heart rate (**D**). The one-dimensional, sustained training of individual muscle groups as commonly practiced by body builders does not represent extreme activity and therefore increases energy use only minimally.

The classic method for measuring energy consumption is **direct calorimetry**. A closed, insulated chamber with controlled air supply represents a closed system in which the law of energy conservation applies: all energy produced must ultimately be transformed into heat. Since measuring this heat energy is expensive and complicated, today, **indirect calorimetry** is used nearly exclusively. This method is based on the fact that a defined amount of oxygen is required to produce a specific amount of energy. One can, therefore, determine energy use by measuring oxygen consumption.

Recently, a new **doubly labeled water technique** (DLW) was developed that allows for very precise BMR measurement through detection of excreted $^{2}H_{2}^{18}O$ molecules. A drawback is the high price of ^{18}O.

A. Energy Metabolism

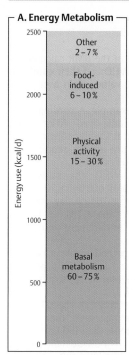

Energy use (kcal/d)

Other	2–7%
Food-induced	6–10%
Physical activity	15–30%
Basal metabolism	60–75%

B. Energy Use and Body Weight

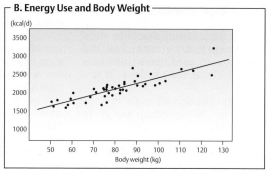

(kcal/d)

Body weight (kg)

C. Energy Use and Activity Levels

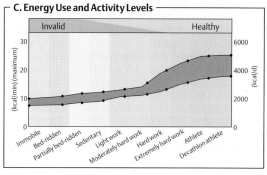

Invalid   Healthy

(kcal/min) (maximum)   (kcal/d)

Immobile, Bed-ridden, Partially bed-ridden, Sedentary, Light work, Moderately hard work, Hard work, Extremely hard work, Athlete, Decathlon athlete

D. Metabolic Rate and Physical Activity

Physical activity	Respiratory rate (l/min)	Oxygen used (l/min)	Heart rate (beats/min)	Calories consumed (kcal/min)	(kcal/kg/h)
Sedentary Sleeping, lying down, sitting, driving, standing up, ironing	< 10	< 0.5	< 80	< 2.5 1.0–1.1 1.1–1.5	1.3–1.5
Lightly active Walking (5 kmh = 3.1 mph), ping-pong, golf	10–20	0.5–1.0	80–100	2.5–5.0 2.5–3.0	2.6–2.9
Moderately active Walking (6 kmh = 3.7 mph), bicycling, tennis, cleaning	20–35	1.0–1.5	100–120	5.0–7.5	4.1–4.3
Very active Hiking uphill with backpack, digging, swimming (3 kmh = 1.9 mph), playing basketball	35–50	1.5–2.0	120–140	7.5–10.0	8.0–8.4
Extremely active Running, climbing	50–65	2.0–2.5	140–160	10.0–12.5	
Unusually and extremely active	65–85	2.5–3.0	160–180	12.5–15.0	
Active to exhaustion	>85	>3.0	>180	>15.0	

Energy Requirements

Energy requirements should be stated as MJ (mega Joule); in reality, kcal (kilocalories) are used more commonly. 1 MJ = 239 kcal, and 1 kcal = 4.184 kJ.

A variety of models are available for the calculation of individual energy requirements.

Here is a **simple formula**: 1 kcal/kg BW/h is required to maintain basic metabolism (BMR). Light physical activity increases this amount by ~1/3 and moderate physical activity by ~2/3. Intense physical activity doubles it.
Here is an example: A 70 kg man would have a BMR of 1 kcal $\times$ 24 h $\times$ 70 kg = 1680 kcal/d. Add 1/3 for light physical activity, for example, no exercise, sedentary occupation. The resulting daily requirement is 2230 kcal. This simple formula disregards differences based on gender, age, or other individual factors.

Using empirical data, the WHO established tables (A) that are commonly used to predict BMR. This calculated BMR is then multiplied by a factor called **Physical Activity Level (PAL)**. To obtain a precise result, the PAL should be used in combination with the duration of the respective activity, e.g. seven hours of sleep at PAL 0.95, three hours housework at PAL 2.4, etc.

The recent introduction of the method using labeled water permits long-term BMR measurements, allowing the establishment of PAL values for defined categories of activity (B). The BMR of various occupational groups was determined, also taking into account various types of leisure activity. The resulting several-day average is more "user-friendly" than the calculation of individual activities.

Simplification of the BMR calculations according to WHO and their combination with PAL values yield a practical table (C).
Let's use our example: According to the table, our middle-aged 70 kg man's BMR is 1740 kcal. Combined with a PAL of 1.4, his daily energy requirement would be 2400 kcal/d.
According to WHO, the same man would have a BMR of $0.048 \times 70 \times 3.653$ = 7.013 MJ or 1676 kcal/day (see Fig. A). Combined with a PAL of 1.4, his daily energy requirement would be 2346 kcal/d.
The simplest method results in a BMR of 1680 kcal/d (add 1/3 for light physical activity) and a total energy requirement of 2240 kcal/d.
The difference between the table, the exact calculation, and the simple method is no more than 160 kcal/d. Due to the large inter-individual differences in energy requirements, this difference is usually irrelevant for practical purposes.

All of these calculations of energy requirements share one property, though: they only apply to healthy individuals of normal weight, and even then, they represent only a guideline. What counts, in the end, is whether the respective caloric intake achieves long-term stable weight.

A. Estimating the BMR (according to WHO 1985)

	Age group	Formula for BMR estimate
Women	10 – 18 y	BMR = 0.056 x kgBW + 2.898
	19 – 30 y	BMR = 0.062 x kgBW + 2.036
	31 – 60 y	BMR = 0.034 x kgBW + 3.538
	> 60 y	BMR = 0.038 x kgBW + 2.755
Men	10 – 18 y	BMR = 0.074 x kgBW + 2.754
	19 – 30 y	BMR = 0.063 x kgBW + 2.896
	31 – 60 y	BMR = 0.048 x kgBW + 3.653
	> 60 y	BMR = 0.049 x kgBW + 2.459

Calculation result represents BMR in MJ/d; multiply by 239 to obtain BMR in kcal/d

B. PAL

Life style and level of activity	PAL	Examples
Chair-bound or bed-ridden	1.2	Elderly, frail
Seated work with no option of moving around and little or no strenuous leisure activity	1.4 – 1.5	Office workers, precision mechanics
Seated work with discretion and requirement to move around but little or no strenuous leisure activity	1.6 – 1.7	Lab technicians, drivers, college students, assembly line workers
Standing work (e.g., housework, shop assistant)	1.8 – 1.9	Housewives, sales persons, waiters, mechanics, craftsmen
Strenuous work or highly active leisure	2.0 – 2.4	Construction workers, farmers, miners, performance athletes

C. Guideline Table

Age Teens and adults	BMR		Activity level (PAL)							
			1.4		1.6		1.8		2.0	
	MJ/d	kcal/d	MJ	kcal	MJ	kcal	MJ	kcal	MJ	kcal
Female										
15 to < 19 y	6.1	1460	8.5	2000	9.8	2300	11,0	2600	12.2	2900
19 to < 25 y	5.8	1390	8.1	1900	9.3	2200	10.4	2500	11.6	2800
25 to < 51 y	5.6	1340	7.8	1900	9.0	2100	10.1	2400	11.2	2700
51 to < 65 y	5.3	1270	7.4	1800	8.5	2000	9.5	2300	10.6	2500
≥ 65 y	4.9	1170	6.9	1800	7.5	1800	8.8	2100	9.8	2300
Male										
15 to < 19 y	7.6	1820	10.6	2500	12.2	2900	13.7	3300	15.2	3600
19 to < 25 y	7.6	1820	10.6	2500	12.2	2900	13.7	3300	15.2	3600
25 to < 51 y	7.3	1740	10.2	2400	11.7	2800	13.1	3100	14.6	3500
51 to < 65 y	6.6	1580	9.2	2200	10.6	2500	11.9	2800	13.2	3200
≥ 65 y	5.9	1410	8.3	2000	9.4	2300	10.6	2500	11.8	2800

Tissue-Specific Energy Metabolism

The **brain** depends almost exclusively on glucose for energy. Since it cannot store compounds for oxidation, it has to receive a constant supply of glucose. To make this possible, a minimum blood glucose level has to be maintained at all times (**A**). The brain uses about 120 g of glucose per day; during phases of prolonged fasting or starvation it can use ketone bodies instead, but only to a limited extent.

Muscle tissue, on the contrary, possesses large glycogen stores. When broken down, it is converted into glucose-6-phosphate, which cannot be further hydrolyzed. It is metabolized exclusively via the glycolytic pathway and cannot pass into the blood as blood glucose. Particularly in cases of sudden spurts of activity, glucose is the predominant energy supply molecule for muscle cells. Under anaerobic conditions, lactate forms, which is then released into the bloodstream.

Triglycerides stored in **fatty tissue** are the most important form of stored energy for humans. To esterify fatty acids, the fatty tissues need activated glycerol. The enzyme glycerokinase, however, which ist required to make activated glycerol, is not available in fatty tissue. The glycerol released during ongoing triglyceride hydrolysis cannot be used to make new fat. Instead, to make new fat, activated glycerol must be provided by glycolysis. Fat synthesis in cells is, therefore, possible only if there is sufficient glucose available—a fact used by many so-called "diets."

The **liver** is the body's metabolic control center. It can take up large amounts of glucose, store it as glycogen, and make it available to stabilize blood glucose levels. As long as there is a sufficient supply of energy nutrients, the liver also synthesizes fatty acids, esterifies them into lipids, and sends them off to the peripheral tissues as lipoproteins.

During **starvation** or **prolonged fasting**, however, the liver increasingly converts fatty acids into ketone bodies (**B**). The liver starts to synthesize them as soon as the supply of acetyl-CoA falls below levels that can be processed in the citrate cycle. These ketone bodies are used as a source of energy in all tissues except the liver itself. At the same time, amino acids resulting from protein breakdown are used for gluconeogenesis in order to maintain the necessary minimum supply of glucose.

Theoretically, human fat stores would supply enough energy for two months. However, only about 3 kg of protein can be mobilized, covering the nervous system's glucose needs for about 15 days. Only due to the flexible nature of nerve cells is fasting beyond that duration possible (**C**). Nerve cells can drastically reduce their glucose use during prolonged fasts, making up for the resulting energy deficit by using ketone bodies. Thus, fewer amino acids are needed for gluconeogenesis, protecting the protein in lean body tissue. This mechanism enables humans to survive several weeks of fasting or starvation .

A. Fuel Reserves of a 70 kg (154 lb) man (kcal)

	Blood	Liver	Brain	Muscle	Fatty tissues
Glucose or glycogen	60 kcal	390 kcal	8 kcal	1200 kcal	80 kcal
Triglycerides	45 kcal	450 kcal	0 kcal	450 kcal	135 000 kcal
Proteins available as fuel	0 kcal	390 kcal	0 kcal	24 000 kcal	37 kcal

B. Fuel Metabolism in the Liver During Prolonged Fasting or Starvation

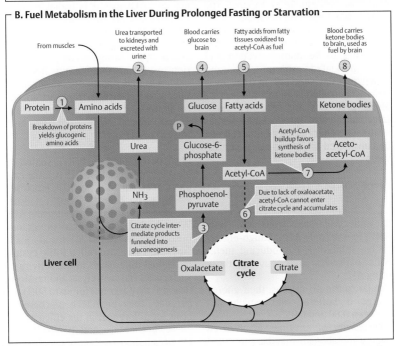

C. Fuel Metabolism During Fasting or Starvation

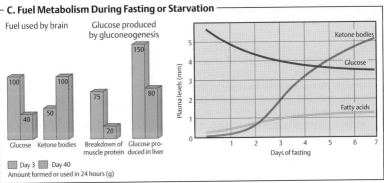

Day 3   Day 40
Amount formed or used in 24 hours (g)

Control of Energy Metabolism

The production of energy-rich ATP is always coupled with its breakdown to ADP (**A**). This is necessary since the body contains only a few grams of ATP, ADP, and AMP. In order to cover the daily caloric requirement of ~2000 kcal, 80 kg of free adenine nucleotides are needed. To achieve this, each ADP molecule has to be phosphorylated and dephosporylated several thousand times per day—and all of that in a strictly controlled fashion.

These processes are regulated via a large number of interlocking mechanisms. The **energy charge** of a cell can be considered to function as a control value:

$$\text{Energy charge} = \frac{[ATP] + \frac{1}{2}[ADP]}{[ATP] + [ADP] + [AMP]}$$

Its value will range from zero (only AMP) to one (only ATP). A high-energy charge inhibits ATP producing metabolic pathways and activates those using ATP.

Similar to the pH of cells, their energy charge is buffered and usually lies between 0.80 and 0.95.

The activity of enzymes involved in energy metabolism may be controlled by a variety of mechanisms. The amount of an enzyme may be regulated via gene expression in the nucleus. For some enzymes, the speed at which they are broken down is regulated. **Reversible modification** is a particularly important mechanism of enzyme control. The following is an example of reversible modification: When glucose is needed, glycogen phosphorylase is activated by phosphorylation of a particular serine R-group in the enzyme. The activated glycogen phosphorylase then catalyzes the breakdown of glycogen, making glucose available.

Although theoretically coupled, ATP-using and ATP-producing processes can be uncoupled at times (**B**). While the cell uses ATP no ADP is available to the mitochondria. This inhibits ATP synthesis, leading to build-up of NADH. The resulting NADH/NAD$^+$ ratio inhibits the citrate cycle, bringing energy production to a standstill. In reality, however, oxidation and phosphorylation can be uncoupled: electron transport in the respiratory chain continues unimpeded, albeit now producing heat instead of ATP.

Phosphofructokinase (PFK) is subject to allosteric inhibition by ATP (**C**). The catalytic reaction uses up ATP. Fructose-1,6-biphosphatase (FBPase) catalyzes the reverse reaction without using ATP. When both reactions occur simultaneously, a net "waste" of ATP results. Such "useless" cycles are called **futile cycles**. Individual differences in the activity of such cycles (fat hydrolysis and reesterification) may account for up to 500 kcal per day. They provide a biochemical basis for differences in the efficiency of energy nutrient use and thereby for differences in body weight of people with identical nutritional habits and environments.

A. Endergonic and Exergonic Processes

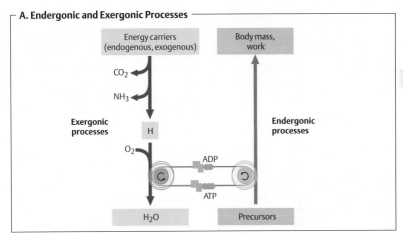

B. Energy Production: Coupled / Uncoupled

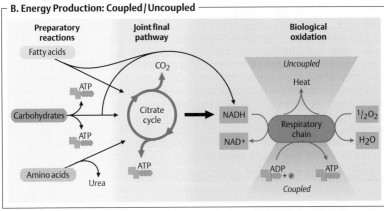

C. Futile Cycle

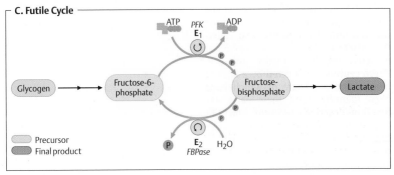

Homeostasis: Hunger and Satiety

The homeostasis of food intake is a complex process involving metabolic, endocrine, and neuronal processes. Due to their complexity this book can only provide a cursory overview (**A**).

Afferent control. Beyond visual and olfactory stimuli, taste plays a major role in regulating food intake. For example, metabolic effects of absorbed nutrients are either mediated directly by nutrient receptors or indirectly through a secondary change in the energy charge of liver cells. A multitude of gastrointestinal hormones plays various, highly significant roles in regulating food intake. The role of cholecystokinin (CCK), which is considered to be an important "satiety hormone," has been researched intensely. Release of these hormones is triggered by receptors in the stomach and duodenum, and the signals passed on either through the blood stream or through vagal afferent nerve impulses. Signals from stretch receptors, indicating stomach fullness, are also transmitted by the vagus nerve. Insulin functions as a satiety signal by regulating central nervous insulin receptors.

Central nervous conduction. We distinguish two centers of importance for nutrient uptake in the hypothalamus: the ventromedial nucleus, also called the **satiety center,** and a ventrolateral nucleus, which regulates **appetite**. These centers are affected by a host of neurochemicals, some of which have been identified and their particular functions described. Serotonin and CCK, e.g., lessen the appetite for carbohydrates, whereas CRF (corticotropin releasing factor) reduces hunger for fats and carbohydrates.

In addition, the complex interplay of CNS neurotransmitters is modulated by higher-level centers. **Psychological influences** have a major impact on food intake regulation. For instance, long-term, sustained stress may lead to lasting weight loss by activating neuroendocrine systems. **Habit**, on the other hand, is a major factor leading to overweight when food is in constant, abundant supply. **Hereditary factors** causing weight gain have also been scientifically confirmed (see p. 38).

Efferent control. Beyond controlling the motor activities directly involved in food intake, the brain can influence peripheral organs via the autonomic nervous system, as well as through hormones released by the adenohypophysis. Often, a high activity level of the sympathetic nervous system correlates with low body weight. In overweight people, decreased secretion of prolactin and growth hormone can be commonly observed. Therefore, efferent control is not limited to processes directly associated with food intake, but its affects also reach deep into cellular metabolism.

A. Homeostasis of Nutrient Uptake

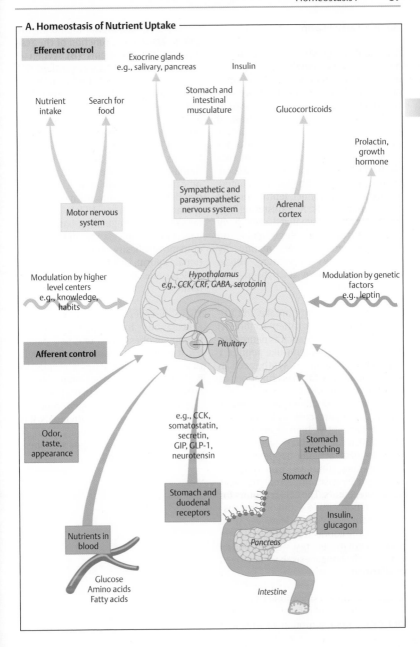

Efferent control

Nutrient intake

Search for food

Exocrine glands
e.g., salivary, pancreas

Insulin

Stomach and intestinal musculature

Glucocorticoids

Prolactin, growth hormone

Motor nervous system

Sympathetic and parasympathetic nervous system

Adrenal cortex

Modulation by higher level centers
e.g., knowledge, habits

Hypothalamus
e.g., CCK, CRF, GABA, serotonin

Modulation by genetic factors
e.g., leptin

Pituitary

Afferent control

Odor, taste, appearance

e.g., CCK, somatostatin, secretin, GIP, GLP-1, neurotensin

Stomach and duodenal receptors

Stomach stretching

Stomach

Insulin, glucagon

Nutrients in blood

Pancreas

Glucose
Amino acids
Fatty acids

Intestine

Homeostasis: Leptin

A person's body weight is determined by the factors hunger/satiation and energy intake/energy use. Ever since hereditary forms of obesity were discovered in mice in the 1950s, researchers have investigated the regulation of these factors. About 20 years ago, it was found that the so-called ob mouse (for obese) is missing a satiety factor that would normally circulate in its blood. Finally, in 1994, the **ob gene** was cloned. The expression product, **leptin**, consists of 167 amino acids. Administering leptin to ob mice normalized their body weight by reducing energy intake and increasing energy use, mainly by increasing body temperature. Leptin and its effects have since been confirmed in humans.

Leptin controls energy uptake and use by regulating various satiety factors (**A**) in the hypothalamus, such as neuropeptide Y (NPY) or glucagon-like peptide 1 (GLP-1). Since leptin is synthesized in white adipocytes, fat mass functions as a sort of central control sensor.

The expression of the ob gene is greatly enhanced by glucocorticoids and insulin. Consequently, high insulin levels should result in low body weight, contrary to what actually happens. These contradictory findings can only be explained by assuming problems with various receptors. The CNS receptors for leptin, neuropeptide Y and other transmitters are now known. However, until recently, the connection between leptin and cellular energy consumption through thermogenesis had not been established.

It has been known since 1994 that there is a protein in brown fatty tissue called **UCP1** (uncoupling protein 1) which, at the inner mitochondrial membrane, is able to assume the function of the respiratory chain proteins (**B**). When it does, the electrochemical gradient (H^+ electron chain) is not used to produce energy in the form of ATP. Rather, free fatty acid anions (FFA^-) serve as proton acceptors—a "nonsensical" cycle that produces only heat and thereby "wastes" energy. Finally, in 1997, **UCP2** was discovered, which, unlike UCP1, is found in many tissues. Neither its significance nor its regulation is known in detail yet. Based on its more widespread occurrence, UCP2 may be responsible for regulating basal metabolic rate and have a role in the development of obesity. Recently, an additional isoform, UCP3, was discovered in skeletal muscle, and traces in all fatty tissues.

These discoveries have raised great expectations for a pharmacological therapy of obesity and of type 2 diabetes. It needs to be pointed out, though, that in humans and animals, regulation is usually polygenic. For instance, it has been shown in humans that a polymorphism of the β3-adrenergic receptor is more common in obese individuals. It is likely that more such genes, each of which contributes a small part to obesity, will be discovered.

A. Homeostasis of Body Weight

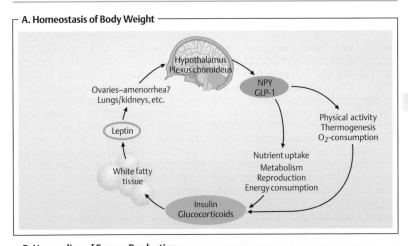

B. Uncoupling of Energy Production

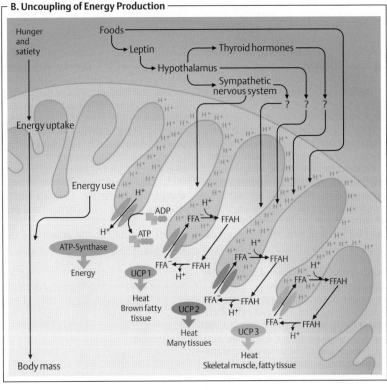

Stomach Function

The stomach stores ingested foods, breaks them down mechanically, alters them chemically, disinfects them with stomach acid, and passes on the resulting **chyme** to the duodenum for further digestion in small portions.

The proximal stomach (**A**), also called **fundus**, develops an active tonus which can adjust to the intragastric pressure. Its primary function is, therefore, storage. Solid food is deposited layer upon layer while liquids run down the stomach wall. The distal stomach sections, **corpus**, and **antrum**, contain within their smooth muscle autonomous pacemaker cells, which produce distally advancing waves of potential (slow waves). Their frequency is 3–4/min. That is, however, below the activation threshold. When needed, contractions with the frequency of **slow waves** are triggered by neuronal and humoral influences. An important stimulus is provided by the stretching of the intestinal wall caused by a full stomach. The peristaltic contractions triggered by the stretching drive the stomach contents towards the **pylorus**, which closes—controlled by a complex interaction of regulatory mechanisms—squeezing and pushing the contents back into the stomach. Due to this maceration, 90 % of all particles leaving the stomach are less than 0.25 mm in size. The close regulatory monitoring of the pylorus' opening and closing is necessary to prevent overburdening of subsequent digestive and absorptive processes.

The 2–3 l of stomach juices are secreted essentially by three types of cells. **Parietal cells** (**B**) actively pump protons into the lumen in exchange for potassium. Potassium and chloride are also transported actively, increasing the H^+ concentration to a level more than a million times higher than in blood. The **protons** are produced in a carboanhydrase reaction. The bicarbonate resulting from this reaction is transported into the blood in exchange for chloride. Pepsinogen, a mixture of protease precursors secreted by the **chief cells**, is converted into protein-digesting **pepsin** when exposed to HCl. Pepsin is an autocatalytic enzyme acting to produce more of itself and needs an acidic environment for its activation. The **surface mucous cells** produce an alkaline secretion which creates an **unstirred layer** on the surface of the mucous membrane. This causes the pH at the cell surface to be near neutral even with extremely acidic pH in the lumen—an essential protection for the stomach wall to prevent self-digestion.

Gastric secretion is divided into several distinct phases (**C**). The **cephalic phase** is triggered by expectation of food, by seeing, smelling, etc. Pavlov discovered that this secretion, mediated by vagal impulses, can be up to 50 % of maximal total secretory activity. The **excitatory phase** is dominated by release of gastrin from G cells of the antrum stimulated by partially digested protein fragments. During the **inhibitory phase** duodenal signals predominate. Signals from stretch-, protein-, fat-, osmo-, and pH-receptors trigger the release of hormones that inhibit the activity of the secretory cells.

A. Peristaltic Contractions

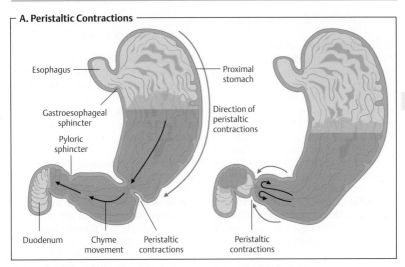

Esophagus
Proximal stomach
Gastroesophageal sphincter
Direction of peristaltic contractions
Pyloric sphincter
Duodenum
Chyme movement
Peristaltic contractions
Peristaltic contractions

B. Parietal Cell (HCl Production)

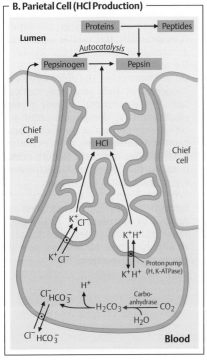

Lumen

Proteins → Peptides

Autocatalysis

Pepsinogen → Pepsin

Chief cell

HCl

Chief cell

K^+ Cl^-
K^+ Cl^-

K^+ H^+
Proton pump (H, K-ATPase)
K^+ H^+

H^+

Cl^-
HCO_3^-

Carbo-anhydrase
H_2CO_3 CO_2
H_2O

Cl^-
HCO_3^-

Blood

C. Phases of Stomach Secretion

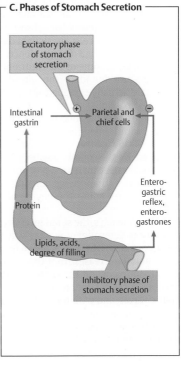

Excitatory phase of stomach secretion

Intestinal gastrin

Parietal and chief cells

Protein

Entero-gastric reflex, enterogastrones

Lipids, acids, degree of filling

Inhibitory phase of stomach secretion

Absorption: Anatomy and Histology

The **small intestine** can be divided into three sections: the **duodenum**, which has important regulatory functions and receptors, with bile and pancreatic ducts leading into it; the **jejunum** (1.5–2.5 m in length); and the **ileum** (2–3 m in length). The intestinal tube is 4 cm in diameter and ~5 m long, which would normally give it a surface area of 0.5 m². Through the addition of **folds**, **villi**, and **microvilli** the absorptive surface increases to 200 m².

Each **villus** makes up a functional unit, together with its neighboring **crypt** (**A**). Initially 16 stem cells per crypt divide into about 150 proliferating cells, which run through a few additional cell cycles. During their migration to the villus tip, they differentiate into various cell types, with secretory or absorptive functions. The tip cells are sloughed off and replaced every 3–6 days. Hence, at any given time, some of the "nutrients" and enzymes found in the intestinal lumen are actually sloughed-off cells of the intestinal lining.

Each villus contains one central blood vessel with subepithelial branching. About 10–15% of the cardiac output is allocated to the small intestine. This blood flow can be increased postprandially to more than twice its original volume, surrounding the chyme after meals.

Like the stomach's, the **small intestine's motility** is determined by slow waves. The frequency of the associated changes in potential decreases from the oral to the anal area, given the orally located sections a trigger function. Also, peristaltic waves, and with them the movement of intestinal contents, can only travel in one direction, i.e., from oral to anal. The intestinal tube is also able to actively mix its contents by separating individual segments.

Analysis of the histology of **enterocytes** (**B**) reveals a multitude of transport pathways within and between the cells, as well as to the outside. Consequently, absorption is not a unified process, but an overarching term encompassing many interlacing processes.

Transcellular transport (**C**) can be active or passive. Electrogenic Na^+ transport plays a central role as the driving force behind many absorptive processes. Na^+ is pumped into the intercellular space by a Na^+ pump located at the basolateral cell membrane. This process is ATP-dependent and creates an extreme difference between the Na^+ concentration inside the cells (15 mmol/l) and the plasma (140 mmol/l). Additionally, this creates a potential difference of about −40 mV between the two media.

On the lumen side, the enterocytes are connected by tight junctions. Particularly in the proximal regions of the small intestine, though, the latter are sufficiently permeable to allow **paracellular diffusion** along a concentration gradient. This can occur in both directions so that water and electrolytes, e.g., can also reach the lumen.

Even small particles are able to pass through the apparently dense intestinal mucosa by **translocation** (leaky gut). These intact, undigested particles play an important role, for instance, in triggering allergic reactions.

A. Villus with Brush Border

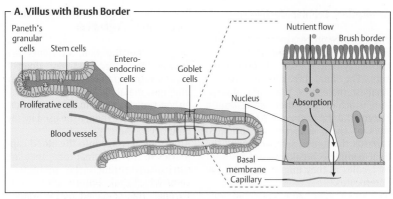

Paneth's granular cells
Stem cells
Entero-endocrine cells
Proliferative cells
Goblet cells
Blood vessels
Nucleus
Nutrient flow
Brush border
Absorption
Basal membrane
Capillary

B. Enterocyte Histology

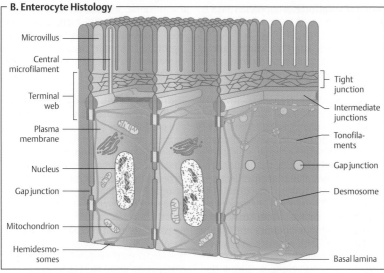

Microvillus
Central microfilament
Terminal web
Plasma membrane
Nucleus
Gap junction
Mitochondrion
Hemidesmosomes
Tight junction
Intermediate junctions
Tonofilaments
Gap junction
Desmosome
Basal lamina

C. Absorption

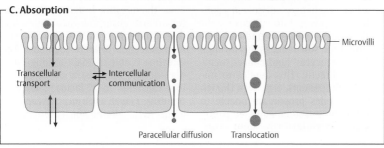

Transcellular transport
Intercellular communication
Microvilli
Paracellular diffusion
Translocation

Absorption: Cellular Mechanisms

The digestive process in the small intestine is induced by free —mostly pancreatic—enzymes, at least for most nutrients. The final breakdown into the smallest molecules, ready for absorption, is achieved by **membrane-bound enzymes** at the microvilli (**A**). The active sites of these enzymes are oriented towards the lumen side, achieving the final complete breakdown of nutrient molecules as they migrate towards the enterocytes.

Actual **absorption** can happen in 3 ways (**B**):

1. **Carrier-mediated transport** is more or less specific to individual atoms or compounds, and may or may not consume ATP.
2. **H_2O-mediated transport** involves water movement through the mucosa, carrying along soluble electrolytes and nonelectrolytes. Permeability to water-soluble substances is relatively high in the upper sections of the small intestine, decreasing gradually towards the distal segments. Therefore, discrepancies between chyme osmolarity and plasma osmotic pressure are rapidly equalized, achieving isotonic conditions between chyme and plasma as early as in the jejunum. During this water exchange, dissolved substances travel into mucosa cells along a concentration gradient.
3. **Lipophilic substances** pass through the enterocytes' lipid bilayer membrane directly. This applies to micelle components, e. g., even though the micelles proper are unable to enter the intestinal cell (see p. 90). Transport through the lipid membrane is simple **passive diffusion** along a concentration gradient.

Once **inside the cell**, nutrients are transported either passively along a concentration gradient or actively. They undergo metabolic processes, which either transform them into transport forms or prepare them to be used by the enterocytes directly.

After their **passage into the blood capillaries** of the intestinal tube, they are carried off through the mesenteric veins which drain into the portal vein. Through this so-called portal system, the nutrients are brought directly to the **liver**. There, they are further metabolized, preventing unnecessary burdening of the systemic circulatory system into which many of the metabolites will finally be released.

The mechanisms of lipid absorption differ from those used for carbohydrates and proteins (see p. 90). Inside the enterocytes, most of the lipids are integrated into chylomicrons and pass into the intestine's lymphatic system and the large veins in this form, entering the systemic circulatory system and bypassing the liver.

Active absorption mechanisms are not evenly available throughout the intestine. Individual nutrients have **preferential absorption sites** (**C**).
Since the intestine is very flexible with regard to its absorptive capabilities, sufficient nutrient uptake is possible even after resection of large segments. The intestine is able to adapt to long-term, high-dosage administration of particular nutrients (e. g., lactose): enzyme patterns, as well as absorptive capacity, adjust to the altered nutrient intake.

A. Absorption

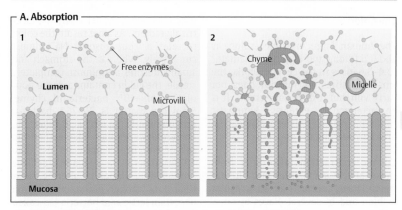

1
Free enzymes
Lumen
Microvilli
Mucosa

2
Chyme
Micelle

B. Absorption Pathways

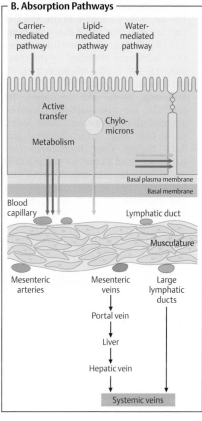

Carrier-mediated pathway
Lipid-mediated pathway
Water-mediated pathway

Active transfer
Chylo-microns
Metabolism

Basal plasma membrane
Basal membrane

Blood capillary
Lymphatic duct
Musculature

Mesenteric arteries
Mesenteric veins
Large lymphatic ducts

Portal vein
↓
Liver
↓
Hepatic vein
↓
Systemic veins

C. Absorption Sites

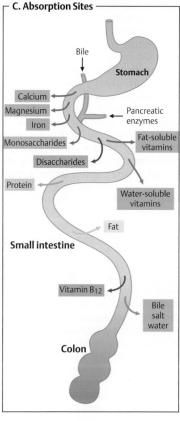

Bile
Stomach
Calcium
Magnesium
Pancreatic enzymes
Iron
Monosaccharides
Fat-soluble vitamins
Disaccharides
Protein
Water-soluble vitamins
Fat
Small intestine
Vitamin B$_{12}$
Bile salt water
Colon

The Colon

The human large intestine (colon) is about 5 ft long and its largest diameter (2.4–3.6 in) is in the cecum. Unlike the small intestine, its mucosa does not carry villi, but it does have crypts. It is characterized by extensive lymphatic tissue and plasma cells, especially in the area surrounding the appendix.

Colonic **contractions** also differ from those of the small intestine. Circular musculature contracts in an irregular fashion and in several places at once, without any net movement of chyme. True peristaltic waves that move the contents along about 8 in at a time are rare. Actual transport occurs through so-called **mass movements**, powerful contractile waves that occur once or twice daily. Like the other types of contractions, they are triggered by food intake—the so-called **gastrocolic reflex**. Chyme from low-fiber foods takes 2–3 days to transit the colon (stool weight 100–150 g), chyme from extremely high-fiber food 1–2 days, with a stool weight of up to 500 g. Larger particles may appear in the stools much faster if transported with the central stream of materials.

The colon reabsorbs 1–1.5 l of water/d. The structure of the pores and tight junctions prevents reflux of Na^+ and water into the intestinal lumen. This allows the colon to absorb Na^+ even from highly hypotonic solutions. The basolateral Na^+/K^+ pump is the driving force here, producing low Na^+ concentrations in the mucosa cells, on the one hand, and on the other, building an electrical gradient (0 mV in lumen, –30 mV inside cells, 20 mV in the interstitium [A]). Cell membrane permeability is increased by aldosterone on the lumen side. K^+ travels back through the tight junctions passively, driven by the electrical gradient. As a net result, the colon secretes K^+ but absorbs Na^+ almost completely. Whereas the stomach and small intestine are almost completely sterile, the colon contains a dense population of ~10^{12} **bacteria/ml chyme**. Stool dry matter is 30–75 % bacteria, predominantly anaerobic *Bifidus* and *Bacteroides*. Aerobes like *Escherichia coli* or enterococci make up less than 1 %. Attempts are being made to achieve immunomod-ulation by altering intestinal flora through oral administration of certain lactic acid bacteria (so-called probiotics, see p. 288).

The anaerobes are able to use ~50 % of the nutrients that come down the pipeline (**B**). They produce **useful metabolites**, which are absorbed by the colon mucosa—the most well-known example is vitamin K (see p. 160).

Resulting gases, like hydrogen, for example, are also partially absorbed and end up in the air we exhale. Short-chain fatty acids, which bacteria produce during fiber breakdown (see p. 80), are used as fuel by mucosa cells and thereby have an impact on cell proliferation. They activate colon motility and improve blood flow inside the mucosa.

A. Electrolyte Absorption in the Colon

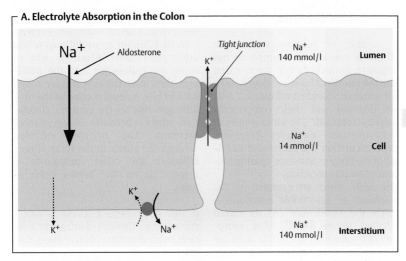

Na$^+$

Aldosterone

Tight junction

K$^+$

Na$^+$ 140 mmol/l **Lumen**

Na$^+$ 14 mmol/l **Cell**

K$^+$

K$^+$ Na$^+$

Na$^+$ 140 mmol/l **Interstitium**

B. The Role of Colon Bacteria

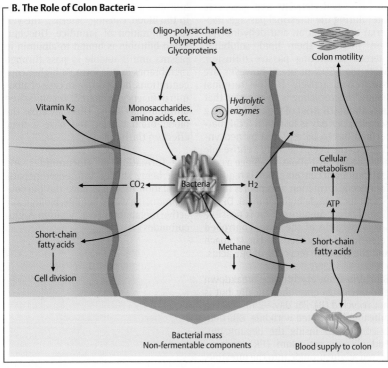

Oligo-polysaccharides
Polypeptides
Glycoproteins

Colon motility

Vitamin K$_2$

Monosaccharides,
amino acids, etc.

*Hydrolytic
enzymes*

CO_2 Bacteria H_2

Cellular
metabolism

ATP

Short-chain
fatty acids

Methane

Short-chain
fatty acids

Cell division

Bacterial mass
Non-fermentable components

Blood supply to colon

Enterohepatic Circulation

A number of substances that are absorbed into blood or lymph do not originate from foods but are released into the intestinal lumen endogenously. For instance, sloughed-off mucosa cells are digested and their components thereby "recycled." The same applies to most intestinal secretions. Enterohepatic circulation is a prominent example of the body's substance-sparing tendency towards recycling.

Bile acids, which are essential for the digestion of fat-soluble compounds, reach the duodenum (**A**) as mixed micelles (see pp. 88–90). After resorption of the micellar lipids, bile acids are left behind in the small intestine. They are absorbed actively and passively later during the intestinal passage. Bacterial deconjugation and dehydroxylation increase their lipid solubility, thereby facilitating passive diffusion. More than 50% of them, however, are reabsorbed actively in the terminal ileum. This recycling is so effective that only about 0.8 g out of the total 20–30 g secreted per day is lost with fecal matter and has to be replaced by neosynthesis in the liver. The body's entire bile acids pool is just about 3 g. Since a critical minimum concentration is required for micelle formation, this pool is insufficient for a single high-fat meal. Digestion of larger amounts of fat is possible solely because of the long, controlled retention of fatty foods in the stomach and the effective recycling of bile acids.

Bilirubin from erythrocyte breakdown also circulates enterohepatically, but is not recycled (**B**). Per day, ~250–300 mg bilirubin is excreted with bile. Bilirubin is conjugated inside the hepatocytes' endoplasmic reticulum (ER) and released as glucuronide into the intestine, where it is only partially re-absorbed. In the terminal ileum and colon, bacteria convert bilirubin to **urobilinogen** and other compounds. About 15–20% of those are reabsorbed into the portal vein, then reach the liver and are added back to bile. A small portion of the urobilinogen reaches the systemic circulation, where it becomes subject to renal excretion. The bilirubin excreted through the stools in the form of urobilinogen and other compounds is responsible for the **brown color of feces**.

If this enterohepatic circle is interrupted, e.g., through damage to liver cells, or obstruction of biliary ducts, discoloration of stools ensues. Also, bilirubin, which is yellow, accumulates in the blood, causing "icterus," the yellow coloration of **jaundice**. Unconjugated bilirubin is bound to albumin in plasma and is unable to pass through membranes in this form. At higher concentrations, however, or in case of albumin deficiency, unbound, unconjugated bilirubin may occur. This may cross the blood–brain barrier and have a toxic effect on the brain.

The **formation of glucuronides** and their being sluiced into enterohepatic circulation may also have the purpose of producing water-soluble, biologically active metabolites (e.g., vitamin A-glucuronides).

A. Portal Circulation

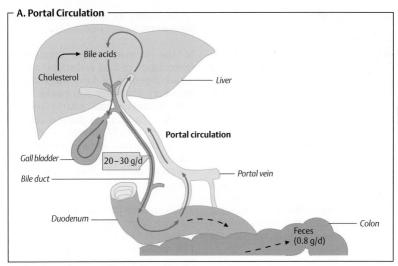

Cholesterol → Bile acids

Liver

Portal circulation

Gall bladder

Bile duct

20 – 30 g/d

Portal vein

Duodenum

Colon

Feces (0.8 g/d)

B. Bilirubin Metabolism

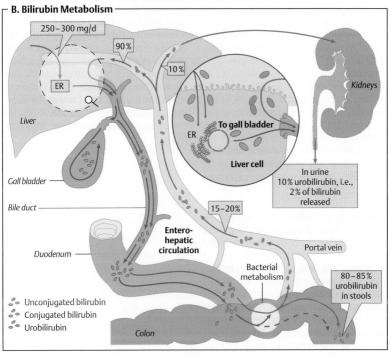

250 – 300 mg/d

90 %

10 %

ER

Kidneys

Liver

ER

To gall bladder

Liver cell

In urine 10 % urobilirubin, i.e., 2 % of bilirubin released

Gall bladder

Bile duct

15 – 20 %

Entero-hepatic circulation

Portal vein

Duodenum

Bacterial metabolism

80 – 85 % urobilirubin in stools

Colon

○ Unconjugated bilirubin
○ Conjugated bilirubin
○ Urobilirubin

Digestion: Control

The gastrointestinal tract has its own **intrinsic nervous system**. It can regulate secretory and motor functions of digestive organs independently of the extrinsic, autonomous nervous system but is nevertheless strongly influenced by the latter. The afferent neurons receive their signals from **mechano-** and **chemoreceptors**; these are most common in the duodenum. Efferent neurons may supply **smooth musculature**, as well as **glands**. Acetylcholine functions as the neurotransmitter for the preganglionic fibers of the vagus nerve. A multitude of bioactive peptides function as neurotransmitters for the postganglionic nerve fibers.

Various cell types embedded in the gastrointestinal mucosa secrete specific **gastrointestinal hormones** and **peptides (A)** upon contact with food components. The classical hormones gastrin, secretin, and cholecystokinin (CCK) are released into the blood in response to their respective stimuli. Some of the peptides diffuse into neighboring tissues and act upon effector cells there. Others are released at the nerve endings and function as neurotransmitters. These substances may have agonistic or synergistic effects on various cell types of different organs.

Hormonal regulation has a decisive influence on all digestive functions and sets in early, i. e., even before actual food intake.
Secretion of saliva, for instance, begins with the expectation of a meal and is not controlled by conditioned (oral or gastrointestinal) reflexes (Pavlov). The function of this early secretion is to enable starch breakdown by salivary amylase and to release antibacterials (thiocyanate), as well as somatostatin and growth factors (IGF, NGF).

In the **stomach**, vagal stimulation (expectation of food and stress) and/or actual ingestion of food triggers **acid secretion**. The latter also causes localized histamine and gastrin release, which in turn causes parietal cells to release H^+ ions. **Pepsinogen** is released by the chief cells in the same fashion, leading to digestion of proteins, enhanced by their denaturation in an acidic environment.

The arrival of fat and proteins in the stomach and upper small intestine stimulates CCK release into the blood. **CCK release** is a preparatory and coordinating step for the digestion of most nutrients in the **duodenum** and **jejunum** and also influences nutrient distribution after their absorption into the bloodstream. CCK quickly reduces the gastric emptying rate and stimulates the secretion of bile and pancreatic fluids into the duodenum. CCK appears to effect gall bladder contractions by stimulating acetylcholine release. CCK also enhances insulin secretion into the blood.

A. Gastrointestinal Hormones: Sites of Production and Effects

Gastrointestinal hormones	Sites of production and effects		
	Site of hormone production	Effects on secretory activity	Effects on motor activity
Gastrin	Stomach and duodenum	Stomach (HCl, pepsin) • • • • Liver (bile) • Pancreas (enzymes) •	Stomach Gall bladder
Cholecystokinin	Duodenum and jejunum	Pancreas (enzymes and HCO₃) • • • • (insulin) • Small and large intestine •	Gall bladder • • • Small and large intestine • • / • Stomach • •
Secretin	Duodenum and jejunum	Pancreas • • • • (HCO₃ and enzymes) Bile duct • •	Small and large intestine • / • Stomach • •
Vasoactive intestinal peptide	Small and large intestine	Pancreas • • • • (enzymes) Liver (bile) • • Small and large intestine • • (enzymes) Stomach • •	Stomach • • • Small intestine
Enteroglucagon	Small and large intestine	Pancreas • (insulin)	Small and large intestine • • •
Gastrointestinal inhibitory peptide	Small and large intestine	Stomach • • • Small and large intestine • (enzymes) Pancreas • (insulin)	
Motilin	Small and large intestine		Stomach • • • • Small and large intestine • • • •
Pancreatic polypeptide		Pancreas • ?	?
Somatostatin	Saliva	GI tract • • Small and large intestine	?
Bombesin	Upper small intestine	GI tract • ? Release of gastrin	?
Neurotensin	Lower small intestine	?	?
Glucagon-like peptide	Lower small intestine and colon	?	Stomach • •
Neuromedin K Substance P	Small intestine (neuronal and endocrine cells)		Small and large intestine • • (atropine-resistant contractions)
Enkephalins	Small intestine	?	?

• Stimulatory effect   • Inhibitory effect   • No effect

Digestion: Principles

Beyond mechanical processing—mixing, maceration, transport—the main function of the digestive tract is to split large food components into small absorbable units (**A**).

During this **enzymatic hydrolysis**, H_2O is reinserted in those places from where it had previously been removed during dehydration synthesis in the animal or plant cells that built the compounds. For all nutrients, this hydrolysis follows the same pattern: first, they are split into larger fragments, and subsequently they are broken down into the smallest, absorbable subunits.

Digestion of foods begins in the **buccal cavity**. The enzyme amylase, produced mostly by the parotid glands is able to hydrolyze complex carbohydrates (starch). In infants, lingual lipase plays an extremely important role, initiating fat digestion. Its role in adults is controversial; in all likelihood, its role in lipid digestion is negligible as long as there is full pancreatic function. Since the buccal cavity is relatively small, the effectiveness of these enzymes depends on how long food is kept in the mouth: the longer it is chewed, the more time for the enzymes to act upon the food.

The macerated food, mixed with saliva, reaches the stomach after passing through the esophagus. At the beginning of a meal, the **stomach** lumen tends to have a neutral pH. Then, HCl is released and mixed with the mass. Once a critical level of acidity is reached, this inactivates the salivary enzymes. Only **proteins** are actively digested in the stomach, and an acidic pH is indispensable for this process. By the time the food leaves the stomach, it usually consists mostly of larger nutrient fragments. Since the same hydrolysis can also be achieved through pancreatic enzymes, digestion without a stomach is possible—within limits.

Small intestine. The most important pancreatic juices are bicarbonate—to neutralize stomach acids—and digestive enzymes for all major nutrients.

Proteolytic enzymes and phospholipase A are secreted as inactive precursors, which are not activated until they reach the duodenum, thus preventing auto-digestion of protein-containing pancreatic membranes. Lipase, amylase, and ribonucleases are secreted in their active form.

These enzymes prevail in pancreatic juice in constant ratios. Adaptation of these concentrations to specific nutrients occurs very slowly, as, for instance, to prolonged high fat intake.

Pancreatic enzymes begin their hydrolytic work in the proximal jejunum, producing either directly absorbable units (lipids) or fragments, which are then further hydrolyzed by specific membrane-bound enzymes located in the intestinal mucosa. The end products of these specific enzymatic reactions are absorbed directly into blood, or into lymphatic fluid, as in the case of lipids.

A. Principles of Digestion

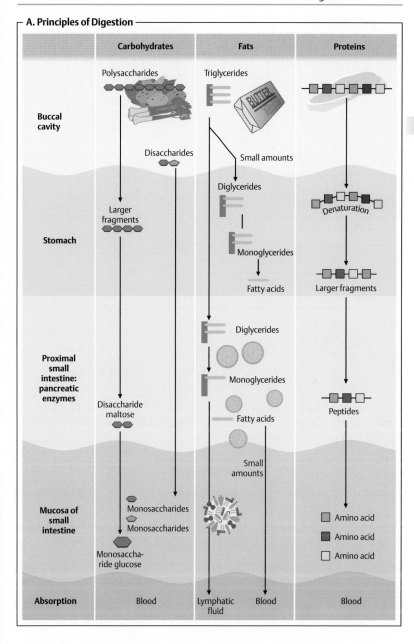

The Nutrients

Structure and Properties

Carbohydrates are hydroxylized aldehydes or ketones and are the most abundant of organic compounds. They serve as fuel, energy storage, basic building blocks in DNA and RNA, and as structural elements of bacterial and plant cell walls. Carbohydrates are bonded to other macronutrients in glycoproteins and glycolipids, which play important roles in cell membranes, as for instance in cell-cell recognition.

Food carbohydrates are built almost exclusively from the **monosaccharides,** glucose, fructose, and galactose. Depending on the number of monosaccharides bonded together, one can distinguish di-, oligo-, and polysaccharides (**A**).

Among the **disaccharides**, **sucrose** (or saccharose) plays a predominant role. It is commonly called "sugar," and can be produced from sugar cane and sugar beets. **Lactose** (milk sugar) is the predominant carbohydrate in milk. It represents a major energy source for infants. **Maltose** (malt sugar) is of lesser significance in foods, but is produced in large amounts when carbohydrate polymers are digested.

Most food carbohydrates consist of **starch**, composed of amylose and amylopectin. These macromolecules (**polysaccharides**) are made exclusively from glucose building blocks—a single amylopectin molecule may consist of hundreds of thousands of glucose molecules. Starch is the energy storage polysaccharide of plants. Cereal grains contain ~75 %, potatoes ~65 % starch (in dry matter). The animal body can store only limited amounts of carbohydrates in the liver and muscle as **glycogen**. Stored carbohydrates bind water, using more space than lipids while containing less energy. This is why the human body uses primarily fats for energy storage. Even though the structure of glycogen is similar to that of starch, it has no role in human nutrition since any stored glycogen is almost completely broken down in foods ready for consumption.

A multitude of other polysaccharides occurs in many plant species. These and others are nowadays added to foods in large amounts during processing. Usually, these additives are derived from starch: on hydrolysis, it is converted to glucose. Through physical, chemical, or enzymatic modification it becomes more water-soluble, and thereby more suitable for food processing.

All carbohydrate polymers are linked by **glycosidic** bonds (**B**). Depending on the OH groups involved in the bonds, different linkage types exist, affecting the digestibility of the various food polysaccharides. The gastrointestinal tract contains specific enzymes able to split α-glycosidic bonds (e.g., maltose, sucrose). The human body also makes an enzyme to split the β-glycosidic bonds in lactose but lacks enzymes specific to any other β-glycosidic linkages (see p. 78).

A. Carbohydrate Classification

Carbohydrate	Occurrence	Structure and Characteristics
Monosaccharides		
D-Glucose (dextrose)	Fruit, honey – traces in most plants	Water-soluble hexose
D-Fructose (fruit sugar)	Fruit, honey – traces in most plants	Water-soluble hexose
D-Galactose	Component of lactose – released during digestion	Water-soluble hexose
Disaccharides		
Sucrose or saccharose (table or cane sugar)	Sugar beets, sugar cane, fruit, maple syrup	Water-soluble disaccharide, consisting of glucose and fructose linked by α-1,2 bonds
Lactose (milk sugar)	Milk, milk products	Water soluble disaccharide, consisting of galactose and glucose linked by β-1,4 bonds
Maltose (malt sugar)	Sprouts, forms during starch digestion	Water soluble disaccharide, consisting of glucose and glucose linked by α-1,4 bonds
Polysaccharides		
Amylose	Starch, cereals, potatoes	Linear glucose polymer with α-1,4 bonds, water soluble
Amylopectin	Starch, cereals, potatoes, thickeners	Branched glucose polymer with α-1,4 and α-1,6 bonds, non-water soluble
Glycogen (animal starch)	Liver, muscle	Branched glucose polymer with α-1,4 and α-1,6 bonds, water soluble
Inulin	Artichokes	Fructose polymer, water soluble
Technical saccharides		
Dextrin	Food additive	Short fragments of an α-1,4 glucose polymer
Invert sugar	Food additive	Hydrolyzed sucrose, equal parts glucose and fructose
Glucose syrup	Food additive	Hydrolyzed starch (glucose)
High fructose corn syrup (HFCS)	Food additive	Hydrolyzed starch, partially isomerized

B. Glycosidic Bonds

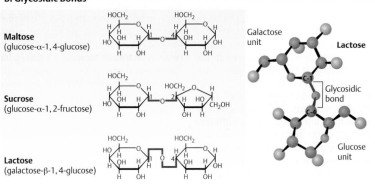

Maltose (glucose-α-1, 4-glucose)

Sucrose (glucose-α-1, 2-fructose)

Lactose (galactose-β-1, 4-glucose)

Galactose unit

Lactose

Glycosidic bond

Glucose unit

Digestion and Absorption

Since only monosaccharides can be absorbed, all carbohydrate polymers must be hydrolyzed during digestion (**A**).

This process is initiated in the mouth by **salivary amylase** and continues in the small intestine under the influence of **pancreatic amylase**. End products of this enzymatic reaction are partially glucose, but also large amounts of maltose and isomaltose. Just like sucrose or lactose, these disaccharides are split into monosaccharides by specific, **membrane-bound disaccharidases**. Since mucosa cells are continuously sloughed off, small amounts of these hydrolases are also found in the intestinal lumen.

Further absorption into **mucosal cells** can occur in several ways (**B**). On the luminal side of the mucosa, glucose and galactose are transported actively against a concentration gradient. The carrier molecule binds Na^+ and glucose in a 1:1 ratio and travels through the membrane. Na^+ is subsequently removed from the cell by Na^+/K^+-ATPase—again against a concentration gradient. Glucose leaves the mucosa cells actively using the GLUT2 carrier protein. About 25% of the glucose reaches the blood by passive diffusion; ~15% is transported back into the lumen by the carrier. Fructose is absorbed passively, with the GLUT5 transport system facilitating diffusion on the luminal side.

Depending on the efficiency of these transport systems, the various monosaccharides are absorbed at different rates. Glucose and galactose are absorbed fastest and compete for the same transport system. Fructose follows about 30% more slowly, while the absorption speed of all the other monosaccharides, including the sugar alcohols used as alternative sweeteners (e.g., sorbit, xylit), is as low as 10–20% of the speed of glucose.

If the individual capacity of one of the digestive/absorptive systems is exceeded, **low molecular weight carbohydrates** reach the **colon**. There, they bind water and can be fermented by intestinal bacteria, causing intestinal gas and diarrhea.

One example is the **lactose/lactase system**: large amounts of lactose always overload the system and cause diarrhea; this is why lactose can be used as a laxative. More important, however, is the occurrence of lactase deficiency. Overall, 30–50 million Americans are lactose intolerant, 90% of Asian-Americans, and 75% of African- and Native Americans. Worldwide, 75% of adults have some degree of lactose intolerance. It is least common among Europeans and constitutes the most common form of intolerance to a disaccharide. Reduced lactase activity is a factor in many diseases of the intestine. Those afflicted ought to be aware that fermented milk products like hard cheeses contain only traces of lactose and rarely cause symptoms. Sour milk products tend to be well tolerated in spite of their lactose content. The increasing use of powdered milk in processed foods, as well as lactose in medical drug preparations and diet products, is problematic for those who suffer from lactose intolerance.

A. Carbohydrate Digestion and Absorption

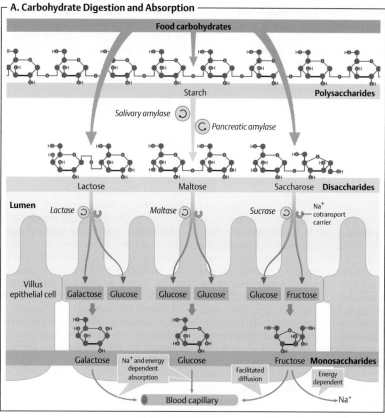

Food carbohydrates

Starch **Polysaccharides**

Salivary amylase

Pancreatic amylase

Lactose Maltose Saccharose **Disaccharides**

Lumen

Lactase *Maltase* *Sucrase* Na⁺ cotransport carrier

Villus epithelial cell

Galactose Glucose Glucose Glucose Glucose Fructose

Galactose Glucose Fructose **Monosaccharides**

Na⁺ and energy dependent absorption Facilitated diffusion Energy dependent

Blood capillary → Na⁺

B. Glucose Carriers

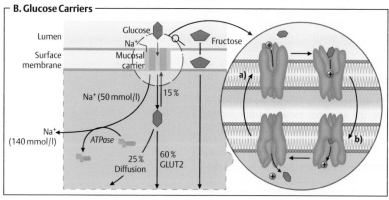

Lumen Glucose Fructose

Surface membrane Na⁺ Mucosal carrier

Na⁺ (50 mmol/l) 15 %

Na⁺ (140 mmol/l) *ATPase*

25 % Diffusion 60 % GLUT2

a)

b)

Metabolism: Distribution and Regulation

Once absorbed, carbohydrates are carried to the liver (**A**). There, fructose and galactose are converted into glucose. Some of the absorbed glucose reaches the peripheral bloodstream, where it is recognized by pancreatic receptors. This triggers increased insulin secretion by the β-cells and reduces glucagon secretion.

These hormonal changes provide a signal which affects the entire metabolism: absorption of glucose into the liver, muscle cells, and fatty tissues is increased, and its conversion into storage forms enhanced. Once inside the liver, glucose is phosphorylated into glucose-6-phosphate (G6P) and trapped since G6P is unable to pass through the membrane. G6P is then metabolized either into energy, into free fatty acids (FFAs) and triglycerides (TG), or into **glycogen**—as long as sufficient storage capacity remains. Due to its hydrated state, glycogen requires lots of space; therefore, the liver can store only about 100 g glucose in this form. Up to 0.5 kg glycogen can be stored in muscle. Hydrolyzed glycogen cannot leave the muscle cells to add to blood glucose and is therefore no longer available to the rest of the body.

Due to this **limited storage capacity**, all carbohydrates consumed beyond energy need are converted to and stored as fat. Fat storage is practically unlimited. Yet, the idea that mostly carbohydrates make people fat is wrong. Basically, all energy nutrients, consumed in excess of energy need, are converted to fat. Since carbohydrates first have to be metabolized for this purpose, their conversion is actually most ineffective. Some of the carbohydrate energy is lost in postprandial thermogenesis. This does not apply to fatty acids, which can be directly integrated into fat cell triglycerides. If any nutrient can be said to be fattening, it tends to be the lipids.

Towards the **end of the absorptive phase** or while **fasting**, when plasma glucose levels drop due to lack of new supplies and/or rapid use, hormonal regulation is reversed (**B**). Plasma insulin levels drop while glucagon secretion increases. Glucagon stimulates liver glycogen breakdown and increases the enzymatic activity required for the reversal of glycolysis (gluconeogenesis from amino acids). The lower plasma insulin causes breakdown of muscle glycogen, making glucose available to the muscles. Catecholamines released during stress or physical activity can have the same effect. Furthermore, increased glucagon levels make fatty acids available through triglyceride hydrolysis. Alternatively, this can be induced by the sympathetic nervous system.

— **A. Distribution and Regulation (Post-absorptive)** —

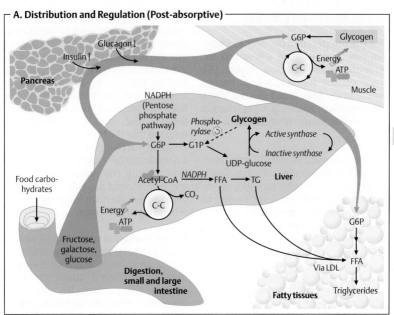

— **B. Distribution and Regulation (Fasting or Starvation)** —

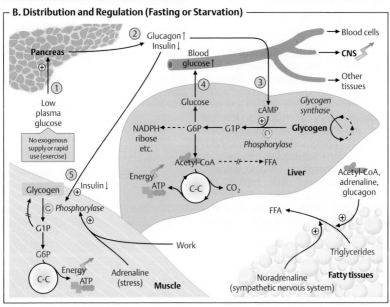

Metabolism: Glucose Storage

The glucose stored in the liver as glycogen can be considered a reservoir for buffering **blood glucose levels** (A). Since glucose is the essential energy source of the CNS, blood glucose levels are regulated within a tight margin through the interplay of glucagon and insulin.

Muscle glycogen is not directly integrated into the blood glucose regulation system. Since muscles lack glucose-6-phosphatase, their cells are unable to convert glucose-6-phosphate formed during glycogen breakdown into glucose, so no glucose can be released into the blood. Rather, muscle glycogen serves as an energy reserve for the muscles. Since stored ATP and other high-energy phosphates last only seconds, while external energy supply through the blood takes some time, muscle glycogen is the sole intermediate energy source.

The storage and breakdown of muscle glycogen are not only influenced hormonally, but also subject to **allosteric regulation** (B). During muscular activity, membrane depolarization and subsequent energy use create high levels of Ca^{2+} and AMP. Both substances activate glycogen phosphorylase, which catalyzes the first breakdown step towards glucose-1-phosphate. Glucose, glucose-6-phosphate, and ATP inhibit this enzyme. Glucose-6-phosphate, on the other hand, which is formed after glucose absorption, activates glycogen synthase.

In extreme situations, the muscle itself may also be used to supply glucose (C). In case of short-term, extreme muscular activity, the oxygen supplied by the blood is not sufficient to completely oxidize the glucose used by the muscle. Nevertheless, to ensure energy supply, glucose is converted to lactate during **anaerobic glycolysis**. Since the muscle has no further use for lactate, it is released into the bloodstream. In the liver, the lactate is used for gluconeogenesis and the resulting glucose released into the blood.

Continued activity, therefore, results in a net transfer of muscle glycogen to the liver. During the recuperation phase, the liver releases more glucose into the blood, which the muscles, in turn, use to rebuild glycogen stores.

During **starvation** or prolonged **fasting** when neither enough glycogen nor lactate is available to maintain adequate blood glucose levels, muscle protein is used for this purpose. Through transamination, specific, so-called **glucogenic amino acids** are converted to alanine, which is released into the bloodstream. Upon reaching the liver, it is metabolized to glucose (gluconeogenesis). Only through this cycle, called "Cori Cycle," is extended survival without food intake at all possible. In any case, it is bound to result in an unavoidable loss of muscle and fatty tissue.

A. Muscle and Liver Glycogen

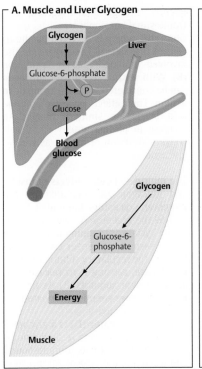

B. Glycogen Synthesis and Breakdown

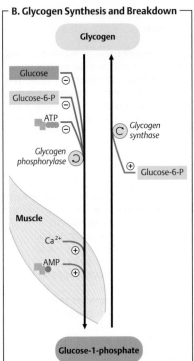

C. Cori Cycle (Glucose-Alanine Cycle)

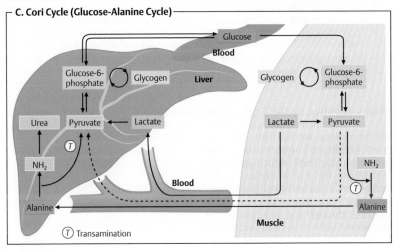

Glucose Homeostasis: Insulin and Glucagon

All cells except brain, active muscle, and liver cells, require membrane transporters for glucose to enter the cells. The transporters are usually present inside the cells and **insulin** makes them available by bringing them to the cell surface; with dropping insulin levels, they recede again.

Insulin has three major metabolic effects:

1. It lowers blood glucose by:
   • Increasing glucose uptake in various tissues,
   • Inhibiting glycogenolysis,
   • Inhibiting gluconeogenesis.
2. It lowers blood fatty acids and enhances fat storage by:
   • Increasing glucose uptake by fat cells,
   • Activating enzymes that catalyze conversion of glucose into fatty acids,
   • Enhancing fatty acid uptake into fat cells from blood,
   • Inhibiting lipolysis.
3. It lowers amino acid levels in blood and increases protein synthesis by:
   • Increasing amino acid uptake into cells,
   • Increasing amino acid use for protein synthesis,
   • Inhibiting breakdown of proteins.

Insulin secretion by the β-cells of the islets of Langerhans is subject to multiple regulatory mechanisms (**A**). The most important control value is the blood glucose level, which fluctuates throughout the day. After food intake and before increased blood glucose levels could even trigger this, insulin is released through the function of the autonomic nervous system, and subsequently through food-triggered, gastrointestinal hormones.

Glucagon, which is secreted by the α-cells of the islets of Langerhans, is also involved in blood glucose regulation (**B**). With regards to glucose, glucagon can be considered to be antagonistic to insulin. Their effects on plasma amino acid levels are similar, though. An increase in plasma amino acid levels triggers secretion of insulin as well as glucagon.

The multiple **cellular effects** of insulin and glucagon are mediated by cell membrane receptors. Binding of glucagon to the receptor (**C**) activates adenylate cyclase (1), leading to formation of the second messenger cAMP. cAMP binds to the regulatory subunit of a protein kinase, causing it to release activated catalytic subunits (2). As a result, target enzymes are phosphorylated (3), altering their activity.

The **insulin receptor** (**D**) is a glycoprotein consisting of two α- and two β-chains. The latter are membrane-bound and reach into the cytosol. After insulin binds to the α-chains, which are located on the cell's exterior, a part of the β-chains is phosphorylated, forming an active tyrosine kinase. Tyrosine kinase phosphorylates tyrosine R-groups of a peptide (insulin receptor substrate, IRS), which in turn triggers a multiple phosphorylation and dephosphorylation cascade. Dephosphorylation of the receptor finally terminates these intracellular effects of insulin.

A. Control of Insulin Secretion

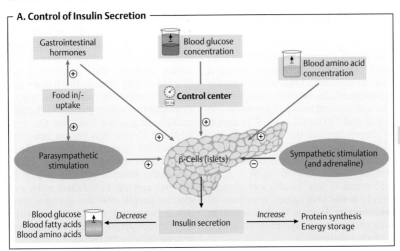

Gastrointestinal hormones

Blood glucose concentration

Blood amino acid concentration

Food in/-uptake

Control center

Parasympathetic stimulation

β-Cells (islets)

Sympathetic stimulation (and adrenaline)

Blood glucose
Blood fatty acids
Blood amino acids

Decrease

Insulin secretion

Increase

Protein synthesis
Energy storage

B. Glucose Homeostasis

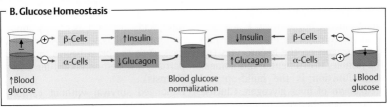

↑Blood glucose

β-Cells → ↑Insulin
α-Cells → ↓Glucagon

Blood glucose normalization

↓Insulin ← β-Cells
↑Glucagon ← α-Cells

↓Blood glucose

C. Signal Transduction: Glucagon

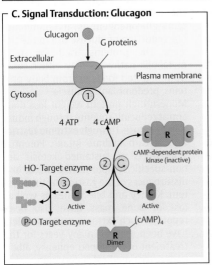

Glucagon   G proteins

Extracellular

Plasma membrane

Cytosol

4 ATP   4 cAMP

C R C
cAMP-dependent protein kinase (inactive)

HO- Target enzyme

Active
C

Active
C

P-O Target enzyme

R
Dimer

(cAMP)₄

D. Signal Transduction: Insulin

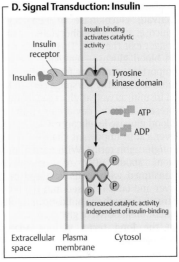

Insulin binding activates catalytic activity

Insulin receptor

Insulin

Tyrosine kinase domain

ATP

ADP

Increased catalytic activity independent of insulin-binding

Extracellular space   Plasma membrane   Cytosol

Glucose Homeostasis: Metabolic Aspects

The blood glucose level of a healthy adult fluctuates between ~70 mg/dl (3.85 mmol/l and ~120 mg/dl (6.6 mmol/l) postprandially. Beyond a certain blood glucose concentration of between 140 mg/dl and 170 mg/dl (~7.7–9.35 mmol/l) (depending on the individual), the kidney tubules are no longer capable of reabsorbing the glucose and glucosuria results. Below ~50–70 mg/dl (~2.75–3.85 mmol/l), the insufficient glucose supply to the CNS causes symptoms of weakness or fatigue. Further lowering may cause seizures, symptoms of shock, and ultimately death.

In the **short term**, the tightly controlled **blood glucose homeostasis** is achieved primarily through the effects of **insulin** and **glucagon** on the hepatocytes (**A**). The primary instrument of this homeostatic function is the build-up and breakdown of liver glycogen. Glucose diffuses freely between blood and liver. Postprandially increased glucose levels activate glucokinase in hepatocytes: glucose, now phosphorylated, can no longer exit the cells. This causes a drop in blood glucose—removing the most important stimulant for insulin secretion. In a healthy person, a certain level of insulin, as well as glucagon, is always present. Minor deviations from the blood glucose level control value, however, cause important changes in insulin/glucagon ratios. With normal nutrition, about 60% of the glucose consumed with foods is stored in the liver and later released into the bloodstream through the build-up and subsequent breakdown of glycogen.

In the **long term**, various adaptive mechanisms are used for blood glucose homeostasis, ensuring a minimum use of 4–5 g glucose/h even with carbohydrate-free nutrition (**B**). Any glucose ingested during the last meal (time 0 hours) is metabolized within a few hours. During this relative high-glucose-supply period, the tissues use glucose exclusively. Subsequent **glycogenolysis** in the liver guarantees further stability of glucose levels for the next 12 hours. During this period, however, glucose use by liver, muscles, and fatty tissues is increasingly curtailed. Simultaneously, **gluconeogenesis** begins in the liver and takes over maintenance of glucose supply after the glycogen storage is exhausted. After 1–2 days without carbohydrate intake, gluconeogenetic activity decreases.

This is a consequence of a metabolic shift in all tissues: increasingly, **free fatty acids** are used as energy supply, minimizing glucose use. After a few days, even the brain begins to at least partially use ketone bodies for energy (**ketosis**).

Prolonged survival without carbohydrate intake is, therefore, possible through synthesis of glucose from proteins (**gluconeogenesis**) and simultaneous reduction of glucose use in the tissues. The proteins used for these metabolic pathways may either come from ingested foods or from body proteins, predominantly muscle.

Modern high-protein weight loss diets aim at reducing appetite through induction of ketosis through extreme restriction of carbohydrate intake. Potential side-effects of sustained ketosis are non-specific symptoms like fatigue and disturbances of the gastrointestinal system. Kidney and bile stones as well as loss of bone mass have also been reported. Such extreme ketogenic diets have been used for many years for the treatment of childhood epilepsy, albeit under strict medical supervision.

A. Glucose Homeostasis—Short-Term

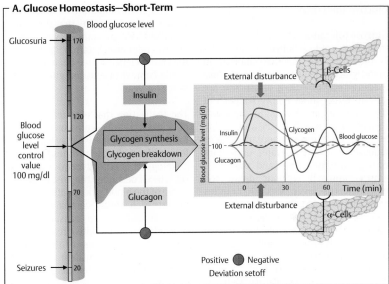

Blood glucose level

Glucosuria

170

120

Blood glucose level control value 100 mg/dl

70

Seizures

20

β-Cells

External disturbance

Insulin

Glycogen synthesis
Glycogen breakdown

Glucagon

Blood glucose level (mg/dl)

Insulin

100

Glucagon

Glycogen

Blood glucose

0   30   60   Time (min)

External disturbance

α-Cells

Positive ● Negative
Deviation setoff

B. Five Phases of Glucose Homeostasis

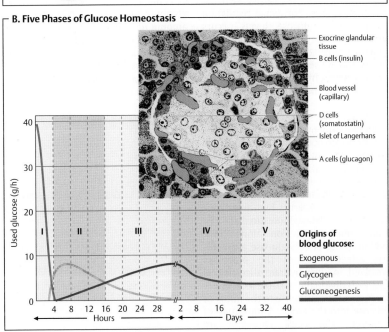

Exocrine glandular tissue

B cells (insulin)

Blood vessel (capillary)

D cells (somatostatin)

Islet of Langerhans

A cells (glucagon)

Used glucose (g/h)

40

30

20

10

0

I   II   III   IV   V

4   8   12   16   20   24   28   2   8   16   24   32   40

Hours   Days

Origins of blood glucose:

Exogenous

Glycogen

Gluconeogenesis

Glucose Tolerance

Glucose tolerance is the body's reaction to an increased carbohydrate supply. It is measured by reactive changes in blood glucose levels. During a **glucose loading test**, 50–100 g of glucose are administered on an empty stomach in 0.5 l of water, and blood glucose levels measured at time 0 (start), and 30, 60, 90, and 120 minutes thereafter. Since glucose dissolved in water undergoes no digestive processes and passes an empty stomach without delay, the blood glucose level peaks 30 minutes after the meal (**A**). In healthy subjects, glucose is taken up by the cells even before peak levels are reached, due to simultaneous onset of insulin secretion, thereby preventing glucose levels from exceeding 120–150 mg/dl (6.6–8.25 mmol/l). The regulatory switch—reversal of the hormonal regulation with sinking glucose levels—occurs with some delay. Rapid flooding with glucose, causing rapidly rising insulin levels and subsequent rapid decline of glucose levels, frequently leads to blood glucose values below initial levels.

However, these statements, derived from experiments with watery glucose solutions, are not applicable to nutritive carbohydrate intakes. **Postprandial glucose concentrations** vary considerably, depending on food composition. For instance, high fat content prolongs gastric retention, whereas high fiber content leads to delayed intestinal absorption. Food preparation alone (raw, boiled, fried) affects glucose availability. Effectiveness of the processes involved in carbohydrate digestion is just as individually variable as is effectiveness of the response to the influx of glucose into the blood. A multitude of vitamins and trace elements are involved in carbohydrate metabolism. It makes sense, therefore, that the availability of those substances would affect glucose tolerance. Vitamin B_6 and chromium deficiencies have been discussed in the context of reduced glucose tolerance for years.

The realization that identical amounts of carbohydrates—consumed in the form of different foods—may lead to different blood glucose profiles led to the development of the **glycemic index (GI)** (**B**). The GI describes the area under the curve of the blood glucose after a carbohydrate-rich meal, compared to the curve resulting from consumption of pure glucose (or white bread, respectively). A disadvantage of the index is that it compares equivalent amounts of carbohydrates. A better measure is the **glycemic load (GL)**, which combines the glycemic index of a given food with the amount of carbohydrate contained in it (**C**). Raw carrots, for instance, have a GI of 71 compared to that of white bread (100). However, since they contain only 4% carbohydrates, each serving has a GL of 4, which is negligible.

A. Postabsorptive Blood Glucose Levels

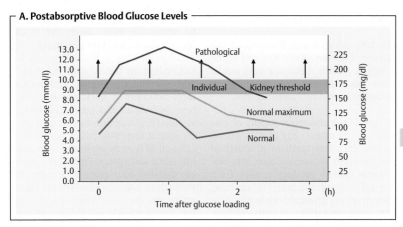

B. Glycemic Index

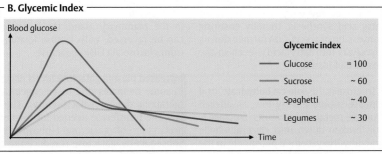

Glycemic index	
Glucose	= 100
Sucrose	~ 60
Spaghetti	~ 40
Legumes	~ 30

C. Glycemic Index vs. Glycemic Load

Food	Glycemic Index	Glycemic Load
		25
Instant rice	91	20
Baked potato	85	21
Corn flakes	84	4
Raw carrots	71	21
White bread	70	19
Whole grain bread	65	17
Muesli	56	16
Spaghetti	41	8
Apples	36	6
Legumes	29	

Fructose and Galactose

Fructose, which has no influence on the release of insulin, is metabolized in the liver (**A**). Which metabolic pathway is used depends on the presence or absence of other monosaccharides.

In case of **simultaneous supply** of glucose and fructose, fructose is transformed into intermediate products of the glycolytic pathway. Since only one phosphorylated product results from the splitting of fructose-1-phosphate, the remaining glyceraldehyde has to be processed via a different pathway first. Like insulin, fructose activates a number of key enzymes required for fatty acid synthesis, thereby ensuring conversion of acetyl-CoA formed during glycolysis into fatty acids—even in the absence of insulin.

If fructose is the **sole carbohydrate**, or if glucose supply is very low, an altered fructose metabolism results; fructose is still broken down into glyceraldehyde and dihydroxyacetone phosphate in the liver. Then, however, these metabolites are used to synthesize glucose or glucose-6-phosphate through reversal of the first part of the glycolytic pathway. This permits blood glucose levels to be maintained and/or to replenish glycogen storage. Since this reverse glycolytic reaction is subject to "strict regulation," the amount of fructose that may be converted to glucose is limited.

One problem with the uptake of large amounts of fructose is the decrease of hepatic ATP due to rapid fructose phosphorylation. This interferes with other important liver biosyntheses, like protein biosynthesis. At the same time, there may be increased AMP breakdown, which may result in an increase of plasma uric acid. Lactate may also be formed, due to the cells' reduced ability to regenerate NAD^+ from the NADH formed during fructose glycolysis.

Depending on the type of nutrition—and particularly during childhood—large amounts of **galactose** from lactose hydrolysis end up in the bloodstream (**B**). Galactose has no influence on insulin secretion either, and practically all of it ends up in the liver after intestinal absorption. From there, it can be shuttled into glucose metabolism through conversion into uridine phosphate glucose (UDP-glucose), or used for the synthesis of glycolipids and other structural polysaccharides as UDP-galactose.

In the mammary gland, this reaction can be reversed, with lactose forming from glucose via UDP-galactose.

Increased plasma galactose levels occur in some neonates due to a congenital metabolic defect (galactosemia). They lack the transferase needed for further processing of galactose-1-phosphate. Subsequently, galactose is reduced to a sugar alcohol, galactitol—a neurotoxin that causes cataracts.

A. Fructose Metabolism

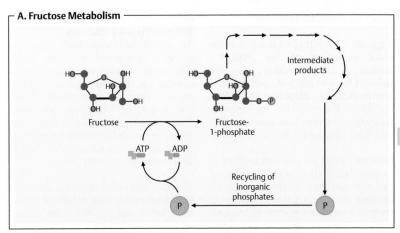

B. Galactose Metabolism

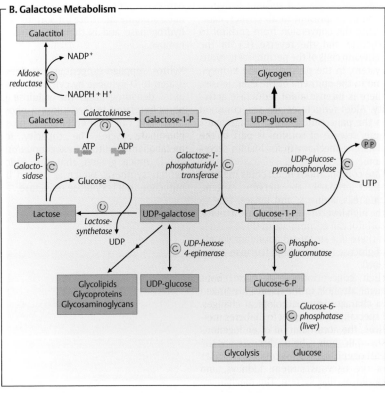

Sugar Alcohols: Metabolism

Sugar alcohols form as a result of enzymatic reduction of the respective mono- or disaccharides (**A**). The reduced form of glucose, **sorbitol** (also known as sorbit), plays a central role in this enzymatic reduction. Its formation is catalyzed by the same alcohol reductase that reduces galactose to **galactitol**.

Sorbitol can be further metabolized to fructose (**B**); if there is excess fructose, this reaction may be reversed. Excess fructose also inhibits the conversion of sorbitol made from glucose to fructose, resulting in an accumulation of sorbitol. Aldol reductase and sorbitol dehydrogenase are present in all tissues, catalyzing the conversion from sorbitol to fructose and the reverse (**C**). In the Schwann cells of the peripheral nervous system, in the papillae of the kidneys, and in the epithelia of the eyes' lenses, there is intense **aldol reductase activity**. Aldol reductases are also common in the pancreatic islets of Langerhans; here, release of sorbitol is part of the signaling mechanism for insulin secretion.

Late complications of diabetes mellitus affect primarily the nervous system, pancreas, kidneys, and lenses. Due to the high level of aldol reductase activity, sorbitol can accumulate in these tissues if there is a sustained abundant supply of glucose (as from high fructose nutrition).

High concentrations of endogenous sugar alcohols in the tissues are linked to characteristic pathological changes. Especially with respect to **diabetes mellitus,** the accumulation of endogenous sugar alcohols is being discussed as the pathogenic cause of secondary diseases of the nervous system, kidneys, and cardiovascular system. The mechanism at the root of these mostly degenerative processes is not yet known.

An additional factor that might be involved here is nonenzymatic glycosylation of proteins, which can also be observed at elevated sugar alcohol levels. Nonenzymatic glycosylation of proteins also occurs when monosaccharide levels are permanently elevated. Since monosaccharides are bonded to peptide chains at random locations, this leads to abnormal glycoproteins (see p. 76).

The formation of excessive amounts of **galactitol** under high galactose conditions takes place in the same tissues where the sorbitol forms. It creates a particular problem since galactitol is not a suitable substrate for sorbitol dehydrogenase and is therefore hard to remove.

Xylitol, supplied exogenously, is dehydrated to D-xylulose by cytoplasmic L-iditol dehydrogenase; the xylulose is phosphorylated to D-xylulose-5-phosphate and can then enter the pentose phosphate cycle. The capacity for metabolizing xylitol of exogenous origin is much greater that the endogenous synthesis, which is limited by mitochondrial L-xylulose reductase.

A. Sugar Alcohols

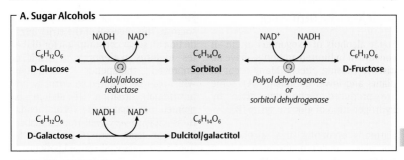

NADH   NAD⁺

$C_6H_{12}O_6$
D-Glucose

Aldol/aldose reductase

$C_6H_{14}O_6$
Sorbitol

NAD⁺   NADH

Polyol dehydrogenase or sorbitol dehydrogenase

$C_6H_{13}O_6$
D-Fructose

NADH   NAD⁺

$C_6H_{12}O_6$
D-Galactose

$C_6H_{14}O_6$
Dulcitol/galactitol

B. Sorbitol Metabolism

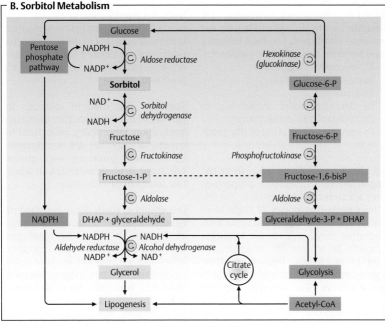

Glucose

Pentose phosphate pathway

NADPH / NADP⁺   *Aldose reductase*

Hexokinase (glucokinase)

Glucose-6-P

Sorbitol

NAD⁺ / NADH   *Sorbitol dehydrogenase*

Fructose-6-P

Fructose

Fructokinase

Phosphofructokinase

Fructose-1-P - - - - → Fructose-1,6-bisP

Aldolase   *Aldolase*

NADPH   DHAP + glyceraldehyde   Glyceraldehyde-3-P + DHAP

NADPH / NADH
Aldehyde reductase   *Alcohol dehydrogenase*
NADP⁺ / NAD⁺

Glycerol   Citrate cycle   Glycolysis

Lipogenesis   Acetyl-CoA

C. Sorbitol Metabolism Under Hyperglycemic Conditions

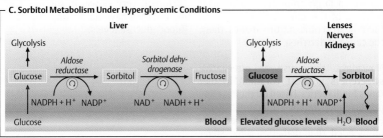

Liver

Glycolysis

Glucose   *Aldose reductase*   Sorbitol   *Sorbitol dehydrogenase*   Fructose

NADPH + H⁺   NADP⁺   NAD⁺   NADH + H⁺

Glucose   **Blood**

Lenses Nerves Kidneys

Glycolysis

Glucose   *Aldose reductase*   **Sorbitol**

NADPH + H⁺   NADP⁺

Elevated glucose levels H_2O **Blood**

Sugar Alcohols: Occurrence

Sugar alcohols of exogenous origin—if consumed in limited amounts—have no disease-causing effects. Many occur in plants and lower organisms (**A**); some are produced technically, often by hydrogenation of glucose syrup (**B**).

Naturally occurring sugar alcohols do not play a major quantitative role in nutrition. However, sugar alcohols added to foods during processing may become significant, depending on the amounts consumed. The **food industry** uses them for the following purposes:

• As alternative sweeteners
• To slow crystallization
• As a softener
• To decrease water availability to microorganisms (preservative)
• To improve rehydration of dry products

All these applications arise from the sugar alcohols' common properties: they are sweet and hygroscopic. The relative **sweetening power** of sugar alcohols is about 60 % compared to sucrose. Therefore, they have to be used in larger amounts to achieve the same perception of sweetness. Because of their hygroscopic nature, this has unwanted consequences for digestive system function. Since many sugar alcohols are poorly absorbed, they may—if consumed in large amounts—reach distal sections of the intestinal tract. There, their hygroscopic nature makes them the cause of diarrhea.

Nowadays, their use as **alternative sweeteners** is most common in diet foods for diabetics, based on their largely insulin-independent metabolic use. However, in recent times, it has been recommended that diabetics avoid sugar alcohols in favor of small amounts of sucrose. This reversal of the strict interdiction on sugar consumption for **diabetes mellitus** patients is a result of improved therapeutic possibilities, which can be adapted to virtually any nutritional situation. It should be pointed out that these recommendations apply to very well-trained diabetics. Sugar alcohols still play a role in the nutrition of less well-trained patients.

Since the energy content of most sugar alcohols (with the exception of maltitol) is equivalent to that of the monosaccharides they are derived from, they have no relevant role in reduced-calorie products.

They are also used in solutions for parenteral nutrition, another important application. Since many indications for parenteral nutrition are accompanied by metabolic problems with glucose use, sugar alcohols represent an attractive source of carbohydrates.

Prevention of tooth decay is frequently cited as a further indication for sugar alcohol use. It should be mentioned here, that the most common representatives like sorbitol are actually rather easily fermented by cariogenic bacteria. Disaccharide alcohols are second generation alternative sweeteners. They are not cariogenic and are hydrolyzed and absorbed very slowly in the intestine; hence, they have hardly any impact on blood glucose levels.

A. Naturally Occurring Sugar Alcohols

Polyalcohol	Occurrence	Characteristics
Erythritol	Algae, grasses, fungi, various bacteria, human urine, fermented syrup	Its vasodilative effect has been investigated. Cariogenicity and physiological significance not sufficiently clear to date
Arabitol	Fungi, lichens, yeasts, higher plants, human body fluids (liquor) and tissue (brain)	Poorly metabolized by mammals (can be used as low-calorie sweetener). Large amounts are excreted with the urine. Cariogenicity studies lacking
Ribitol	Lichens, fungi, yeasts, higher plants, human body fluids, nectar; component of various liposaccharides and of riboflavin	Involved in pentose phosphate cycle. Less antiketogenic and metabolized more slowly than xylitol
Xylitol	Various microorganisms, lower and higher plants (much higher concentrations then sorbitol or D-mannitol), animal tissues	Absorbed very slowly in human gastrointestinal tract. Precursor of liver glycogen. Used in enteral and parenteral feeding and as alternative sweetener for diabetics and for noncariogenic nutrition
Sorbitol	Algae, fungi, many higher plants, animal tissues	Absorbed more slowly than glucose and used as alternative sweetener for diabetics. Precursor in of liver glycogen. Used preferentially in food processing and as sweetener. Fermented by cariogenic bacteria
D-Mannitol	Bacteria, algae, grasses etc., including higher plants	Absorbed more slowly than sorbitol and xylitol; precursor of liver glycogen. Stronger laxative effect than sorbitol and xylitol. Most ingested mannitol reaches the urine unchanged. Cariogenic effect similar to that of sorbitol
Galactitol Dulcitol	Algae, fungi, higher plants	Precursor of liver glycogen. Poorly absorbed. Cariogenic effects not investigated

B. Synthetic Sugar Alcohols

Polyalcohol	Occurrence	Characteristics
Lactitol	Natural occurrence not proven	Hydrolyzed to galactose and sorbitol in gastrointestinal tract by duodenal glucosidases. Its carbon skeleton may be broken down completely in the small intestine. Apparently noncariogenic; human long-term studies lacking
Maltitol	Natural occurrence not proven	Slowly hydrolyzed to glucose and sorbitol in small intestine. Noncariogenic. Used as sweetener in various foods (~ 2 kcal/g)
Isomaltitol	Natural occurrence not proven	Lower-level caloric utilization observed in rats. Cariogenicity studies lacking; behaves like lactitol and maltitol
Palatinite	Natural occurrence not proven	Caloric utilization ~ 50%. Metabolism and cariogenic effects like lactitol and maltitol
Maltotriitol Maltotetraitol	Not found to occur naturally to date	Intestinal breakdown. Inhibit amylase

Glycoproteins

Glycoproteins are proteins with covalently bonded oligosaccharides. The carbohydrate content of these molecules varies considerably. For instance, more than 4 % of the molecular mass of immunoglobulin G (IgG) is carbohydrate; more than 20 % of glycophorin, found in erythrocyte membranes, and more than 60 % of the mucin of the stomach mucosa are carbohydrate.

Membrane-bound glycoproteins are involved in a multitude of cellular phenomena (**A**). These include cell-surface recognition by other cells, hormones, or viruses, as well as antigenic characteristics (e. g., blood groups).

Inside the extra-cellular matrix and in the mucins of the gastrointestinal and urogenital tracts, glycoproteins serve as protective, biologically active **lubricants**.

Nearly all of the globular plasma proteins as well as the secreted enzymes, are actually glycoproteins—albumin is one of the few exceptions.

The carbohydrates are either bonded to the O atom of the serine or threonine R-groups with O-glycosidic bonds or to the N atom in the asparagine R-group with N-glycosidic bonds. The basic structure of the sugars consists mainly of N-acetyl-glucosamine (GlcNAc), fucose, and mannose. At their ends they have galactose (gal), mannose, and/or sialic acid (sia) attached.

Since these carbohydrates can be linked in different ways, the resulting multitude of combinations can have different information contents.

For instance, the life span of the entire **sialoglycoprotein** (**B**) molecule depends on the sialic acid residue at its end. Many immunoglobulins and peptide hormones that circulate in the bloodstream are equipped with this residue. The point at which the sialic acid is enzymatically removed is encoded in these proteins. The asialoglycoprotein receptor in the plasma membrane of liver cells then recognizes the galactose released during the removal reaction and endocytoses the entire protein. This mechanism allows proteins to be so equipped that their life span, depending on specific physiological requirements, may range from a few hours to several weeks.

When aldoses (e. g., glucose) bond with the amino groups of proteins, instable **glycosylamines** form. These can rearrange themselves into stable products in so-called **Amadori reactions** (**C**). However, the alkaline nitrogen introduced thereby now favors enolization within the molecule. The resulting radical anion can react with oxygen and other glycoproteins and lead to the formation of hydroxyl radicals. These radicals may cause polypeptide chain breaks, ultimately resulting in the loss of functional units. Such processes are being discussed in the literature pertaining to late consequences of diabetic hyperglycemia.

Amadori products also form between collagen polypeptide chains. They cross-link the chains and may thereby enhance the aging of connective tissue.

A. Glycoprotein Functions

Cell surface recognition

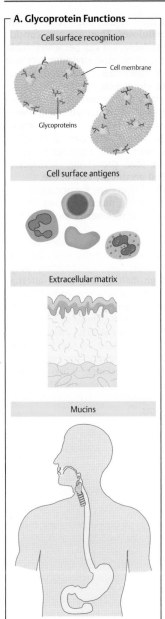

Cell membrane

Glycoproteins

Cell surface antigens

Extracellular matrix

Mucins

B. Lectins

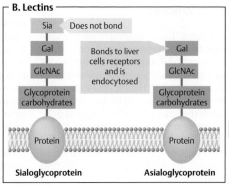

Sia	Does not bond
Gal	
GlcNAc	
Glycoprotein carbohydrates	

Bonds to liver cells receptors and is endocytosed

Gal
GlcNAc
Glycoprotein carbohydrates

Protein

Protein

Sialoglycoprotein   **Asialoglycoprotein**

C. Amadori Product

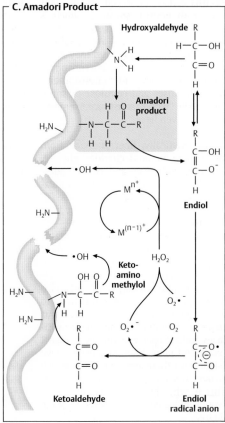

Hydroxyaldehyde

$$H-C-OH$$
$$R$$
$$C=O$$
$$H$$

Amadori product

$$H_2N-N-C-C-R$$

$$R$$
$$C-OH$$
$$C-O^-$$
$$H$$

Endiol

$\cdot OH$

M^{n+}

$M^{(n-1)+}$

H_2O_2

$\cdot OH$

Keto-amino methylol

$$H_2N-N-C-C-R$$

$O_2\cdot^-$

$O_2\cdot^-$ O_2

$$C=O$$
$$C=O$$
$$H$$

Ketoaldehyde

$$R$$
$$C-O\cdot$$
$$C-O$$
$$H$$

Endiol radical anion

Fiber: Structure

The term "fiber" encompasses a multitude of carbohydrates and lignin, which by current definitions escape hydrolysis by digestive enzymes completely or at least partially. Hence, they are not absorbed in the small intestine and reach the colon. This physiological definition cannot be transferred to a uniform chemical standard. The attempted classification is based on different degrees of solubility under different treatments (**A**).

Pectins can be dissolved out of plant cells with **neutral solvents**, which is why they are classified as soluble fiber. Cell wall components are insoluble under these conditions, and they make up the largest share of fiber consumed with foods. In an **acidic environment**, **hemicelluloses** and **cellulose** dissolve. Lignin, the "woody substance," remains resistant even here.

Characteristically, fiber is made from the simple monosaccharides glucose, fructose, arabinose, and ribose; additionally, it may contain certain derivatives of various monosaccharides (**B**) and, in lignin, some non-carbohydrate structures.

Cellulose, the most abundant organic compound in our biosphere, is made only from glucose. It differs from starch and glycogen in that the glucose subunits are linked with β-1,4 bonds. This β-linkage causes long, straight chains to form, making it suitable as a fibrous material. Mammals do not have cellulases and are therefore unable to digest wood and plant fiber. Ruminants have bacteria in their digestive tract, which make β-1,4 linkage-breaking enzymes. This is why these animals can digest woody plant parts like straw, to some degree.

By far most wheat and rye fibers are **hemicelluloses**. They are also considered insoluble, but can become soluble in acidic or alkaline environments due to their short-chain, branched nature. **Pectins**, the soluble fibers in fruit, are a chemically heterogeneous mix. Galacturonic acid is their main component, besides a number of other monomers. They form characteristic gels when mixed with water, a property that is used in food processing. Technically modified pectins are also in use.

Additional fibers are, for instance: gum arabic, seed mucilage, sea weed extracts, and technically modified cellulose.

The above definition of fiber applies increasingly to new products, most of which are produced synthetically: polyoles, high-melting fats, or fat alternatives. Starch, which was considered to be completely digestible until recently, also has a fiber component. This so-called "**resistant starch**" either results from the structure of the food—e.g., coarsely ground grains—or from altered amylose. For instance, when potatoes are cooked and subsequently left to cool, indigestible, "retrograded" amylose forms.

A. Fiber

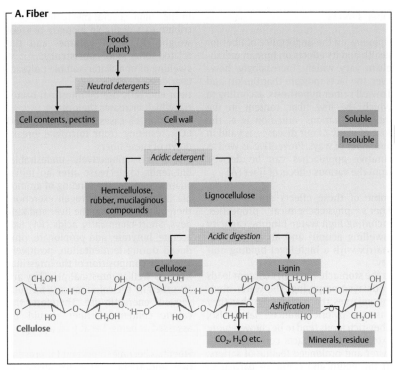

B. Other Important Components of Fibrous Compounds

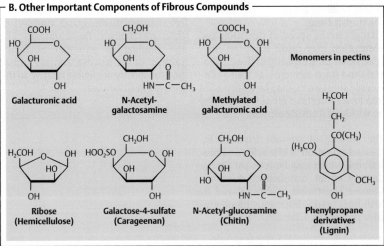

Fiber: Effects

Opinions on the importance of fiber for health and its effects on human metabolism vary widely. Increasingly, however, the facts indicate that Burkitt and Trowell's **fiber hypothesis**, according to which the low fiber content in the industrial nations' nutrition is at the root of many of our diseases, is valid in a number of ways. Preventive as well as curative approaches can be derived from the various effects of fiber (**A**).

Some of these effects are based on fiber's physicochemical properties, including high water-binding capacity (swelling action) and an indigestible matrix with a high-level binding ability.

In the **stomach**, high fiber content leads to **delayed emptying**. The water-binding enlarges the particles so that they pass the pyloric sphincter later. Also, fiber-rich foods tend to be chewed more extensively. Both facts contribute to a faster and prolonged feeling of **satiety**. In the ileum and colon, in particular, strong swelling action of fiber shortens the **transit time**.

Changes in the **speed of digestion and absorption** may result from the nonspecific binding capacity of fibers. Minerals and trace elements, as well as fat-soluble substances, may be transported into lower intestinal areas this way and be withheld from absorption.

The binding of steroids leads to increased **excretion** of **bile acids** and **cholesterol**, which may be relevant for the therapy of fat metabolism disorders. Glucose absorption is also delayed by high fiber intake, improving **blood glucose profiles** in diabetics.

In the colon, several mechanisms contribute to a desirable increase of **stool weight** (**B**), **stool volume**, and the related softer **stool consistency**:
swelling of non-water-soluble polysaccharides;
their energetic use by intestinal bacteria, which increases their mass;
formation of gases like methane and CO_2, resulting from microbial breakdown of these fibers.
The latter is—subjectively—undesirable, but tends to decrease after an initial adaptive period. The binding of ammonia increases fecal nitrogen excretion, thereby unburdening the liver and kidneys. Short-chain fatty acids (FA) like acetate, butyrate, and propionate, produced during fermentation, positively affect the **composition of the intestinal flora,** as well as intestinal pH. They are absorbed by the colon mucosa for subsequent energetic use. Therefore, the caloric content of fiber should be assessed as being 2 kcal/g on average.

Fiber has become important for prevention and therapy of many diseases: obstipation, diverticulosis, colon cancer, diabetes mellitus, and disorders of lipid metabolism. Disadvantages like the binding of essential nutrients, changes of the mucosa, and gas formation are mostly negligible relative to the long-term advantages.

A. Fiber: Effects

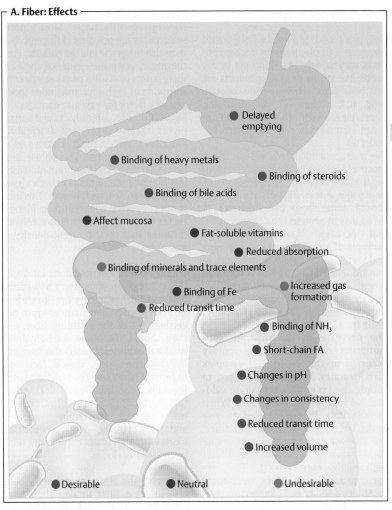

- Delayed emptying
- Binding of heavy metals
- Binding of steroids
- Binding of bile acids
- Affect mucosa
- Fat-soluble vitamins
- Reduced absorption
- Binding of minerals and trace elements
- Increased gas formation
- Binding of Fe
- Reduced transit time
- Binding of NH_3
- Short-chain FA
- Changes in pH
- Changes in consistency
- Reduced transit time
- Increased volume

● Desirable   ● Neutral   ● Undesirable

B. Stool Weight

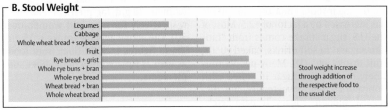

Legumes
Cabbage
Whole wheat bread + soybean
Fruit
Rye bread + grist
Whole rye buns + bran
Whole rye bread
Wheat bread + bran
Whole wheat bread

Stool weight increase through addition of the respective food to the usual diet

Occurrence and Requirements

Only plant foods provide carbohydrates. Absolute carbohydrate in foods contents vary widely (**A**). Contents in dry goods like grains or grain products are relatively high, whereas fruits contain only 10 % weight in carbohydrates. Vegetables, with the exception of legumes, tend to be rather low in carbohydrates.

The average adult needs at least 200 g glucose/d for use by glucose-dependent organs. The brain alone needs 140 g/d. At any age, at least 25 % of caloric intake should come from carbohydrates to avoid loss of protein (gluconeogenesis) and increased lipolysis. Using the example of a middle-aged man of normal weight, that means a minimum of 147 g/d. The **AMDR**, as which the most recent intake recommendations for energy nutrients are expressed, is 45–65 % of energy (265–380 g/carbohydrate for a 2345 kcal/d intake).

The **decrease in carbohydrate consumption** during the past century occurred at the expense of complex carbohydrates. Grains, which used to supply the bulk of carbohydrate calories, were the big losers (**B**). When carbohydrate intakes started to rise again, largely due to the fat-free craze, the increase came mostly from simple sugars, sucrose in particular, and later high fructose corn syrup (**C**). The average consumption of caloric sweeteners in America today is 72 kg/person/year. This is not just an American issue. Since 1960, sugar consumption worldwide has increased by a factor of >2.5. Most of the U.S. sugar intake comes from "hidden sugars" in soft drinks, baked goods, fruit drinks, etc. (**D**). Many people routinely replace the sugar in coffee with noncaloric "diet" sweeteners, but disregard "hidden" sugars. Tomato ketchup or mustard, for example, may contain up to 30 % sugar. Most caloric sweeteners are not only cariogenic, but may also upset the energy balance. Furthermore, scientific evidence increasingly points to insulin peaks due to consumption of high-glycemic index foods as a risk factor for vascular damage.

Some other commonly raised arguments against sugar lack a scientific basis. For instance, sugar is often said to "rob you of vitamins." This phrase suggests that sugar consumption increases the vitamin requirements to such a level that they can no longer be met. This idea is not supported by scientific evidence. Fact is that sugars are "empty calories," meaning that their nutrient density is low or zero.

If more than 20 % of the caloric intake, as it is common in youngsters nowadays, derives from sugar, they are—to state it in a very simplified manner—just not getting 20 % of the vitamins, fiber, etc. they should. Therefore, **carbohydrate intake recommendations** should specify that consumers should focus on unrefined plant sources (whole grains, legumes, fruit, and vegetables). Additionally, foods rich in carbohydrates are major sources of vitamins, minerals, and fiber. Finally, high-carbohydrate foods with high water content are relatively low in calories.

Following the above guidelines would also increase **fiber** intake. The **AI** for total fiber in the U.S. is 25 g/d for women, 38 g/d for men (21 and 30 g, respectively for men and women over 50). The actual average intake is 15 g/d. These figures include fiber from foods as well as isolated functional fiber supplements.

A. Carbohydrate Content of Foods (per 100 g)

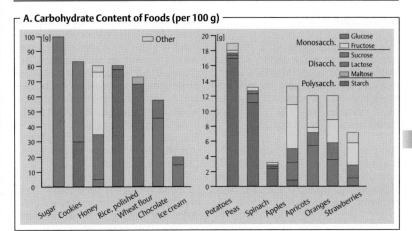

B. U.S. Flour and Cereal Consumption

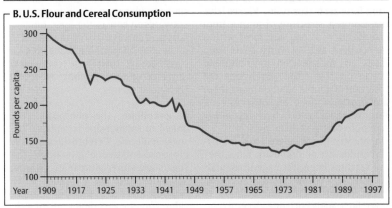

C. Sugar Consumption

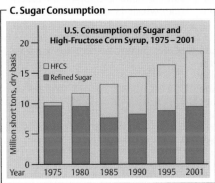

D. Sources of Added Sugar

Source	kg/year
Soft drinks	24
Baked goods	10
Fruit drinks	7
Dairy desserts	4
Candy	4
Breakfast cereals	3
Tea	2
Other (includes most table sugars)	18
Total	**72**

Classification

The term "lipids" refers to a group of substances that are insoluble in water and soluble in organic solvents. The easiest way to classify lipids is to divide them into classes according to structural characteristics (**A**). Chemically, these classes differ considerably.

The **polyprenyls** class is based on the **isoprene** building block. They include **steroids** (e. g., cholesterol), **fat soluble vitamins** (vitamins A, D, E, K), and other **terpenes** (e. g., menthol).

The largest branch of lipids is derived from fatty acids (see p. 86). **Waxes** have the simplest structure, resulting from esterification of one fatty acid with a monovalent alcohol. Fatty acids from foods are metabolized to **eicosanoid** precursors by chain extension and insertion of double bonds. Among them are prostaglandins, leukotrienes, and thromboxanes, which have regulatory functions on the cellular level.
Quantitatively, **triacylglycerols** (or **triglycerides**) are predominant. Since they are used for energy storage in animals they are also termed storage lipids (**B**). They are formed by esterification of three fatty acids with one glycerol (glycerin). The resulting molecules are nonpolar, hence the name, neutral fats.

The **phospholipids** class contains an additional phosphate group. If glycerin is their base component, they are called **glycerophospholipids**. The phosphate group can be esterified with various alcohols like phosphatidylethanolamine, -serine, and -choline (lecithin), to name a few important representatives.

Sphingosine, an amino alcohol with a long side chain, represents another basic building block. When sphingosine bonds to a fatty acid with an amide bond, it forms ceramide. Sphingolipids result from linkage with additional R-groups. If that linkage occurs via a phosphate group, the resulting compounds are called **sphingophospholipids**, of which large amounts are found in the brain and nervous system. Their most important representative is **sphingomyelin**, in which choline is attached to the phosphate group.

To build biological membranes (e. g., cell and organelle membranes), polar lipids are needed. In biological membranes, the polar group (alcohol, choline, glucose, etc.) is always oriented outwards, whereas the long, nonpolar fatty acid chains make up the core of the membrane bilayer. Membrane lipids are classified by their base components (glycerol or sphingosine), as well as their polar groups.

In **glycolipids,** the phosphate group linked to sphingosine is replaced by a sugar molecule. **Cerebrosides** are simple representatives of glycolipids: their sugars are either glucose or galactose. Sulfatides have an additional sulfate R-group attached to the sugar. **Gangliosides** contain a complex oligosaccharide, which in turn contains N-acetyl neuraminic acid. Glycolipids are found in all tissues on the outside of cell membranes. Some have receptor functions.

A. Classification

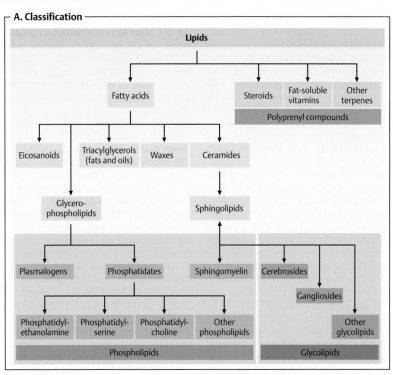

B. Storage and Membrane Lipids

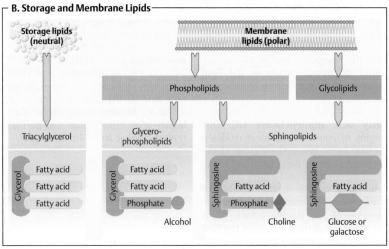

Fatty Acids

Fatty acids not only **provide energy** but are also important **structural** components of lipids. Chemically, they are organic acids (carboxylic acids) with long hydrocarbon chains (**A**). Usually, the carboxyl group is esterified with alcohols like glycerol, sphingosine, or cholesterol. Free, nonesterified fatty acids (free fatty acids, FFA) are dissociated at physiological pHs.

Fatty acids may contain **double bonds** (i. e., **unsaturated** fatty acids) that occur in **cis-configuration** under physiological conditions. If they contain only one double bond, they are called **mono-unsaturated** fatty acids (**MUFA**). Double bonds put a "kink" into the otherwise straight molecular chain, making the molecule more flexible. They also lower the melting point of a molecule, rendering the lipid more liquid. Technologically, the opposite path is used: hydrogenation of double bonds leads to firmer products, which are contained in many industrially produced foods as "hydrogenated (or hardened) fats."

Hydrogenation, as well as other intensive heat treatments, can cause changes in the configuration of double bonds, leading to **trans-configurations**. Their potential negative health effects are under discussion—whatever the final outcome, they are definitely undesirable.

Fatty acid nomenclature (**B**). One begins to count at the most oxidized carbon atom; hence the C atom of the carboxyl group is designated as "1." An accurate description of a fatty acid contains at a minimum the number of C atoms and the number as well as the position of any double bonds. An ω (or n) indicates the position of the first double bond, counting from the methyl end. The correct spelling of linoleic acid, an 18 C atom fatty acid with two double bonds in C9 and C12 is: linoleic acid (18:2; 9, 12, ω-6).

Longer, naturally occurring fatty acids always have an even number of carbon atoms. This is due to their synthesis from C2 units.

The following applies to fatty acids in general: the longer the chain and the fewer double bonds, the harder the fat. The shortest fatty acid contained in lipids is butyric acid (4:0). When released from fats such as butter during aging, due to its short-chain nature, it is not just liquid but sometimes gaseous (smell of butyric acid). The long-chain, saturated fatty acids occur exclusively in solid fats or as a result of the hydrogenation of unsaturated fatty acids.

The animal body is able to synthesize its own fatty acids but unable to introduce double bonds beyond C9. Long-chain, **polyunsaturated fatty acids** (**PUFA**) are therefore **essential** and must be obtained from foods. The most important essential fatty acids are **linoleic acid** (18:2; 9, 12, ω-6) and α-**linolenic acid** (18:3; 9, 12, 15, ω-3). The human body can make longer, polyunsaturated fatty acids from these two precursors by chain extension and desaturation (e. g., **arachidonic acid, (ARA)** 20:4; 5, 8, 11, 14; ω-6, **eicosapentaenoic acid (EPA)**, 20:5; 5, 8, 11, 14, 17; ω-3, **docosahexaenoic acid (DHA)**, 22:6; 4, 7, 10, 13, 16, 19; ω-3). Nutritional supply of these higher-level homologues can partially replace linoleic and α-linolenic acid.

A. Fatty Acid Structure

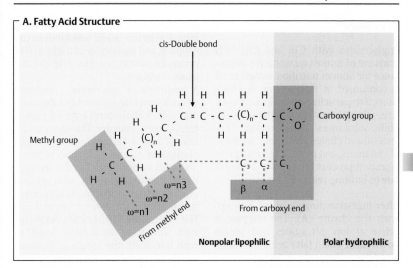

B. Fatty Acids

Fatty acids		Number of C atoms		Number of double bonds		Double bond positions from carboxyl end
Saturated	(	x	:	y	;	a, b, c, d...)
Butyric acid		4		0		
Valerianic acid		5		0		
Caproic acid		6		0		
Caprylic acid		8		0		
Capric acid		10		0		
Lauric acid		12		0		
Myristic acid		14		0		
Palmitic acid		16		0		
Stearic acid		18		0		
Arachidic acid		20		0		
Behenic acid		22		0		
Monounsaturated	(	x	:	y	;	a, b, c, d...)
Oleic acid		18		1		9
Erucic acid		22		1		13
Nervonic acid		24		1		15
Polyunsaturated	(	x	:	y	;	a, b, c, d...)
Linoleic acid		18		2		9, 12,
α-Linolenic acid		18		3		9, 12, 15,
Arachidonic acid		20		4		5, 8, 11, 14,

Lipid Digestion

Triglycerides with C16 and C18 fatty acids are of utmost quantitative importance for human nutrition. Whether fat is consumed in isolation or in emulsions, fat particles, regardless of their size, always contain additional lipophilic substances: phospholipids, cholesterol and cholesterol esters, fat-soluble vitamins, and more. The subsequent digestion process takes up to 24 hours, due to limiting reactions.

After ingestion, lingual lipase is mixed with the chyme (**A**). The enzyme is active at low pH values and breaks down short-chain fatty acids from milk fat triglycerides preferentially. The literature also describes a gastric lipase which may be specific to short- and medium-chain fatty acids from milk fat. Gastric motility ensures thorough mixing with the enzymes and a breakdown of fat into smaller particles. Even initially large proportions of fat are, therefore, emulsified by the end of their passage through the stomach. Short-chain fatty acids freed up in the stomach by hydrolysis at C1 or C3 can be directly absorbed into venous blood through the stomach wall. Opinions on the significance of this gastric fat digestion vary. In infants pancreatic function is not fully developed, so that the activities of lingual and gastric lipase may contribute to fat digestion in an important way. In adults, these gastric processes are of minor importance.

Controlled by the gastric pylorus, the emulsified lipids are released into the duodenum where **pancreatic juices** and **bile** are added. Bile acids attach to the fat particles, causing their surface to become negatively charged, which allows colipase to attach to the triglycerides. Pancreatic lipase, which is inhibited by bile acids, now binds to the colipase, and hydrolysis of triglycerides occurs in positions 1 and 3 at the oil/water interface.

A multitude of additional pancreatic enzymes operate according to the same principle. A **cholesterol esterase** hydrolyzes cholesterol ester. The same can be achieved by a carboxylesterase. **Phospholipases** A_1 and A_2 hydrolyze phospholipids in positions 1 and 2, respectively. Phospholipase A_2 with its end product lysophospholipid is of greater significance of the two.

The size of the fat particles decreases with advancing hydrolysis. Together with bile acids, the resulting lypolysis products assemble spontaneously into negatively charged particles once they exceed critical concentrations. Ca^{2+} enhances this process. Since all lipophilic particles are included in this spontaneous aggregation, the aggregates are termed **mixed micelles**.

This digestive process produces, by hydrolysis, absorbable molecules, on the one hand; on the other hand, particle sizes are reduced by a factor of 100 from fat emulsion to micelle. The resulting maximized surface area is crucial for the subsequent contact with the intestinal mucosa.

A. Digestion of Non-Water-Soluble Substances

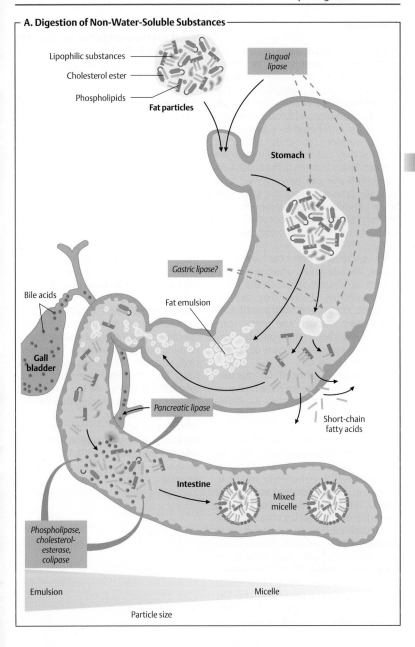

Lipophilic substances
Cholesterol ester
Phospholipids
Fat particles

Lingual lipase

Stomach

Gastric lipase?

Bile acids

Fat emulsion

Gall bladder

Pancreatic lipase

Short-chain fatty acids

Intestine

Mixed micelle

Phospholipase, cholesterol-esterase, colipase

Emulsion

Micelle

Particle size

Absorption

The products of hydrolysis (**A**) reach the brush border membrane as mixed micelles where they are passively absorbed into the mucosa cells. The **micelle uptake** mechanism into the cell is not fully understood to date. In particular, it is questionable whether the micelles enter the cells whole or whether they just deliver their contents to them. The transition to the brush border membrane can be imagined as a massage process across the UWL (see below). Reduced intestinal motility may severely impede fat absorption since lipids are unable to passively cross the UWL.

After secretion into the intestinal lumen, the bile acids, which are essential for fat absorption, reach the lower small intestine. There, they are reabsorbed in part and transported back to the liver through the portal vein. From there, they return into the gall bladder, completing the cycle of hepatic circulation (see p. 42).

The subsequent **intracellular metabolism** produces lipoproteins, which pass into the lymphatic system as **chylomicrons**.

The contents of the intestine are in constant motion due to peristalsis. Only the interface immediately adjacent to the intestinal wall is completely still. It is, therefore, called **unstirred water layer (UWL)**. Diffusion through the UWL and subsequent permeation through the membrane depend on a concentration gradient (C2 > C3 > C4) (**B**). This gradient is achieved through concentration in the micelles (step A, C1 > C2) on the one hand, and through quick intracellular removal (step D) on the other hand. The last step requires **fatty acid binding protein (FABP)**, which ensures fat removal and thereby a low concentration (C4) of free fatty acids on the inside of the brush border membrane. FABP has greater affinity to unsaturated fatty acids.

FABP also increases fatty acid activation (Acyl-SCoA synthesis), which represents the first step towards **intracellular resynthesis (C)**. The esterification of monoglycerides and fatty acids, as well as phospholipid and cholesterol ester resynthesis, occurs in the endoplasmic reticulum (ER). The latter is catalyzed by an enzyme identical to the pancreatic cholesterol esterase that operates in the intestinal lumen. At the pH range (6.6–8) that prevails in the intestine, the enzyme favors hydrolytic activity, whereas it catalyzes esterification at the pH range (5–6.2) that prevails inside cells.

Subsequently, lipids migrate through the cisterns of the smooth ER to the rough ER, where apoproteins are added, forming **prechylomicrons**. The prechylomicrons are transported to the Golgi body for final assembly. Glycosylation initiated inside the rough ER is completed here, providing them with a glycoprotein surface.

After fusion of the chylomicrons with the lateral plasma membrane, they are released into the intercellular space by exocytosis and from there enter the lymphatic vessels.

A. Fat Absorption

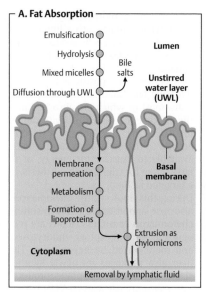

- Emulsification
- Hydrolysis
- Mixed micelles
- Diffusion through UWL

Bile salts

Lumen

Unstirred water layer (UWL)

Basal membrane

- Membrane permeation
- Metabolism
- Formation of lipoproteins
- Extrusion as chylomicrons

Cytoplasm

Removal by lymphatic fluid

B. Fat Absorption

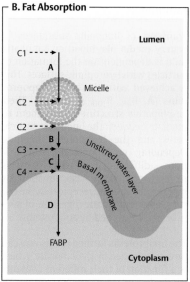

Lumen

C1 ····> **A**
C2 ····>   Micelle
C2 ····>
C3 ····> **B**   *Unstirred water layer*
C4 ····> **C**   *Basal membrane*

D

FABP

Cytoplasm

C. Fat Absorption

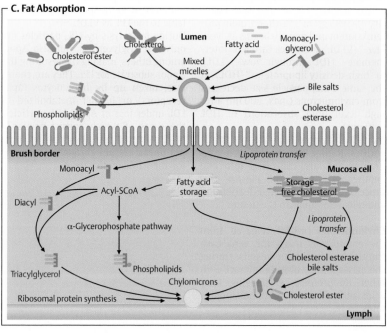

Lumen

Cholesterol ester — Cholesterol — Fatty acid — Monoacyl-glycerol

Mixed micelles

Phospholipids

Bile salts

Cholesterol esterase

Brush border

Monoacyl

Lipoprotein transfer

Mucosa cell

Diacyl — Acyl-SCoA

Fatty acid storage

Storage free cholesterol

α-Glycerophosphate pathway

Lipoprotein transfer

Triacylglycerol

Phospholipids

Cholesterol esterase bile salts

Chylomicrons

Ribosomal protein synthesis

Cholesterol ester

Lymph

Transport

Transport of lipophilic substances in watery media like blood or lymphatic fluid is dependent on the formation of particles with hydrophilic surfaces. This is achieved with the help of **apoproteins** (A, B_{48}, B_{100}, C, and E). Their amphipathic structure allows them to mediate between the lipophilic particle cores and the hydrophilic medium. Depending on apoprotein compositions, different transport particles result. Apoproteins also function as markers for specific receptors in the tissues. Even enzymatic digestion of particles is determined by apoproteins.

The **lipoproteins** formed in this way can be distinguished by their density, which is a function of their different contents in lipids and proteins. **Chylomicrons** consist mostly of lipids and have a density of <0.95 g/cm^3. The lipoprotein protein content and density begins at "very low-" (**VLDL**), increases through "intermediate-" (**IDL**) through "low-" (**LDL**), to "high-density lipoproteins" (**HDL**). At the same time, particle size decreases from chylomicrons (max. 600 nm after high level lipid absorption) to HDL (~10 nm).

Individual lipoproteins are not static entities. Rather, they represent a continuum and are converted into one another (**A**). Inside the plasma, this process ensures controlled distribution and release of lipids to the tissues.

Chylomicrons (n-CM) released from the enterocytes reach the vena cava through the lymphatic vessels. During this passage they already interact with other lipoproteins, exchanging fatty acids and taking up additional apoproteins.

The resulting **mature chylomicrons** (CM) make contact with a **lipoprotein lipase** (LPL), which is bound to the surface of blood vessel endothelial cells via heparan sulfate. The LPL hydrolyzes triglycerides in positions 1 and 3, releasing fatty acids from the lipoproteins, most of which are absorbed into the endothelial cell. LPL activity can be regulated via insulin and catecholamines so that fatty acids can be made available to muscles for energy, or to fatty tissue for triglyceride synthesis, in a targeted fashion.

During this lipolysis, the chylomicrons also lose apoprotein C_{II}. The resulting **chylomicron remnants** (REM) are recognized (ApoE receptor), endocytosed, and metabolized by hepatocytes. The liver also packages its newly synthesized or recycled lipophilic products into transport particles (n-VLDL); after enrichment with ApoC, they are available to the LPL as **VLDL**.

During hydrolysis by LPL, particles not only lose triglycerides, but also ApoC, among others, making the resulting **IDL** a poor substrate for LPL. They are, therefore, taken up by hepatocytes (aporeceptors) or further metabolized to LDL under loss of ApoE. **LDL particles**, the cores of which consist primarily of cholesterol, are absorbed by most **peripheral tissues** through LDL-receptor-mediated endocytosis.

A. Lipoproteins

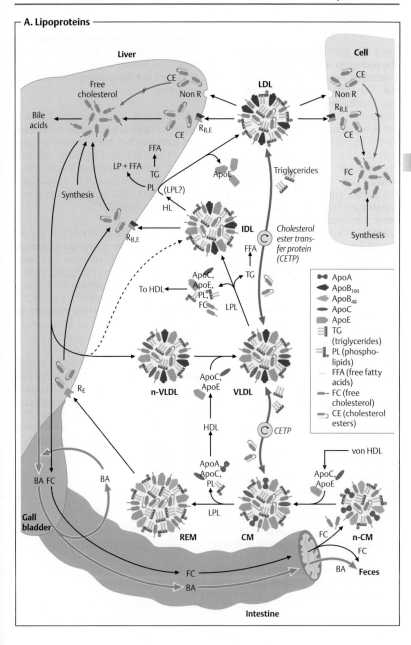

LDL

Since LDL particles primarily represent the **transport form of cholesterol**, their controlled uptake by the cells is essential. This occurs through an $ApoB_{100}$- and ApoE-specific **receptor (A)**. The interaction between ligand and receptor is based on their different charges: on the ligand side, the apoproteins provide the alkaline amino acids lysine and arginine (positive charge), while the active center of the receptor contains the acidic amino acids glutamic and aspartic acid (negative charge). The carboxy terminal end of the receptor reaches through the plasma membrane. On the inside of the membrane, the protein **clathrin** causes the membrane to cave in and form vesicles that cinch off.

After LDL binds to the receptor, the entire LDL-receptor-complex is endocytosed into the cell **(B)**. Lysosomes digest the LDL particles into fatty acids, amino acids, and nonesterified cholesterol. The receptor, as well as the clathrin involved, can be reused.

The uptake of LDL particles elevates **intracellular free cholesterol** concentration, triggering a cascade of further events:

- The activity of the enzyme hydroxymethylglutaryl-(HMG)-CoA reductase, which determines the speed of cholesterol biosynthesis, is inhibited.
- At the same time, acyl-CoA cholesterol acyl-transferase (ACAT) is stimulated; it converts cholesterol to cholesterol esters and thereby makes it storable.
- Also, synthesis of further LDL receptors is inhibited, limiting further LDL uptake into the cell.

These mechanisms control the concentration of unesterified cholesterol in cells. In the liver, endocrine glands, lungs and kidneys, ~90% of the LDL are taken up via these **receptor-mediated** activities.

However, in the small intestine and possibly the spleen, a **receptor-independent pathway** has been shown to exist. Here, the LDL's binding to the cell surface triggers absorptive endocytosis. Apparently, however, this uptake neither inhibits HMG-CoA-reductase nor does it stimulate ACAT.

An additional possibility of LDL uptake exists through the **scavenger** or **acetyl-LDL receptor**. This receptor has been shown to exist in macrophages, smooth muscle cells, and endothelial cells. It seems to be responsible primarily for the uptake of lipoproteins modified by oxidative processes (e.g., lipid peroxidation).

This receptor ensures cholesterol supply to the cells even in case of hereditary LDL receptor deficiency (familial hypercholesterolemia). This receptor cannot be down-regulated, so that cholesterol-loaded LDL may accumulate in the cells. This is considered to be a first step towards atherosclerosis.

A. LDL Receptor

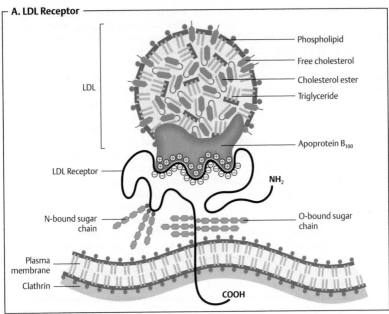

LDL	Phospholipid
	Free cholesterol
	Cholesterol ester
	Triglyceride
	Apoprotein B$_{100}$
LDL Receptor	NH$_2$
N-bound sugar chain	O-bound sugar chain
Plasma membrane	
Clathrin	COOH

B. LDL Catabolism

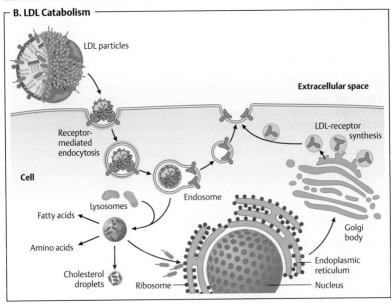

LDL particles

Extracellular space

Receptor-mediated endocytosis

LDL-receptor synthesis

Cell

Lysosomes

Endosome

Fatty acids

Amino acids

Cholesterol droplets

Golgi body

Endoplasmic reticulum

Ribosome

Nucleus

HDL

HDL particles can be distinguished into discoidal (disk-shaped) and spherical ones. The discoidal ones are termed **nascent** (n-HDL), the spherical ones **mature HDL particles**. Plasma contains mostly spherical particles with a hydrophilic core, consisting of triglycerides and cholesterol esters surrounded by phospholipids and apoproteins. The transition of the nascent to the spherical form is a result of cholesterol esterification and uptake of cholesterol esters from the surroundings.

Inside the plasma, **n-HDL (A)**, which is secreted by the liver, encounters the enzyme lecithin cholesterol acyl-transferase (LCAT), which catalyzes the esterification of cholesterol in the n-HDL's core. The resulting **HDL-3** continues to take up cholesterol and cholesterol esters. Additionally, an intensive exchange takes place between chylomicrons (CM) and VLDL. The additional ApoA required comes from a pool of free ApoA that results from breakdown of the CM surface. Peripheral cell receptors recognize this ApoA on the surface of HDL particles and trigger the release of intracellular cholesterol to them.

This continuous process of **cholesterol uptake**, cholesterol esterification through LCAT, and modification of the apoprotein surface particles results in the formation of **HDL-2** and **HDL-1**. These may, on the one hand, be taken up and metabolized by hepatocytes, either through receptors, or through receptor-independent mechanisms. On the other hand, they may also yield just parts of the lipophilic core and subsequently parts of the surface, converting them back into their respective precursor stages. Through this continuous cycle, **HDL** fulfills its essential function: the **transport of cholesterol and triglycerides** back from the peripheral tissues to the liver, where they are converted primarily into bile acids.

It is not yet fully understood how HDL particles remove cholesterol from cells. For monocytes (macrophages), trans-cellular transport of the HDL-HDL receptor vesicle has been proposed, during which HDL gets enriched by cholesterol from lipid droplets (**B**). Other theories assume the binding of HDL-ApoA to a receptor and subsequent (unexplained) permeation of intracellular cholesterol into the HDL. Since various apoproteins themselves can serve as cholesterol acceptors, even an uptake of ApoA, e.g., into cells and subsequent intracellular formation of pre-HDL (n-HDL) might be possible.

Transfer proteins (active in the plasma) may play important roles in regulating lipoprotein metabolism, for instance, when controlling the efflux of cholesterol from peripheral cells. Besides cholesterol ester transfer protein (CETP), which enables the exchange and net transfer of cholesterol esters (CE), triglycerides (TG) and phospholipids (PL), there is a phospholipid transfer protein (PTP), which is limited to transporting PL and TG. This way, TG and CE may be swapped between HDL and triglyceride-rich particles such as chylomicrons or VLDL.

A. HDL Metabolism

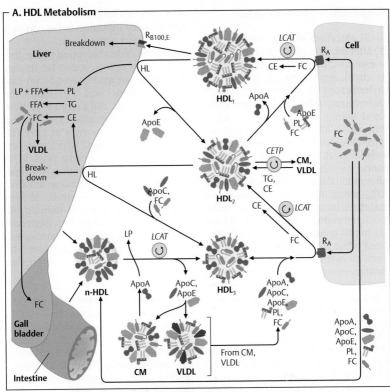

B. Cholesterol Uptake in Monocytes/Macrophages

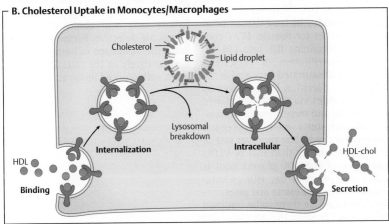

Postprandial Lipid Distribution

Lipids absorbed into the mucosa cells (1) after intraluminal hydrolysis (**A**) are re-esterified inside the cells and reach the circulatory system (2) in the form of **chylomicrons** via the lymphatic system. Chylomicrons (CM) can be found in the blood within 1–2 hours after a meal. With a half-life of 4–5 minutes, they are extremely short-lived; however, after a high-fat meal, their influx continues for hours.

After modification by **lipoprotein lipase** (LPL, see p. 100), the **remnants** are absorbed into the liver by receptor-mediated endocytosis and metabolized (3). In this process, all esters are hydrolyzed while the remaining compounds form an available pool, together with substances synthesized endogenously by the liver (e. g., fatty acids from glucose). Lipids in this pool that the liver does not need are immediately packaged with apoproteins again and released into the bloodstream as **VLDL** (4). VLDL as well are subject to constant hydrolysis by LPL. However, VLDL, with a half-life of 1–3 hours, are much more long-lived than CM. Most of the fatty acids released from VLDL serve as storage triglycerides in fatty tissues or as energy sources for muscle. LCAT converts the remaining **IDL** into **LDL** (5) through esterification of cholesterol with a polyunsaturated fatty acid at the C2 position of lecithin. LDL are taken up by most tissues via receptor-mediated endocytosis and serve primarily as supply of cholesterol esters for cellular cholesterol needs. The turnover rate of LDL is much lower than that of VLDL: only 45 % of the LDL plasma pool is eliminated in a given day. **HDL** picks up excess cholesterol esters and phospholipids (6), causing them to be returned to the liver (7). Since HDL also interacts with other lipoproteins, it can be considered a key substance in the complex lipid transport system.

During the **early absorption phase**, levels of enzymes involved in **fat storage** rise. These are mainly acetyl-CoA carboxylase, fatty acid synthase, the malate enzymes, and a series of pentose phosphate cycle enzymes. Extracellular lipoprotein lipase activity in fatty tissues increases as well, which is necessary for fatty acid uptake from VLDL coming from the liver. At the same time, the activity of hormone-sensitive lipase, catalyzing the release of fatty acids from adipocytes, is reduced. All these events are subject to hormonal control (insulin and thyroid hormones), regulating necessary enzyme levels by up- or down-regulating transcription and translation.

The different absorption behavior of the **middle chain triglycerides** (MCT = short- and mostly medium-chain fatty acids) is exploited for dietetic purposes. Since MCT are not reesterified inside the mucosa and are bound to and transported with albumin in the blood directly, they often represent the only option for fat absorption in patients whose fatty acid absorption mechanisms are defective. Furthermore, they have the advantage of being absorbed quantitatively in the intestinal lumen, even with reduced lipase activity.

A. Postprandial Lipid Metabolism

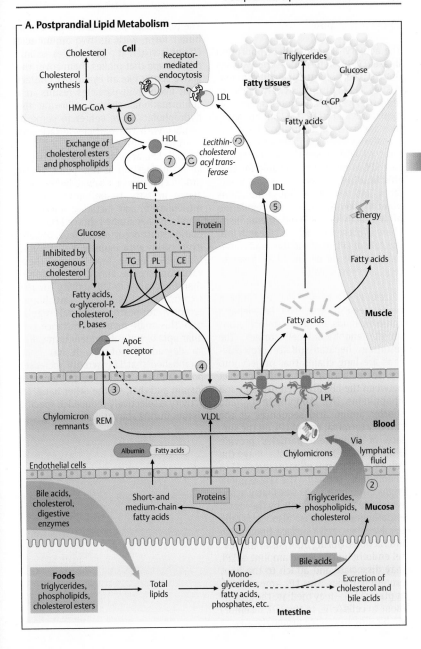

Lipoprotein Lipase

The activity of endothelial **lipoprotein lipase** (LPL) determines the various uptake levels of fatty acids in different tissues. LPL **hydrolyzes** triglycerides in high-triglyceride lipoproteins like chylomicrons and VLDL to 2-monoglycerides and fatty acids. It also effects the **transfer** of phospholipids and apoproteins to HDL. Recent research shows that LPL is further responsible for **specific binding** of lipoproteins to cell surfaces and receptors. These functions point to a central role of the regulation of LPL activity for lipid metabolism. There is presently intense research into the role of LPL malfunctions and mutations in the development of diseases (e. g., atherosclerosis).

LPL can only attach to the cell wall if it binds heparin first. The LPL-heparin complex binds to glycosaminoglycans on the endothelial cell surface. The resulting heparan-sulfate proteoglycans are long chains that project into the vessel lumen and enable contact between the LPL attached to them and lipoproteins (**A**). Apoprotein C_{II} and shorter amino acid sequences at the carboxy terminal end of LPL on the surface of lipoprotein particles provide binding sites. In this, $ApoC_{II}$ plays the role of a cofactor (colipase) required to enable LPL activity. The subsequent triglyceride hydrolysis frees fatty acids, which are taken up locally by the vessel endothelium. LPL is also generally involved in cell surface-lipoprotein interactions. During lipolysis at the vessel endothelium, a small amount of LPL may dissociate and attach to the lipoprotein particles. This LPL—measurable as plasma LPL—may mediate the attachment to cells (e. g., to the LDL receptor) via binding to surface proteoglycans.

The potentially active LPL is present in dimer form, with its two amino acid chains (twisted at a 180° angle) assuming a shape that makes them cover the active center like an eyelid (**B**). Contact with lipoprotein particles results in a conformational change, allowing the hydrophobic active center to come in contact with the particle surface and exert its catalytic effect.

Overall, **LPL activity regulation** is still an open question at this point. LPL is produced in most tissues, being most active in fatty tissue, heart muscle, musculature, and lactating mammary glands. Earlier studies showed that regulation must occur on the level of gene expression with subsequent varying LPL-mRNA tissue levels. Since these variations come about more slowly than the change in LPL activity, greater significance has been attributed, recently, to posttranslational regulation. This might mean, for instance, cellular uptake and subsequent intracellular degradation of LPL. It has been established that LPL activity increases postprandially under the influence of insulin and that, on the other hand, its activity is selectively reduced in specific tissues during starvation or fasting.

A. LPL-Lipoprotein Bonding

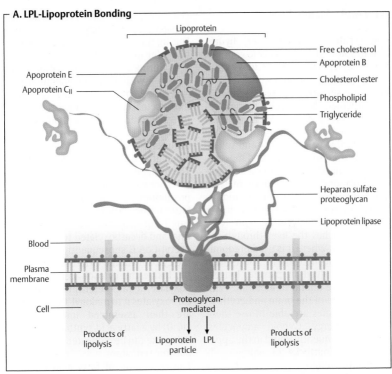

Lipoprotein

Free cholesterol
Apoprotein B
Cholesterol ester
Phospholipid
Triglyceride

Apoprotein E
Apoprotein C$_{II}$

Heparan sulfate proteoglycan
Lipoprotein lipase

Blood
Plasma membrane
Cell

Proteoglycan-mediated

Products of lipolysis

Lipoprotein particle   LPL

Products of lipolysis

B. Triglyceride Hydrolysis by LPL

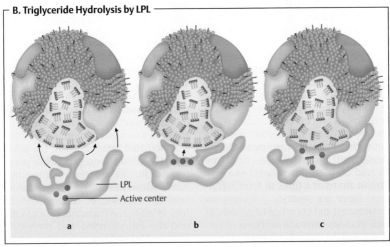

LPL
Active center

a   b   c

Fatty Acids: Metabolism

Triglyceride (= triacylglycerol) hydrolysis in adipocytes is subject to complex hormonal regulation (**A**). Besides by glucagon, growth hormones, and others, **hormone-sensitive lipase** is activated, in particular, by catecholamines released during times of heightened energy need. Hormone-sensitive lipase is activated via a β-receptor and subsequent formation of the second messenger cAMP in the adenylate cyclase system. Hormone-sensitive lipase releases free fatty acids (FFA) from tri- and diglycerides; there is a separate lipase specific to monoglyceride hydrolysis. Glycerol reaches the liver through the blood stream where it is used predominantly for gluconeogenesis. Short-chain FFA are dissolved in plasma, longer-chain FFA are bound to albumin. With the exception of the brain and erythrocytes, all tissues are able to use these FFA for energy. Gynoid adipocytes, which are frequently found in the upper thighs and buttocks of women additionally contain α2-receptors that inhibit cAMP synthesis. Consequently, lipase activation through catecholamines occurs at a greatly reduced rate in those adipocytes.

Fatty acid breakdown is intensified in the liver while FFA plasma levels are elevated (**B**). After being brought into the cells, fatty acids are activated to form acyl-CoA—a process that requires ATP—and are transported to the mitochondria with the help of **carnitine**. During subsequent β-oxidation, sections are cleaved off from the carboxyl end, two carbon atoms at a time, to form acetyl-CoA. There are separate pathways for unsaturated and branched fatty acids, as well as those with odd numbers of carbon atoms. A similar breakdown of long-chain fatty acids takes place inside the hepatocyte peroxisomes.

During times of high acetyl-CoA availability, for instance from increased lipolysis during fasting or starvation, or in patients with diabetes mellitus, two acetyl-CoA molecules may condense into acetoacetyl-CoA. Acetoacetyl-CoA is used to form **ketone bodies** (e. g., acetacetate), an energy source for the tissues that even the brain is able to use, albeit after a short adaptation phase.

The biosynthesis of fatty acids, **lipogenesis**, occurs in many tissues, however, postprandially primarily in liver and fatty tissues. During glycolysis pyruvate is formed, taken to the mitochondria, and decarboxylated to acetyl-CoA. Acetyl-CoA is subsequently returned to the cytosol via the citrate-malate shuttle. Inside the cytosol acetyl-CoA carboxylase, a rate-determining enzyme, carboxylates it to malonyl-CoA. C2 units are then assembled into palmitate (16:0) by a fatty acid synthase complex. Palmitate can be elongated in the endoplasmic reticulum.

The **regulation of fatty acid metabolism** is determined primarily by the ratio of available FFA compared to the size of the mitochondrial acetyl-CoA pool—besides being subject to a multitude of hormonal influences. At elevated FFA levels (e. g., during fasting or starvation) carnitine palmitoyl-transferase is activated, enabling the transport of activated fatty acids (acyl-CoA) into the mitochondria with subsequent elevated β-oxidation, more acetyl-CoA, and increased ketogenesis. At the same time, FFA inhibit lipogenesis while postprandial insulin secretion, on the other hand, stimulates acetyl-CoA carboxylase. The increase of malonyl-CoA in turn inhibits the transport of acyl-CoA into the mitochondria and therewith fatty acid breakdown.

A. Lipolysis in Adipocytes

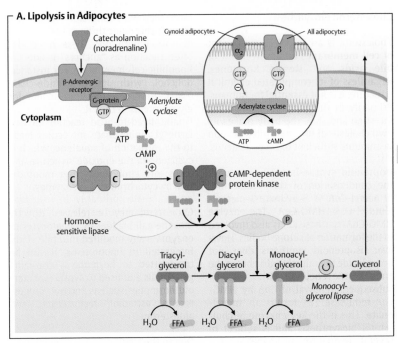

B. Fatty Acid Metabolism in Hepatocytes

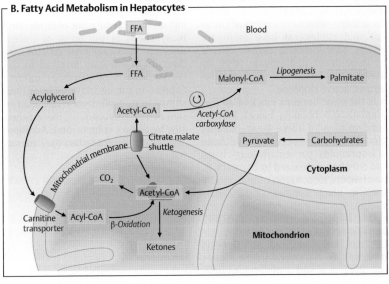

Cholesterol: Biosynthesis

Cholesterol is an essential component of **cell membranes** and a precursor of **bile acids** and **steroid hormones**. Regardless of its complicated chemical structure, it is **not essential** for humans. Primarily in the liver, but also in the intestine and skin, the body makes its own cholesterol in a controlled fashion in amounts sufficient to cover its needs.

Isoprenoid synthesis (A) begins with the condensation of three molecules of acetyl-CoA to 3-hydroxy-3-methyl-glutaryl-CoA (**HMG-CoA**). The enzyme HMG-CoA-synthase (1) is also involved in the formation of ketone bodies. However, isoprenoid synthesis does not occur inside the mitochondria but in the endoplasmic reticulum (ER).

Subsequent removal of CoA by HMG-CoA-reductase (2) results in **mevalonate**. This is the key enzyme of cholesterol biosynthesis and is subject to several regulatory mechanisms. For instance, insulin and thyroxin stimulate its activity, whereas exogenous glucagon and cholesterol have inhibitory effects. Mevalonate is decarboxylated to isopentenyl diphosphate (**IPP**) by mevalonate kinase (3). IPP is also termed **active isoprene**.

It is the basic building block of all isoprenoids (C5 building block). Further condensation of these basic building blocks is species-specific. A multitude of **isoprenoids** (particularly long-chain) can only be synthesized by plants (e. g., carotenoids, tocopherols), some only by specific plant families (e. g., caoutchouc). For animals, synthesis of the cyclic isoprenoid cholesterol (6 IPP-units) is of utmost importance.

IPP can be converted to **farnesyl diphosphate** via several intermediates (4). Since it is still a molecular chain, molecules with long side-chains may form at this point through further condensation with IPP. These molecules often function as "anchors" inside the lipophilic cell membrane. For instance, dolichol, with its long side-chain (~90 C-atoms), is the lipid anchor for glycoproteins in the ER.

Finally, head-to-head reaction of two farnesyl diphosphate molecules leads to the formation of **squalene**, which is cyclized via the epoxide structure and turns into **cholesterol** after modification by cytochrome P_{450} enzymes.

Cholesterol may be released directly into the gall bladder by hepatocytes or enzymatically modified into bile acids. Integrated in lipoproteins, it can be transported to hormone-synthesizing gland cells and used to synthesize steroid hormones such as cortisol, progesterone, estradiol, testosterone, and aldosterone.

Due to the significance of hypercholesterolemia for the pathogenesis of various diseases, **regulation of cholesterol biosynthesis** is the focus of intense research. Transcriptional control of a diversity of enzymes involved in this biosynthesis is of particular interest. Expression can be triggered by various stimuli, e. g., cholesterol levels, expression of LDL receptors, or, more generally, by dietary composition. Additionally, these different factors may interact with one another.

A. Cholesterol Biosynthesis

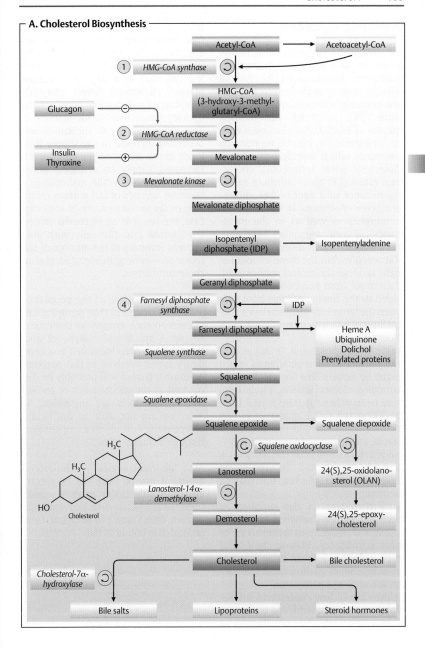

Cholesterol: Homeostasis

Intracellular transport and distribution processes have a major influence on cholesterol homeostasis (**A**). Animal cells can obtain free cholesterol through **neosynthesis in the endoplasmic reticulum** (ER), in which the limiting enzyme is HMG-CoA-reductase. Cellular cholesterol can also be supplied by **lysosomes**, which hydrolyze exogenous cholesterol esters. Intracellular cholesterol esters (CE) also contribute to the maintenance of a pool of free cholesterol. Free cholesterol is stored in cell membranes as well as in the membranes of cell organelles. Different **membranes** contain different amounts of it; even within the same membrane high- and low-cholesterol regions exist. Cholesterol from exogenous sources is added to the freely available pool only when the latter is depleted below a critical limit or when membrane capacity is exceeded.

Inside cells cholesterol is subject to transportation, the regulation of which might be responsible for cellular and pathophysiological effects. Cholesterol from neosynthesis is transported from the ER to the Golgi apparatus to cell membranes inside lipid-rich vesicles in a rapid, energy-consuming process. Lysosomal cholesterol from LDL particles is probably transported by the same route. Hence, it reaches the plasma membrane quickly.

Since cholesterol is also supplied by foods, interactions between exogenous supply and endogenous synthesis are of great significance. Plasma cholesterol levels, which have been established as an independent pathogenetic risk factor, are used as a parameter.

In the case of **low cholesterol intake**, which can only be achieved by a strict dietary regimen, the contribution of food cholesterol to total cholesterol metabolism is minor (**B**). Assuming 55 % absorption, the cholesterol supplied by foods makes up only 10–15 % of the cholesterol used in a day. In this case, plasma cholesterol levels and LDL receptors (responsible for cellular uptake) remain in a "steady-state."

The body can react to the **commonly occurring increase in the supply** from foods in two ways: compensate for the increased supply by reducing endogenous synthesis while maintaining a constant number of LDL surface receptors, or fail to compensate. In the latter case, the result is an increased cholesterol influx into the cells with subsequent lowering of the number of LDL receptors—leading to elevated plasma cholesterol levels.

In fact, a subsection of the population (~20–25 %) reacts in this "pathological" manner to such exogenous cholesterol supply. A specific phenotype of apoprotein E has been identified as a hereditary factor involved in this reaction. Additional factors will probably be discovered as the mechanisms of cholesterol homeostasis are unraveled. To date, we are not able to distinguish compensators from noncompensators through a clinical test.

At **"pharmacological" cholesterol doses**, as can be achieved by dietary measures only under extreme conditions (carbohydrate-free high-fat/high-protein diets), any physiological compensation is bound to fail.

A. Regulation of Cholesterol Homeostasis in Macrophages

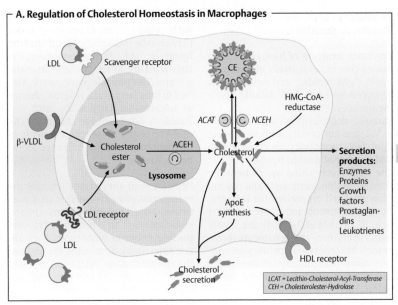

B. Influence of Exogenous Cholesterol Supply

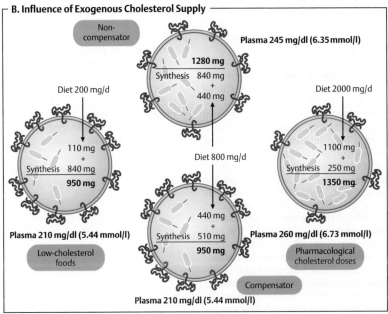

Regulatory Functions: Membrane Structure

The basic structure of biological membranes consists essentially of phospholipids, glycolipids, and cholesterol. Triglycerides are not found inside membranes.

Partially dependent on nutrition (see p. 112) and hormonal status, membrane lipid fatty acids vary in chain-length and number of double-bonds.

The lipid composition varies between tissues, within each cell, and within individual cell organelles. For instance, the plasma membrane of nerve cells is rich in glycolipids, which are rarely found in erythro- and hepatocyte membranes. Mitochondrial membranes contain more phosphatidyl-ethanolamine and -choline than the plasma membrane. There are additional differences between inner and outer mitochondrial membranes. Apparently, the **membrane-specific lipid composition** is essential for differential membrane function.

The **fluid-mosaic model** of the membrane (A) best represents the functional condition of cell membranes. In the watery medium provided by cytoplasm and the interstitium, amphipathic lipids form a **lipid bilayer** ~5 nm thick. The polar, hydrophilic component, consisting of glycerol, phosphate group, R-groups and/or sugars point to the "water side," while the nonpolar fatty acids, the lipophilic components, cling to each other. This way, a bilayer forms, which may be called "fluid." The lipid molecules can "float" within their respective layers, whereas their ability to switch between the two layers is limited. This behavior, termed "**membrane fluidity**," is strongly influenced by the fatty acid composition of the membrane lipids. Due to the character of the bond with glycerol, rotation is possible between the hydrophilic "head" and the lipophilic "tail." At the same time, the fatty acids are able to "dangle" from the glycerol. This possible movement is limited in long fatty acids, whereas shorter or unsaturated fatty acids with cis-double-bonds increase fluidity. The cholesterol and protein components of the membrane further influence membrane fluidity.

Embedded in the bilayer are specific **membrane proteins**, each with a particular task. Integral proteins are the globulins, each of which may traverse the bilayer one or more times. They are asymmetrically distributed throughout the cell membrane. Peripheral proteins "float" on the membrane and are equipped with a lipid anchor or just loosely associated with a membrane component. Most receptor- and channel proteins are integral proteins. Glycoproteins involved in cell-cell recognition tend to be peripheral proteins. It is not fully understood at this time how membrane lipids influence the function of membrane proteins. It is imaginable that a change in the fluidity of the phospholipid bilayer might affect the conformation of the embedded proteins and thereby alter their function.

A. Membrane Fluidity

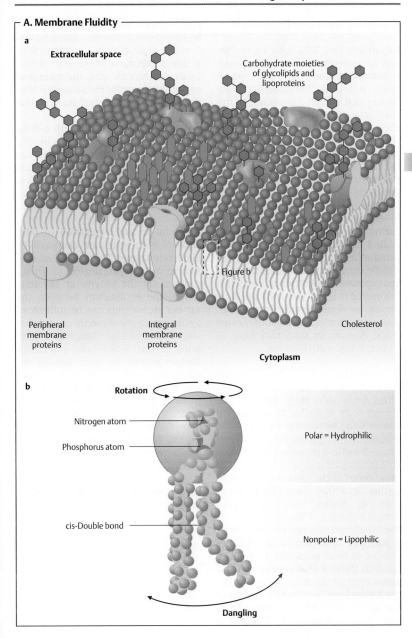

a

Extracellular space

Carbohydrate moieties
of glycolipids and
lipoproteins

Figure b

Peripheral
membrane
proteins

Integral
membrane
proteins

Cholesterol

Cytoplasm

b

Rotation

Nitrogen atom

Phosphorus atom

Polar = Hydrophilic

cis-Double bond

Nonpolar = Lipophilic

Dangling

Regulatory Functions: Eicosanoids

Polyunsaturated fatty acids are precursors and intermediates of endogenous **eicosanoid synthesis**. The term eicosanoids refers to hormone-like substances that exhibit a multitude of frequently antagonistic, mostly localized effects.

The major classes of **prostaglandins** are named PGA to PGI; an index indicates the number of C-C double-bonds outside of the ring (**A**). Prostaglandins with two double bonds, e.g., PGE_2, are synthesized from arachidonic acid (20:4; n-6)—the other two double-bonds are lost during cyclization. **Thromboxanes** are related compounds with a six-membered ether ring. Arachidonic acid can also be converted into leukotrienes by lipoxygenase. **Leukotrienes** were first discovered in leukocytes and have three conjugated double bonds. Prostaglandins, thromboxanes, and leukotrienes are called eicosanoids since they have 20 (Greek: eikosi = 20) C-atoms.

Eicosanoid biosynthesis requires exogenous fatty acids of the n-6 and n-3 series from alimentary sources. The human body is unable to introduce a double bond between the 6th and 3rd C-atom, counting from the methyl end (the ω-3 and ω-6 positions). The body is able to elongate incoming fatty acids of these series at the carboxyl end and to further desaturate them (**B**); however, incoming higher level homologues remain n-6 and n-3 fatty acids.

The most important precursor for the **n-6 pathway** is **linoleic acid**, which is present in most plant oils. It is designated as the essential fatty acid of this series, even though it can be replaced by the higher level homologues. Desaturation of C6 (counting from the carboxyl end) yields γ-linolenic acid, which is rare in foods, with the exception of a few plant oils. Chain elongation by two C-atoms yields dihomo-γ-linolenic acid, a direct precursor of several eicosanoids. Arachidonic acid, the main precursor substance for eicosanoid synthesis, can also be obtained from animal foods.

The **n-3-pathway** begins with α-linolenic acid, which is ubiquitous in very small amounts. Larger amounts are found, for example, in flaxseed oil and to a lesser extent in canola and soy oil. Higher level homologues are abundant in fish oils.

Desaturation and elongation of fatty acids of both series are catalyzed by identical enzymes. Due to this, two substances with varying degrees of affinity compete for the enzyme at any step. Hence, the equilibrium between the various eicosanoids can be influenced by dietary supply of specific, metabolizable intermediates. Exogenous fatty acids of this series from alimentary sources cannot be used directly for eicosanoid synthesis, however, regardless of their position in the synthesis pathway. They may be stored long term in fatty tissues or are inserted into phospholipids (at C2), which are used for cell membranes. From there they can be released by phospholipase A_2, if needed. Hence, the cell membrane constitutes an available pool of fatty acids, the composition of which also has an impact on which eicosanoids are made.

A. Eicosanoid Synthesis

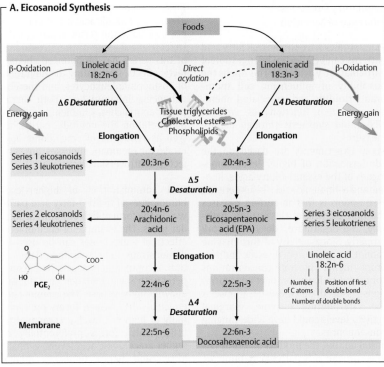

B. Arachidonic Acid Metabolism

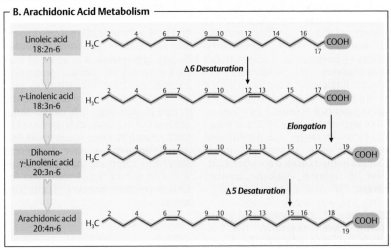

Regulatory Functions: Influence of Nutrition

Many studies have shown that fatty acid patterns can be affected by ingestion of particular fatty acids (**A**). This opens the possibility of influencing **cell membrane fluidity** and associated membrane protein functions as well as **eicosanoid synthesis** through dietary measures.

Many experiments are based on the administration of higher level homologues of the essential fatty acids, linoleic and α-linolenic acid. The underlying assumption is that in certain diseases the first enzyme of the enzyme pathway, δ-6-desaturase, does not work properly. Since activity of this enzyme cannot be measured directly, indirect proof—higher substrate concentrations compared to lower product concentrations—is used. Since δ-6-desaturase is the rate-limiting enzyme, marginal activity levels could have wide-ranging consequences.

Based on this, the product of δ-6-desaturase in the n-6 pathway, γ-**linolenic acid,** is supplemented in the form of specific plant oils. When high levels of γ-linolenic acid are supplied, amounts of mainly the next intermediary, dihomo-γ-linolenic acid, are elevated predominantly in membranes. Dihomo-γ-linolenic acid can be converted to arachidonic acid, but it is also the direct precursor of series 1 eicosanoids. Since eicosanoids have effects in nano- and picogram ranges, and the different series are often antagonistic, minor changes in their balance are often sufficient to achieve clinically relevant effects.

Restriction of **arachidonic acid** intake through purely vegetarian nutrition, which has been practiced for a long time, is founded on a similar basis. It lowers arachidonic acid metabolite levels, especially the series 4 eicosanoids. Leucotriene B_4, one of the eicosanoids of this series, has pronounced chemotactic effects, stimulating the migration of eosinophile leukocytes, and thereby enhancing inflammation. Both therapeutic approaches, γ-linolenic acid supplementation for neurodermatitis, as well as reduction of arachidonic acid intake for rheumatic illnesses, are subject to controversial discussion.

Oral administration of higher-level homologues of the n-3-fatty acid pathway in the form of **fish oils** aims at similar goals. The example of chemotactic effects of leukotrienes can be used to demonstrate their role in inflammation: eicosapentaenoic acid (n-3) competes with arachidonic acid (n-6) for the enzyme lipoxygenase. The chemotactic effect of LTB_5 (which forms preferentially at high n-3 levels) compared to LTB_4 (which forms preferentially at higher arachidonic acid levels) is much lower and hence tends to inhibit inflammation.

N-3 fatty acids have also become known for another effect: **inhibition of thrombocyte aggregation**. It is assumed that native Greenland Eskimos' propensity to bleed, combined with their low incidence of coronary artery disease (CAD) is due to their high fish intake. Large amounts of n-3 fatty acids are found in wild ocean fish. Farm-raised ocean fish and freshwater fish have a different fatty acid spectrum than wild ocean fish. Oral fish oil supplementation for CAD prevention, however, is still controversial.

A. Nutritional Modification of Fatty Acid Composition

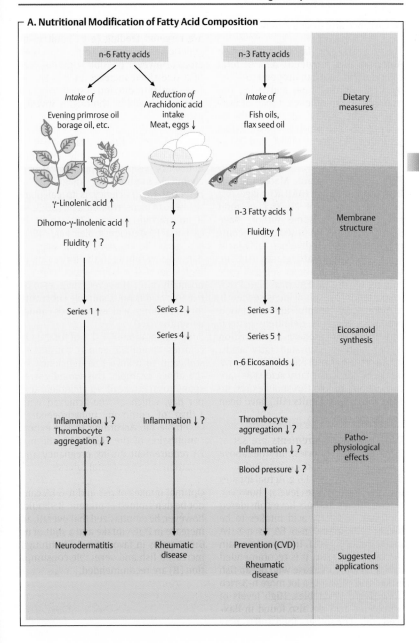

n-6 Fatty acids		n-3 Fatty acids	
Intake of	*Reduction of*	*Intake of*	Dietary measures
Evening primrose oil borage oil, etc.	Arachidonic acid intake Meat, eggs ↓	Fish oils, flax seed oil	
γ-Linolenic acid ↑		n-3 Fatty acids ↑	Membrane structure
Dihomo-γ-linolenic acid ↑	?	Fluidity ↑	
Fluidity ↑ ?			
Series 1 ↑	Series 2 ↓	Series 3 ↑	Eicosanoid synthesis
	Series 4 ↓	Series 5 ↑	
		n-6 Eicosanoids ↓	
Inflammation ↓ ? Thrombocyte aggregation ↓ ?	Inflammation ↓ ?	Thrombocyte aggregation ↓ ? Inflammation ↓ ? Blood pressure ↓ ?	Patho-physiological effects
Neurodermatitis	Rheumatic disease	Prevention (CVD) Rheumatic disease	Suggested applications

Occurrence and Requirements

Thirty years ago, fat in the average American diet provided ~42% of total calories. This rate had dropped to ~33% by 1998. At that rate, and using the example of a middle-aged man of normal weight (**A**), fat intake would be ~86 g/d, 36% of which is consumed as saturated FA, 42% as MUFA, and 7% as PUFA.

The current **Acceptable Macronutrient Distribution Range (AMDR)** suggests a fat intake range of 20–35% of total energy. Recently, some authors have discussed ranges up to 40%. The recommendations for individual fatty acid types reflect **Adequate Intakes (AI)**. The latest recommendations suggest consuming mostly MUFA since high PUFA intake tends to result in increased levels of potentially harmful lipid oxidation products. There is definitely general agreement that modern-day nutrition is too high in saturated fatty acids. Because the harmful effects of excessive intake of particular fatty acid types are cumulative, and no threshold exists, no **Tolerable Upper Limits (UL)** have been set for any of them.

Daily n-3 FA **requirements** are set at 0.7% of total calories. In the above example this would correspond to a daily supply of ~1.1–1.6 g. Actual intakes usually reach these levels; however, recently many authors have considered "optimal" n-3 fatty acid intakes to be higher. The actual n-6 FA to n-3 FA intake ratio is ~10:1. In order to attain the target 5:1 ratio, it is recommended to significantly increase wild ocean fish intake and consume a lot more n-3-rich (i.e., green) vegetables. High levels of α-linolenic acid are also found in flax-seed oil. For other foodstuffs, new options for enrichment with n-3 FA are targeted feeding (e.g., poultry) or genetic engineering (e.g., oil seed crops). However, possible consequences of a one-sided increase in n-3 FA intakes and introduction of such enriched products should be thoroughly investigated.

Unlike n-3 FA deficiency, lack of **n-6 FA intake** results in clinically apparent deficiency symptoms. The classical, biochemical method for diagnosis of essential FA deficiency is to calculate the ratio of eicosatrienoic acid (20:3; n-9) to arachidonic acid (20:4; n-6). In essential FA deficiency, oleic acid (18:1; n-9) uses the enzymes of the enzyme pathway—resulting in the formation of higher level n-9 homologues that are normally rare. However, since eicosatrienoic acid is not a suitable substitute for arachidonic acid, eicosanoids cannot be synthesized.

Supplementation of 1–2% of total daily calories as linoleic acid is considered sufficient to relieve this deficiency. In the above example, this would correspond to an intake of 5 g of linoleic acid per day, which can be achieved with 1 tbsp of common, unhydrogenated vegetable oil. According to the expert commission of the FAO/WHO, the n-6 FA requirement during pregnancy and lactation is 5–7% of total calories.

Optimal intakes of n-3 and n-6 FA cannot be determined at present. It should, however, be emphasized that overall, an increase in PUFA intake and a shift of n-6:n-3 ratios in favor of n-3 FA through increased fish and vegetable consumption (**B**) are recommended.

A. Actual Supply vs. Recommendations

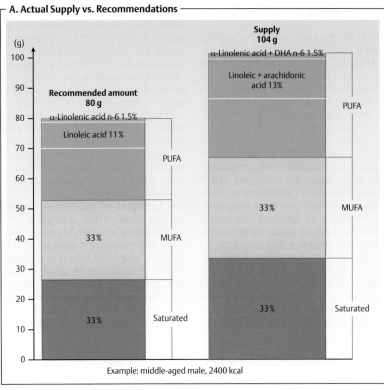

Supply 104 g

α-Linolenic acid + DHA n-6 1.5%

Linoleic + arachidonic acid 13%

PUFA

Recommended amount 80 g

α-Linolenic acid n-6 1.5%

Linoleic acid 11%

PUFA

33%   MUFA

33%   MUFA

33%   Saturated

33%   Saturated

33%   Saturated

(g)

Example: middle-aged male, 2400 kcal

B. Fatty Acid Composition

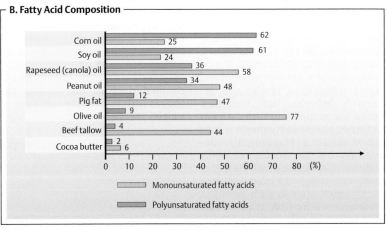

	Monounsaturated	Polyunsaturated
Corn oil	62	25
Soy oil	61	24
Rapeseed (canola) oil	58	36
Peanut oil	48	34
Pig fat	47	12
Olive oil	77	9
Beef tallow	44	4
Cocoa butter	6	2

□ Monounsaturated fatty acids

■ Polyunsaturated fatty acids

Proteins as a Source of Nitrogen

The term "proteins" is derived from the Greek "proteno," which means "I take first place." Berzelius and Mulder, who coined this term during the first half of the nineteenth century, meant proteins to be nitrogen-containing compounds in foods, without which life is impossible. In fact, proteins are the sole source of usable nitrogen (N) for humans. Plants obtain N from nitrogenous organic or inorganic soil compounds (**A**). When plants are harvested, that N is lost to the soil. It therefore needs to be replenished regularly from exogenous sources such as fertilizer, composted plants, and animal waste. Bacteria associated with legumes that are able to fix atmospheric N and release it into the soil (when they are decomposed) import N into this otherwise closed circuit. Plants use N to synthesize amino acids from which they make their species-specific proteins.

All living things use the same mechanism to bond amino acids together: during protein biosynthesis, the carboxyl group of one amino acid forms a bond with the amino group of the next one. Water is removed in this process (dehydration synthesis). The resulting peptide bond (**B**) can be rehydrolyzed, during digestion, for example. During hydrolysis, the water that was removed during dehydration synthesis is re-inserted between two molecules. Unlike the synthesis of carbohydrates and lipids, **protein biosynthesis** is not a tightly regulated, enzymatically catalyzed process. The bonding of amino acids occurs exclusively with the help of RNA (translation). The exact sequence of the amino acids in each protein is predetermined by DNA, with its species- or cell-specific sequence. There-

fore, as opposed to carbohydrates and lipids, the proteins of different species may be similar but are rarely identical.

Endogenously synthesized proteins (several thousand) can be divided into several large groups according to **function**. The mechanical stability of organs and tissues is due to **structural proteins**. Most of them consist of the long amino acid chains of so-called fibrous (structural) proteins. Approximately a third of the total human protein mass is made up of a single structural protein, **collagen**.

The **transport** of substances through plasma, inside cells, and across cell membranes is another function of proteins. The transported substances may be gases, reversibly bound to a protein (O_2 to hemoglobin in erythrocytes), substances with poor water-solubility (e. g., fat-soluble vitamin A bound to RBP), or polar molecules carried across nonpolar barriers (e. g., ion channels in lipid bilayers).

The body uses the immune system (e. g., immunoglobulins) and the blood-clotting system (e. g., fibrinogen) as **defense and protective mechanisms**.

Hormones and their cellular receptors (e. g., insulin and insulin receptor) are essential for **control and regulation**.

Other metabolic processes would be unthinkable without DNA-encoded **enzymes**. It is the controlled catalysis of chemical reactions that enables the body to react to changing conditions in a highly specific manner.

A. Nitrogen Cycle

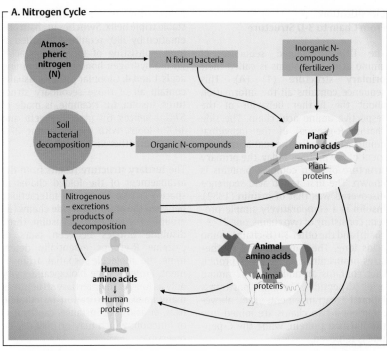

B. Peptide Bonds

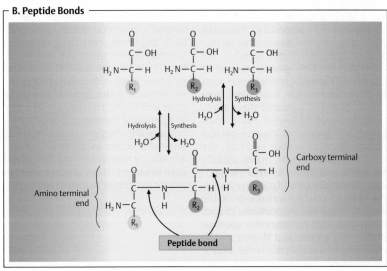

Classification:
From Chain to 3-D Structure

The DNA-determined sequence of amino acids in proteins is called their **primary structure** (1) (**A**). This sequence contains all the information about the further behavior of the respective amino acid chain. The side chains (**R-groups**) of the individual amino acids predict the spatial arrangement of the protein. Today, the primary structure of even complex proteins is known. The first amino acid sequence discovered was that of **insulin** (1952). Insulin is a comparatively simple protein, consisting of two chains, one 21 (A-chain) and the other 30 (B-chain) amino acids long. The pancreas first synthesizes proinsulin, a single-chain protein that contains an additional 33 amino acids (C-peptide). Then, in a posttranslational rearrangement, the above-mentioned two chains are joined into the finished protein, while the C-peptide is removed.

The folding of the amino acid chain (2) determines its **secondary structure**. Folding is achieved through the formation of hydrogen bonds between the –C=O and the HN– groups involved in the peptide bonds. Certain amino acids (e.g., tyrosine, valine, isoleucine) favor the formation of a **pleated sheet** structure, the result of several chains combined in a parallel or counter-parallel arrangement; its peptide grid folds like a harmonica with side chains sticking out below and above. Another energetically favorable secondary structure is the **helix**. In a right-handed α-helix, the peptide shape spirals clockwise in such a way that each turn includes approximately 3.6 amino acid R-groups. The collagen of the connective tissue matrix, for instance, consists of left-handed

helices, three of which combine into a stable triple helix. Switches in chain orientation by 180° require a so-called β-**loop**, consisting of four amino acids with a hydrogen bond between amino acids 1 and 4. Globular proteins usually contain all of those secondary structures. Insulin, for example, is made of 57% α-helices, 6% pleated sheets, and 10% β-loops, with the remaining 27% structured otherwise.

The **tertiary structure** results from the arrangement of the folded chains in space (3) that is due to interactions between the amino acid side chains (R-groups). For instance, in insulin, three disulfide bridges between pairs of cysteine R-groups essentially determine the molecule's spatial arrangement. Proteins have biological activity only as long as their tertiary structure is maintained. **Denaturation** by ethanol, heat, or acids, for instance, causes loss of function, which may or may not be reversible.

Quarternary structures result from an assembly of several tertiary structures. Such oligomers, consisting of several subunits or monomers, are common in large, globular proteins. The monomers may have independent biological activity, whereas some become functional units only inside a quaternary structure (e.g., enzyme complexes). Insulin, too, forms quarternary structures: in blood, some of it occurs as dimers. A pancreatic storage form consists of Zn^{2+}-stabilized hexamers. Those are used as slow-release insulins in diabetes therapy.

A. From Chain to 3-D Structure

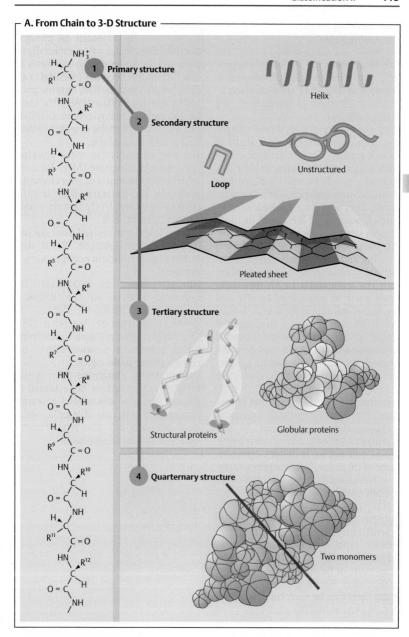

1 Primary structure

Helix

2 Secondary structure

Loop

Unstructured

Pleated sheet

3 Tertiary structure

Structural proteins

Globular proteins

4 Quarternary structure

Two monomers

Basic Building Blocks:
The Amino Acids

The 20 amino acids (AA) used for protein synthesis are the **proteinogenic amino acids (A)**. They are exclusively L-amino acids; their D-enantiomers are biologically inactive.

They can be divided into four categories, according to the chemical nature of their R-groups (exception: glycine). **AA with nonpolar side chains** consist of a straight or branched hydrocarbon chain, or—in methionine—of a thioether group. They make up the hydrophobic core of proteins or are found in those protein sites that touch membrane lipids. **Polar AA** can engage in hydrogen bonding and other bonds and thus stabilize or contribute to the tertiary structure. The **acidic** and **basic AA** are usually dissociated at physiological pHs and are, therefore, able to form ionic bonds. Results of recent research challenge the classic distinction between essential and nonessential AA. Of the eight AA termed "essential," six can be synthesized endogenously from the respective keto acids—they are, therefore, not truly essential. Only **lysine** (Lys) and **threonine** (Thr) are truly essential since their transamination is irreversible.

The other AA used to be considered simply as nonspecific N donors. However, some of them may become temporarily, or at least conditionally, essential under specific pathological conditions.

Consensus exists that **histidine** (His) is essential in children as well as in case of chronic renal failure. In case of prolonged His deficiency, plasma His levels drop even in healthy people and normalize after His supplementation. His must, therefore, be essential to a certain degree even in healthy adults.

Tyrosine (Tyr) is synthesized endogenously from the essential AA **phenylalanine** (Phe). In neonates, especially in preemies, endogenous Tyr synthesis is insufficient. Tyr becomes essential in all diseases affecting the liver enzyme phenylalanine hydroxylase (PAH). The classic example is phenylketonuria (PKU) but sepsis and cirrhotic diseases should also be mentioned here.

The liver of adults can make **cysteine** (Cys) from **methionine** (Met). Patients with homocysteinuria or liver cirrhosis, preemies, and neonates have insufficient or are completely lacking endogenous Cys synthesis.

Serine (Ser) is synthesized from **glycine** (Gly) and formaldehyde. Renal disorders impair sufficient endogenous Ser synthesis.

Nitrogen monoxide (NO) with its numerous effects on the vascular, nervous, and immune systems is derived from **arginine** (Arg, see p. 128). This suggests that arginine supplementation may have positive effects on certain severe pathologies.

Quantitatively, **glutamine** (Gln) is the body's most important nonessential N source. There is substantial research indicating that in case of trauma, intestinal disorders etc., Gln requirements exceed endogenous synthesis.

A. Proteinogenic Amino Acids

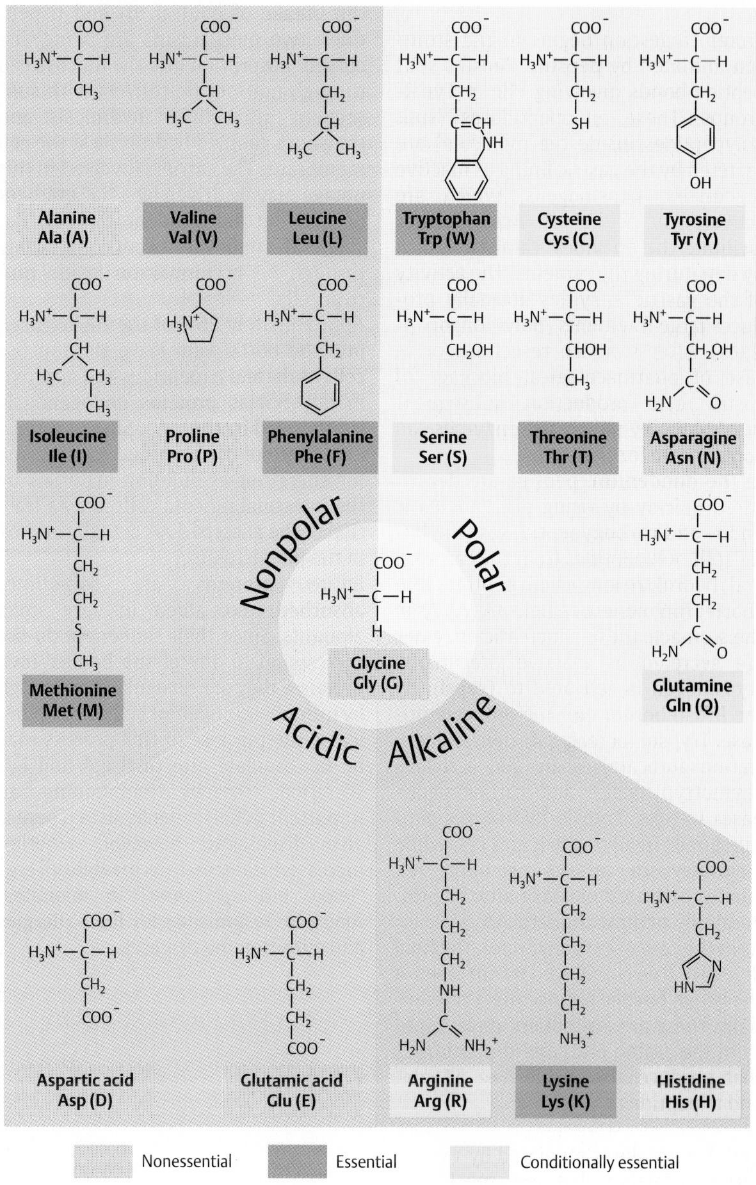

Alanine Ala (A)	Valine Val (V)	Leucine Leu (L)
Tryptophan Trp (W)	Cysteine Cys (C)	Tyrosine Tyr (Y)
Isoleucine Ile (I)	Proline Pro (P)	Phenylalanine Phe (F)
Serine Ser (S)	Threonine Thr (T)	Asparagine Asn (N)
Methionine Met (M)	Glycine Gly (G)	Glutamine Gln (Q)
Aspartic acid Asp (D)	Glutamic acid Glu (E)	Arginine Arg (R)
Lysine Lys (K)	Histidine His (H)	

Nonpolar

Polar

Acidic

Alkaline

Nonessential   Essential   Conditionally essential

Digestion and Absorption

Protein digestion begins in the **stomach**, initiated by **pepsins**. Pepsins split peptide bonds involving Phe or Tyr R-groups. These endopeptidases (split polypeptides inside the molecule) are secreted by the gastric lining as inactive precursors, pepsinogens, which are activated at acidic pH. Acids further facilitate the enzymes' catalytic attack by denaturing the proteins. The activity of the gastric enzymes normally produces large fragments (poly-, oligopeptides). After stomach resections or in case of pharmacological blockage of gastric acid production, subsequent breakdown by pancreatic enzymes can compensate for that step.

In the **duodenum**, pepsins are deactivated quickly by rising pH. Pancreatic **endo- and carboxypeptidases** (the latter split polypeptides from the carboxyl end) hydrolyze long-chain peptides into shorter fragments or single AA (**A**). As in the stomach, these pancreatic enzymes are secreted as inactive precursors: trypsinogen is activated to **trypsin** by the brush border enzyme **enteropeptidase**. Trypsin increases its own concentration autocatalytically and activates chymotrypsinogen and carboxypeptidases in turn. Trypsin hydrolyzes peptide bonds involving Arg and Lys, while **chymotrypsin** attacks aromatic AA. Finally, activated **elastase** attacks preferentially neutral aliphatic AA.

As in the case of carbohydrates, the final digestive step is achieved by enzymes of the **brush border membrane**. Preferentially, these are **aminopeptidases** (split from the amino end) and **dipeptidases** that produce absorbable free AA, di-, and tripeptides.

Cellular uptake is mediated by various carrier proteins that are specific to particular AA groups (**B**). With regard to the uptake of neutral di- and tripeptides, two mechanisms are being discussed: absorption into the mucosa cell through nonspecific carriers with subsequent intracellular hydrolysis and transport-coupled hydrolysis at the cell membrane. The carriers involved in this uptake may be driven by a Na^+ gradient or may be independent thereof. Basolateral removal occurs passively through AA accumulation inside mucosa cells.

Approximately 25 % of the AA released into the portal vein leave the mucosa cells as di- and tripeptides and approximately 5 % as proteins endogenously synthesized by the cells. Since a significant share of the absorbed AA are used for energy or as building materials by the intestinal mucosa cells, only a fraction of the absorbed AA actually end up in the bloodstream.

Entire **proteins** are sometimes **absorbed**, too, albeit in very small amounts. Since their sequences do not correspond to any of the bodies' own proteins, they are recognized as foreign by immune-competent cells. Physiologically, the purpose of this process may be to stimulate intestinal IgA and IgG secretion, thereby maintaining an important defense mechanism. There is also discussion, however, whether increased intestinal permeability (e. g., "leaky gut syndrome" in neonates) might be responsible for food allergies and autoimmune diseases.

A. Digestion and Absorption

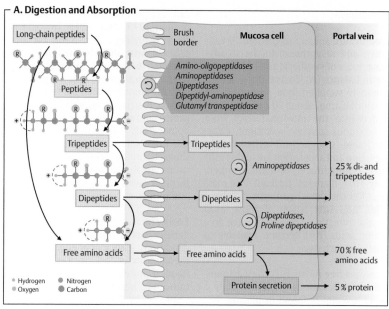

B. Mechanisms of Absorption

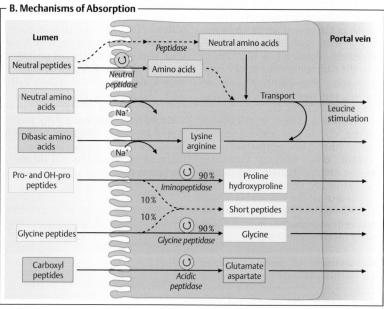

Metabolism

Proteins are subject to constant breakdown and resynthesis. In the **steady-state**, rates of synthesis and breakdown are in balance (**A**). To any 100 g of exogenously supplied food protein in the small intestine, about 70 g of protein is added into the intestinal tract from endogenous sources: secretions, enzymes, and sloughed-off cells. Protein digestion and absorption are highly efficient. Approximately 95 % are absorbed, only ~10 g/d are lost through fecal matter. After complete hydrolysis of all peptides, and subtraction of those used by the intestinal mucosa, ~150 g free amino acids (AA) become available to the body each day.

Incoming free AA are first compartmentalized into various **AA pools**. Only a small amount is found in plasma, 70–80 % of the free AA are found in skeletal muscle. **Intracellular accumulation** of free AA in the respective tissue constitutes a first controlled step in AA metabolism. Assuming a 10 g loss to feces, the daily exogenous protein supply is only ~90 g. Highly efficient AA recycling provides so many additional endogenous AA that the total protein turnover rate is as high as 300 g/d. For instance, of ~75 g of skeletal muscle protein that is synthesized and degraded, only ~10 % is exchanged between skeletal muscle and plasma pool as free AA. Constant replacement of the intestinal mucosa, and synthesis and breakdown of plasma proteins and blood cells also contribute to the high protein turnover rate.

An **assessment of protein turnover rates** can be achieved by measuring the turnover rates of short-lived proteins. Plasma proteins with a high breakdown rate like prealbumin or retinol-binding protein (27 % and 120 % breakdown, respectively/day) are useful for purposes of detecting latent malnutrition. **Nitrogen balance** is more commonly used for this purpose. Nitrogen (N) is easy to determine: after oxidation of the organic matrix, the mass is converted to protein, using a factor. N balance is in homeostasis when the amount supplied by foods corresponds to that lost through urine, feces, and skin. Additional small amounts of N are lost through sweat, hair, menstrual blood, and semen.

Energy intake significantly influences N balance. Under **reduced energy supply** conditions, sufficient energy for protein metabolism is lacking. On the other hand, if protein supply is below a certain limit, nitrogen balance cannot be improved by high energy supply. Even with **adequate energy supply**, a multitude of diseases, protein energy malnutrition (PEM), or poor protein quality can nevertheless cause negative N balance. If adequate energy but no protein is supplied, daily N losses decrease to approximately 2–3 g/d within a few days. This daily loss persists even after prolonged protein-free diets. It can be deduced from this that a daily protein loss of 16–17 g is obligatory and has to be compensated in the long term to maintain body proteins and therewith life function.

A. Protein Turnover in the Steady State

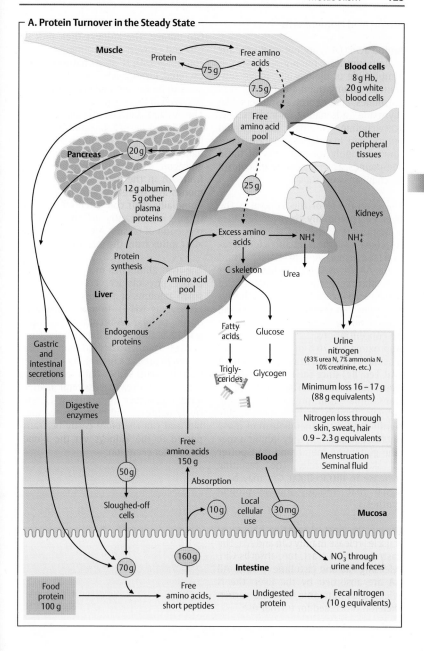

Amino Acid Homeostasis

Amino acids (AA) are not only used for protein synthesis, but are precursors of a multitude of biologically active substances. Among them are, for instance, hormones and neurotransmitters like thyroxine, adrenaline, noradrenaline, acetylcholine, glutamate, and γ-amino butyric acid. In order to maintain a continuous supply for synthesis of these compounds, as well as proteins, control mechanisms are crucial.

The central site of this control is the **liver. Postprandially**, the liver degrades a significant portion of the incoming AA, converting the N into urea for excretion (see below). Approximately a third of the AA are used for synthesis of liver and plasma proteins. Regulation of these catabolic and anabolic pathways is so tight that even a protein-rich meal leads to only a slight increase in plasma AA concentrations.

Approximately 70% of the increase in plasma AA is due to **branched-chain AA** (Val, Leu, Ile) since the liver is unable to transaminate them. These AA can be transaminated in muscle, brain, and kidneys, though, making them highly significant for the metabolism of those organs. For instance, they inhibit a specific glutamine membrane transporter in skeletal muscle. The resulting increase in intracellular Gln may be a signal that initiates muscle protein synthesis.

During the **post-absorptive phase** (**A**) muscles release mainly Gln and Ala. The gastrointestinal tract, too, absorbs Gln, releasing Ala and cirtulline in turn. All AA are absorbed by the liver, the N released as ammonia, and the carbon skeleton processed for further use.

Acidosis causes inhibition of hepatic Gln uptake. The kidneys then pick up Gln and convert it to ammonia, which combines with H^+ ions that need to be excreted, forming NH^{4+}. All H^+ ions that need to be excreted due to acidosis are removed in this form.

The AA Arg and Leu stimulate insulin secretion, others (e.g., Asn, Gly) stimulate glucagon secretion. Insulin enhances muscle protein synthesis, while glucagon enhances gluconeogenesis from AA in the liver. Since both hormones are, therefore, stimulated postprandially, their concerted effects contribute significantly to the effective reduction of plasma AA concentrations after influx from the intestine.

The liver eliminates most of the N (**B**). Under physiological conditions, only small amounts of it are excreted by the kidneys as NH^{4+}. Ammonia produced during cellular AA breakdown is transported as Gln. In the liver, all the NH^{4+} derived from AA degradation is converted to urea at a high energy cost. The body uses this somewhat wasteful urea cycle since urea has several distinct advantages over ammonia: it is relatively nontoxic and highly water-soluble, and can therefore easily be transported to the kidneys via the bloodstream for excretion.

A. Postabsorptive Amino Acid Metabolism

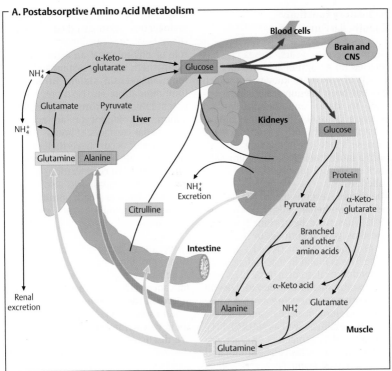

Blood cells

Brain and CNS

α-Keto-glutarate

Glucose

NH_4^+

Glutamate   Pyruvate

NH_4^+

Liver   **Kidneys**

Glutamine   Alanine

Glucose

Citrulline

NH_4^+ Excretion

Protein

Pyruvate   α-Keto-glutarate

Intestine

Branched and other amino acids

α-Keto acid   Glutamate

Renal excretion

Alanine NH_4^+

Glutamine   **Muscle**

B. Hepatic N Elimination

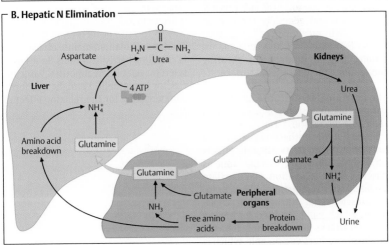

Aspartate

$$H_2N - \overset{\overset{\textstyle O}{\|}}{C} - NH_2$$
Urea

Kidneys

Liver

4 ATP

Urea

NH_4^+

Glutamine

Amino acid breakdown   Glutamine

Glutamate

Glutamine NH_4^+

NH_3 Glutamate

Peripheral organs

Free amino acids   Protein breakdown

Urine

Regulatory Functions:
Endothelial Functions

During recent years, research has focused on an amino acid product the effects of which are known, but which has not been unequivocally characterized to date: **endothelium-derived relaxing factor (EDRF)**. At this point, it is assumed that EDRF is probably identical with nitrogen monoxide (NO) or with a more stable NO-containing substance like S-nitrosocysteine (also called NO-R).

The enzyme responsible for NO synthesis in endothelial cells, NO synthase (NOS), has since been cloned and the encoding gene identified. In the brain, there is one isoform (type I); another (type II) was found in macrophages.

The endothelial isoform (type III) is predominantly membrane-bound. Like all NO synthases, it uses Arg as a substrate (**A**). In addition, it needs molecular O_2, Ca-calmodulin, as well as NADPH, BH_4, FAD, and FMN as cofactors. NOS activity and hence NO release can be stimulated by a series of agonists: acetylcholine, histamine, serotonin, ADP, substance P, bradykinin, and generally through an increase in intracellular Ca^{2+} concentrations. Expression of this enzyme is, among others, induced by shearing forces along the endothelial surface.

The **functional significance** of EDRF for various organ systems is a subject of intense discussion. Until recently, endothelial NO synthesis was discussed only with regard to its **relaxing effects** on vascular tone (**B**). Vascular tone is based on the activation of guanylate cyclase with subsequent cGMP increase in muscle cells. Nitroglycerin treatment, which has been used for angina pectoris attacks for a long time, is based on the same effective principle, which is why EDRF (NO) has also been called an endogenous nitro-vasodilator. Today, the NO system is considered to play the role of physiological antagonist to the sympathetic nervous system and to the renin-angiotensin system in **vascular tone regulation**. Furthermore, NO is a potent inhibitor of **thrombocyte aggregation** and **leukocyte adhesion** to endothelial surfaces. Should platelet aggregation occur nevertheless, ADP and serotonin released from thrombocytes trigger NOS activation, causing increased NO release. NO also inhibits **smooth muscle cell proliferation** through stimulation of guanylate cyclase.

These three factors—leukocyte adhesion, proliferation, and subsequent platelet aggregation—are of great significance in the **initial phase of arteriosclerosis**. The weakening of the Arg-NO system seems a likely pathogenetic factor in vascular lesions. Several variables are discussed as triggering factors for defects in NOS activity (**C**): reduced receptor coupling of the agonists, marginal substrate (Arg) or cofactor availability, or inactivation of EDRF (NO) on its way to the site of its intended activity. The latter is blamed mainly on oxidized LDL and/or peroxide anions. In arteriosclerotic vessels, an abnormal vasoconstrictor (endothelin 1) might also form, compensating for the relaxing effect of NO.

A. NO Synthesis

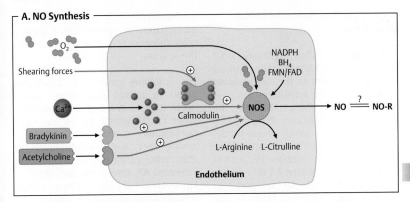

B. NO Effects on Smooth Musculature

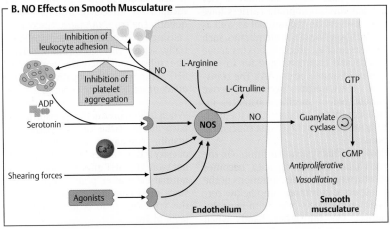

C. Interfering Factors

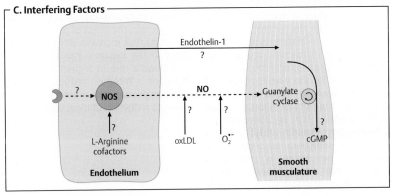

Regulatory Functions: The Blood–Brain Barrier

In the brain, so-called "tight junctions" between the endothelial cells of blood capillaries represent the **blood–brain barrier**. Lipophilic substances can pass this barrier, moving through the endothelial lipid bilayer. Also, O_2–CO_2 diffusion occurs along their partial pressure gradient. Water can diffuse through the tight junctions because of its small molecular size. All other polar substances need special transport systems to pass the blood–brain barrier (**A**). For this, appropriate carriers have to be present on the luminal as well as on the brain side of the membrane. Such carriers exist for glucose, ions (as active pumps and channels), and for various groups of amino acids (AA). The transport mechanisms permit selective enrichment of specific substances inside the brain, rendering it theoretically independent of plasma concentrations.

However, this system has limits. On the one hand, carrier capacity becomes insufficient when concentrations of the transported substance drop below certain plasma levels (e.g., with hypoglycemia). On the other hand, when several substances use the same transport system, they compete for the carrier. This makes the system indirectly dependent on substrate supply in the plasma. This situation applies, for instance, to large, neutral AA.

Competition for the carrier is particularly significant between tryptophan (Trp) and long-chain neutral amino acids (LNAA). Trp is converted to **5-hydroxytryptamine** (5HT) better known as **serotonin** in serotonergic neurons. The latter is stored in intraneuronal vesicles and released after neuron depolarization. A classic neurotransmitter, it binds to a specific postsynaptic receptor (5HT receptor) with subsequent active reuptake into the neuron.

The following model was developed based on animal experiments and it might explain **seasonal affective disorder** (SAD), which causes increased carbohydrate cravings during winter, among others. **Rising insulin levels** (**B**) after carbohydrate consumption trigger increased AA absorption into muscles. Trp levels are not affected by this since it easily binds to albumin and thereby escapes the effects of insulin. Consequently, the Trp/LNAA ratio is increased, causing Trp to be transported preferentially across the blood–brain barrier. The subsequent increase in neuronal 5HT synthesis has a negative feedback effect on carbohydrate cravings.

When insulin production is insufficient, particularly in the case of **peripheral insulin resistance** (type 2 diabetes, obesity), this satiety mechanism does not work (**C**). 5HT effects remain below normal even after pure protein meals since, due to the lacking insulin release, the Trp/LNAA ratio is not changed in favor of Trp.

5HT neurons have significant carbohydrate consumption-limiting effects. For example, the effect of pharmaceutical drugs that increase 5HT concentrations in the synaptic gap shows that 5HT plays a role in regulating feeding behavior. Weight reduction—albeit transitory—can be achieved mainly through reduction of meal sizes.

A. Transport Systems

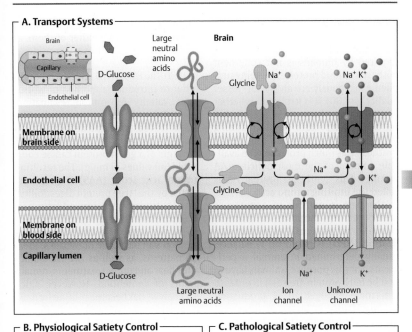

B. Physiological Satiety Control

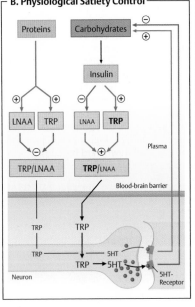

C. Pathological Satiety Control

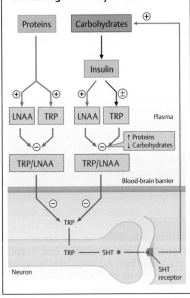

Protein Quality

Since the pattern of the essential AA required by humans is not congruent with that of food proteins, proteins supplied exogenously are always of "lesser quality" (<1.00). It is irrelevant whether large amounts of several AA are found in the respective protein; the determining factor is that the body can only newly synthesize as much protein as the available amount of the most deficient AA permits. This synthesis-limiting AA is called the **limiting amino acid**.

In the past, a number of approaches were used for purposes of practical evaluation of proteins. **Net protein utilization** (NPU) is based on N balance, usually determined in animal experiments. For this purpose, animals have to first be fed a protein-free diet in order to determine endogenous N production via mandatory N losses in feces and urine. Subsequently, the protein to be investigated is supplied at increasing levels until homeostasis of N balance is reached. With a protein of "high-value" this is achieved more quickly than with a protein of a lesser NPU.

Biological value (BV) represents a refinement compared to NPU. The protein supplied is no longer assessed solely via its N content, but its digestibility is taken into account as well.

Protein efficiency ratio (PER) used to be the prescribed standard procedure, especially in the U.S. For its determination, weight gain in young rats is related to their protein intake.

Each of these methods has its disadvantages: the transferability of the animal experiments' results is not always insured, N balances do not capture all parameters, and they are costly and work-intensive. Additionally, each of these methods yields different results. Sometimes in the literature only one of these methods is mentioned, but values listed are derived by either of them, at times causing them to vary considerably.

In 1990, the FAO/WHO issued a report in order to introduce a method of worldwide validity for protein evaluation, specifying an exact method. The method is based on the definition of an **ideal AA pattern** (A), to which the AA contents of a given protein can be compared (all values in mg/g). The resulting **amino acid score** (AAS) is then corrected by the "true protein digestibility" that continues to be derived from animal experiments and has to be looked-up in the respective tables. Even this method still has some drawbacks: ideal AA patterns, as well as AA availability after heat and other treatments, remain points of contention. However, since AA analysis has become routine by now, it provides a fast and cost-effective method, particularly for developing countries.

Comparison of the resulting **protein digestibility-corrected amino acid scores** (PDCAAS) with commonly used BV values (B) show that animal products and soy achieve better values with PDCAAS, while other plant foods get lower scores. In plants, Lys tends to be the limiting AA. Requirements for Lys are set relatively high and will probably be adjusted downward for adults.

A. PDCAAS for Protein Evaluation

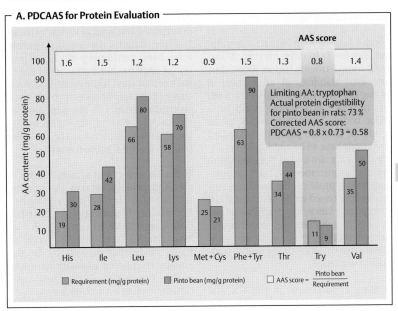

AAS score

| 1.6 | 1.5 | 1.2 | 1.2 | 0.9 | 1.5 | 1.3 | 0.8 | 1.4 |

Limiting AA: tryptophan
Actual protein digestibility for pinto bean in rats: 73%
Corrected AAS score:
PDCAAS = 0.8 × 0.73 = 0.58

AA content (mg/g protein)

	His	Ile	Leu	Lys	Met + Cys	Phe + Tyr	Thr	Try	Val
Requirement	19	28	66	58	25	63	34	11	35
Pinto bean	30	42	80	70	21	90	44	9	50

■ Requirement (mg/g protein)   ■ Pinto bean (mg/g protein)   □ AAS score = $\dfrac{\text{Pinto bean}}{\text{Requirement}}$

B. BV vs. PDCAAS

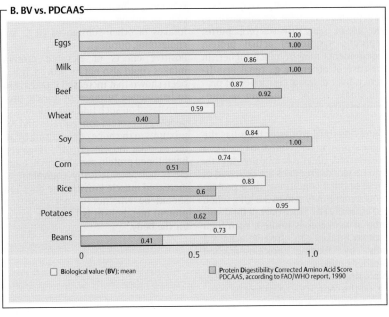

	Biological value (BV)	PDCAAS
Eggs	1.00	1.00
Milk	0.86	1.00
Beef	0.87	0.92
Wheat	0.59	0.40
Soy	0.84	1.00
Corn	0.74	0.51
Rice	0.83	0.6
Potatoes	0.95	0.62
Beans	0.73	0.41

□ Biological value (BV); mean   ■ Protein Digestibility Corrected Amino Acid Score PDCAAS, according to FAO/WHO report, 1990

Occurrence and Requirements

When a healthy man (**A**) eats a protein-free diet for 7–10 days, his daily N loss in all compartments (urine, feces, skin, hair, etc.) stabilizes at an average of 54 mg/kg. This corresponds to a daily loss of 0.34 g protein/kg (24 g/d for a 70 kg body). To include 97.5% of all people of this age group two standard deviations have to be added: the resulting 0.45 g/kg are called the **minimum protein requirement**. This (approximately 31 g protein/d), however, is sufficient only based on an assumed 100% absorption. Since, in practical terms, this can be achieved only under standardized dietetic conditions, an additional safety margin for the overall population is needed.

In many countries, as in the U.S., the presently **recommended intake** for adults is 0.8 g/kg body weight (see also AMDR for proteins, on this page). In the case of many diseases (e.g., burns, nephrotic syndrome) actual protein requirements may be much higher; in the case of others (e.g., renal insufficiency, liver disease) restriction of protein intake to the minimum requirement may be indicated.

A growing third trimester fetus has the highest protein need but also receives a preselected, ideal AA mixture directly into its blood. Preemies are deprived of these optimal conditions; their protein requirement may rise to 3.8 g/kg when fed enterally (**B**). Since overall fluid volume of neonates is limited, such high protein intakes can often be achieved only by feeding protein-enriched mother's milk.

A nursing infant's requirement of 2.2 g/kg, on the contrary, can be met by feeding mother's milk alone.

Actual intakes are often far above recommended amounts in Western industrialized nations. In the U.S., people have been consuming 80–125 g protein/d since the beginning of the twentieth century and those intakes have not changed. Protein sources, though, have changed: whereas in the past most of the protein was of vegetable origin, today, animal proteins make up more than 70% of total protein intake.

There has never been proven toxicity of **elevated protein intakes**. Accounting for this fact, the recently established **Acceptable Macronutrient Distribution Range (AMDR)**, lists 10–35% of total calories from proteins, with an upper range that exceeds by far the amount considered adequate according to the existing RDA (~10% of total calories, depending on activity levels).

However, a high intake of animal protein is always associated with high intakes of other substances (e.g., fat, cholesterol, purines).
Positive effects of elevated protein intakes could also not be proven. It has been shown that increased intakes lead to heightened turnover of muscle protein. Based on such findings, millions of people eat protein concentrates and AA mixtures in the hope of benefiting by an increase in muscle growth. However, heightened protein metabolism in muscle is not automatically equivalent to increased muscle growth. The question should be whether or not increased protein metabolism is better or worse for the body.

A. Requirements and Intake

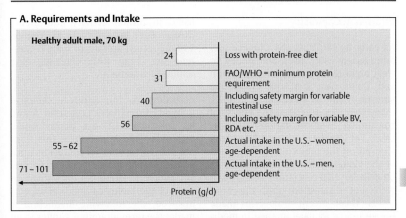

Healthy adult male, 70 kg

24	Loss with protein-free diet
31	FAO/WHO = minimum protein requirement
40	Including safety margin for variable intestinal use
56	Including safety margin for variable BV, RDA etc.
55–62	Actual intake in the U.S. – women, age-dependent
71–101	Actual intake in the U.S. – men, age-dependent

Protein (g/d)

B. Recommendations by Life Stage and Gender Groups (DRI, 2001)

Life Stage and Gender Group	Age	AI (g/kg/d)	EAR (g/kg/d)	RDA (g/kg/d)	RDA (g/d)
Infants	0– 6mo	1.52			
	7–12mo	1.52	1.1	1.5	17
Children	1– 3y		0.88	1.1	13
	4– 8y		0.76	0.95	19
Boys	9–13y		0.76	0.95	34
	14–18y		0.73	0.85	52
Girls	9–13y		0.76	0.95	34
	14–18y		0.71	0.85	46
Men	>19y		0.66	0.80	56
Women	>19y		0.66	0.80	46
Pregnancy	14–50y		0.88 or + 21 g	1.1 or + 25 g	
Lactation	14–50y			1.05 or + 21.2 g	
Physical activity	No evidence of increased requirements				

C. Protein Content in Food

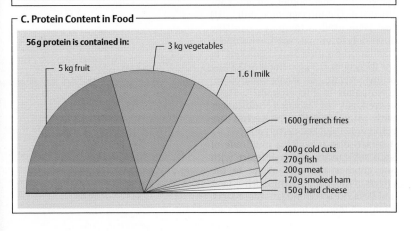

56 g protein is contained in:

- 5 kg fruit
- 3 kg vegetables
- 1.6 l milk
- 1600 g french fries
- 400 g cold cuts
- 270 g fish
- 200 g meat
- 170 g smoked ham
- 150 g hard cheese

Vitamin A: Chemistry

As early as 1500 BC, the Chinese recommended using liver and honey to treat night blindness. Before McCollum and Davis described the fat-soluble vitamin A and its significance in 1913, many treatises described the effects of consuming liver on various eye diseases. For long time, vitamin A research focused on the molecular mechanisms of the **visual cycle**. Vitamin A's effects on **cellular differentiation** and **growth** were not discovered until the early 1980s. These recent discoveries made the vitamin a focus of interest in medical and molecular biological vitamin research.

The term vitamin A applies to all compounds with biological activity similar to that of vitamin A. Chemically, these substances are similar, while the functions on which the vitamin A-like effects are based are quite diverse.

Particularly the analytical distinction between the various carotenoids, precursors of vitamin A, used to be very difficult. It is, therefore, not surprising that the mutual conversion of these substances into one another remains controversial. The **international units (IU)** that were used in the past essentially apply only to animal experiments under standardized nutritional conditions. In the IU system, 0.3 µg retinol (or 0.34 µg retinyl acetate, or 0.6 µg β-carotene) corresponds to 1 IU vitamin A. These conversions of **isolated substances with vitamin A-like properties** are commonly used and permissible.

A **mixed diet** provides a multitude of such substances, which interact with one another and are subject to the effects of exogenous factors such as heat and light. To accommodate these facts, vitamin A requirements and intakes are listed in **retinal activity equivalents (RAE)**. For instance, 1 mg retinol, 1.15 mg retinyl acetate, or 6 mg β-carotene are 1 mg RAE. One mg RAE $\approx$3000 IU vitamin A.

According to international chemical nomenclature (IUPAC), vitamin A and its derivatives (**A**) are jointly called **retinoids**. The definition of this term has caused substantial confusion since it fails to differentiate between natural and synthetic vitamin A derivatives. In view of the biological/medical aspects involved, the following distinction is made: the term vitamin A applies to all compounds that retain all effects of the vitamin (retinol, retinyl ester). Distinguished from those are the retinoids, which show only some of the effects of the vitamin in the body (no influence on spermatogenesis and visual cycle). This definition applies to synthetic, exogenously supplied retinoic acid and its derivatives. Retinoic acid no longer has the same effects as retinol since it is the end product of an irreversible metabolic pathway and can therefore not be re-metabolized to retinol.

A. Chemistry

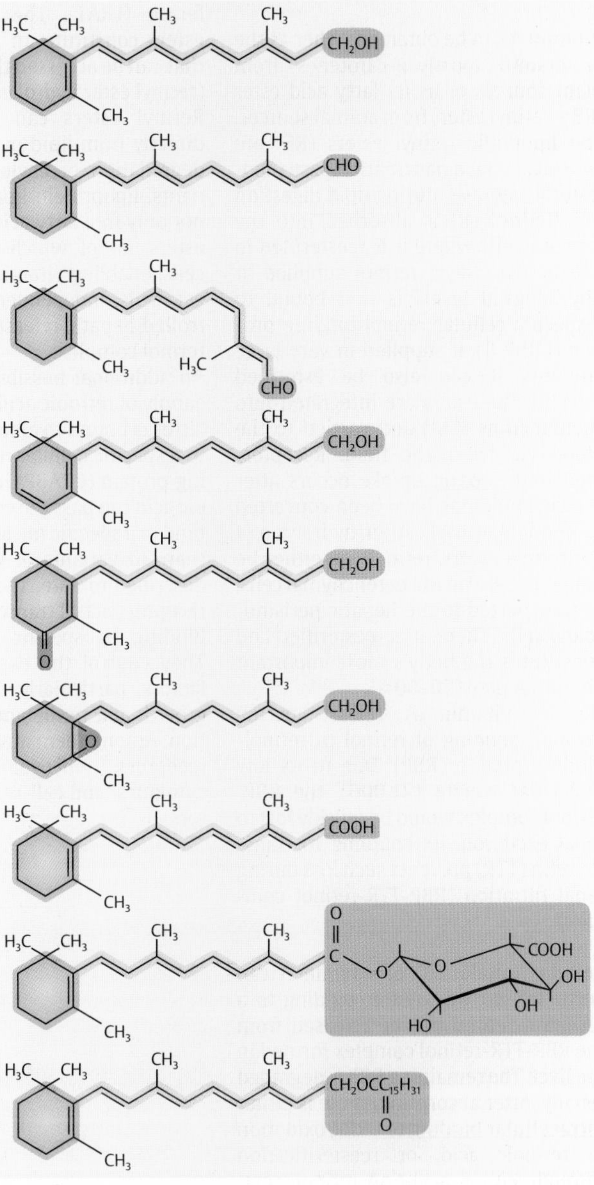

Retinol	H_3C CH_3 CH_3 CH_3 CH_2OH
Retinal	H_3C CH_3 CH_3 CH_3 CHO
11-cis-Retinal aldehyde	H_3C CH_3 CH_3 H_3C CHO
3-Dehydroretinol	H_3C CH_3 CH_3 CH_3 CH_2OH
4-Ketoretinol	H_3C CH_3 CH_3 CH_3 CH_2OH O
5,6-Epoxyretinol	H_3C CH_3 O CH_3 CH_3 CH_2OH
Retinic acid	H_3C CH_3 CH_3 CH_3 COOH
Retinol-β-glucuronide	H_3C CH_3 CH_3 CH_3
Retinyl palmitate	H_3C CH_3 CH_3 CH_3 $CH_2OCC_{15}H_{31}$ O

Vitamin A: Uptake and Metabolism

Vitamin A can be obtained either as the provitamin (mostly β-carotenes) from plant sources or as its fatty acid ester (RE = retinyl ester) from animal sources. The lipophilic retinyl esters (RE) are hydrolyzed by a pancreatic lipase (cholesterol esterase) during lipid digestion (**A**). **Retinol (R)** is absorbed into the **mucosa cells** where it is reesterified in one of two ways: retinol supplied at physiological levels is first bound to a specific cellular retinol-binding protein (CRBP II). If supplied in very large amounts it can also be esterified directly. The esters are integrated into chylomicrons (CM) and carried to the blood via lymphatic fluid. Receptor-mediated **hepatic** uptake occurs after the chylomicrons have been converted to remnants (REM). After hydrolysis of the retinyl esters, retinol can either be bound to CRBP in the parenchymal cells, or transported to the hepatic perisinusoidal cells. There, it is reesterified and constitutes the body's most important vitamin A pool (50–80 %).

Hepatic vitamin A release occurs through bonding of retinol to retinol-binding protein (RBP). Due to its low molecular weight (21 000), the RBP-retinol complex would be quickly lost to renal excretion. Its coupling to transthyretin (TTR) prevents such loss during renal filtration (RBP-TTR-retinol complex).

Cellular uptake (B) of vitamin A can occur in two ways. After binding to a receptor, retinol can be released from the RBP-TTR-retinol complex formed in the liver. The remaining RBP is degraded renally. After absorption, there is either **intracellular** binding to CRBP, oxidation to retinoic acid, or reesterification through either acyl-CoA-retinol acyltransferase (ARAT) or retinol acyltransferase (LRAT). The resulting retinyl esters constitute an intracellular pool that can be accessed through hydrolysis (retinyl ester hydrolases – REH).

Retinyl esters can also be derived directly from lipid metabolism: during degradation of chylomicrons to remnants, lipoprotein lipase (LPL) releases not only free fatty acids but also retinyl esters, all of which are absorbed by cells, enabling vitamin A supply to target cells independently of the controlled hepatic release of the RBP-TTR-retinol complex.

An additional possibility is direct oral supply of **retinoic acid**. In the blood, the latter is bound to albumin and attaches to a specific cellular retinoic acid-binding protein (CRABP) inside cells. Retinoic acid can pass the cell membrane and bind to a specific nuclear receptor, more than 30 variants of which have been described to date. The nuclear retinoid receptors act as transcription factors by binding to specific DNA sequences. They control the expression of many factors, particularly factors regulating growth and tissue and cell differentiation. Among them are growth hormone receptors, oncogenes, interleukins, cytokines, and cell-cell interaction factors.

A. Absorption

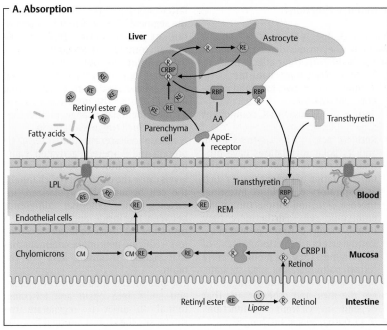

B. Metabolism

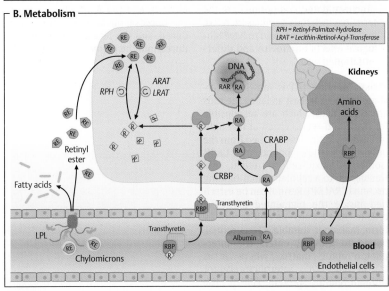

RPH = Retinyl-Palmitat-Hydrolase
LRAT = Lecithin-Retinol-Acyl-Transferase

Vitamin A: Functions

Vitamin A does not act in a uniform manner. The various derivatives found in the body exert their effects through different functional mechanisms:

• **Retinol** is a transport form and metabolic intermediate.

• **Retinal** is an essential component required for vision.

• **Retinoic acid**, in its cis-trans form, and its polar metabolites have pronounced effects on proliferation and differentiation of various tissues such as respiratory epithelium, intestinal mucosa, skin, and various tumor and embryonic cells. Furthermore they inhibit a range of tumor promoters.

• **Retinyl esters** are the storage forms of this vitamin. They are predominantly retinyl palmitate, but also stearate, oleate and others. Main storage sites are the liver and other organs that depend on vitamin A's functions (e. g., retina, testes, and lungs).

• **Glucuronidated compounds** are the form in which the vitamin is excreted, but have also been found to have biological effects on growth and differentiation in vitro.

Visual function (A) is mostly understood by now, at least as far as the rods are concerned, which are responsible for black-and-white vision at low light intensities. Retinol is absorbed from the outer capillaries, bound to CRBP, isomerized, oxidized to retinal, and transferred to a cellular retinal-binding protein (CRALBP). Retinol can be esterified inside the pigmented epithelial cells to the all-trans- as well as the cis-form, making it storable. 11-cis-retinal, bound to CRALBP, enters the interphotoreceptor matrix where it is transferred to interphotoreceptor retinoid-binding protein (IRBP). The latter transports the 11-cis-retinal to the segment disks where it is bound to the apoprotein opsin. This protein-retinal complex, **rhodopsin**, absorbs light within the 400–600 nm range. Incoming light isomerizes 11-cis-retinal to all-trans-retinal, thereby separating it from opsin. The separation causes a conformational change in the rhodopsin, which triggers a cascade.

A phosphodiesterase binds to a G-protein and is thereby activated, causing cGMP hydrolysis. Declining cGMP levels cause the closing of Na^+ channels; the cell becomes hyperpolarized, increasing the potential difference between the inside and outside. As a result the cell releases fewer transmitters, reducing neuronal excitement and that signals "incoming light" to the brain.

The photolyzed rhodopsin is unstable, and splits into opsin and all-trans-retinal. In order to regenerate the rhodopsin, the all-trans-retinal first has to be isomerized to 11-cis-retinal. For this purpose, the all-trans-retinal is reduced, and the retinal is then reintroduced into the pigment cells' cycle.

A. Vision

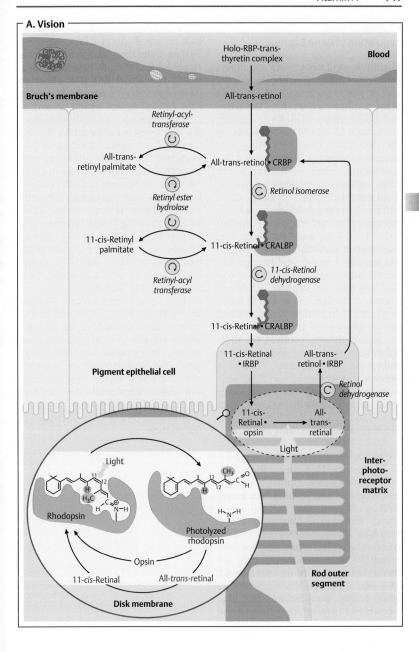

Vitamin A:
Regulation of Gene Expression

Vitamin A regulates growth and differentiation of many types of cells and tissues. It affects particularly the **mucosa of the respiratory tract** (A): if the active metabolite retinoic acid (RA) is missing, patchy lack of cilia (A1–A3) results. At the same time, mucus-secreting cells increase in numbers. This disturbed differentiation causes a reduction in the lungs' ability to expel particles, making them more susceptible to infections.

Sustained vitamin A deficiency leads to metaplasia of the respiratory epithelium (**B, C**), a precancerous stage. This may explain the relationship between low vitamin A supply and lung cancer. Since compounds in cigarette smoke like benzopyrene deplete the lungs' vitamin A storage, the resulting localized vitamin A deficiency may enhance the development of lung cancer.

RA apparently also controls the morphogenesis of several tissues during **embryonic development**. Vitamin A deficiency as well as use of RA (as acne medication) during early pregnancy results in typical malformations: open back (spina bifida), cleft lips or palate, and malformations of arms and legs.

The **biological effects** of the active forms of RA are based on their interactions with two subfamilies of nuclear retinoic acid receptors and retinoid X receptors (RAR and RXR with their respective subtypes). RAR bind all-trans-retinoic acid with high affinity, altering gene expression through direct interaction with the ligand (**D**). RXR, even though they are also activated by **all-trans-retinoic acid**, have low affinity to this ligand. Other retinoids like **9-cis-retinoic acid** bind much better here. Hence, isomerization of the all-trans- to the 9-cis form favors RXR-mediated effects of RA.

To date, more than 30 different nuclear receptors for retinoids have been identified. The actual RAR/RXR effect on gene expression requires the binding of RXR (including its ligand-cis-RA) to another receptor (heterodimerization) (**E**). This receptor can be an RA, thyroid, vitamin D, estrogen, androgen, or progesterone receptor. Different types of **heterodimerization** can result in different forms of binding to DNA resulting in different gene expression. The retinoid receptor works as a transcription factor, increasing transcription in proportion to the amount of RA present. RA has an inhibitory effect on other transcription factors like AP-1 (activation protein 1), which enhances gene expression of various proteins. It is thought that this occurs through heterodimerization of RAR and/or RXR with the subunits of AP-1, fos, and jun, which are proto-oncogenes. Since receptors for growth hormone, oncogenes, interleukins, cytokine, and cell-cell interaction factors like laminine and fibronectin interact with retinoid receptors, RA is an important regulator of growth as well as cell and tissue differentiation.

A. Epithelial Changes Due to Vitamin A Deficiency

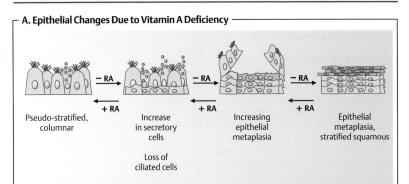

Pseudo-stratified, columnar — RA → +RA — Increase in secretory cells

Loss of ciliated cells

Increasing epithelial metaplasia

Epithelial metaplasia, stratified squamous

B. Healthy Respiratory Epithelium

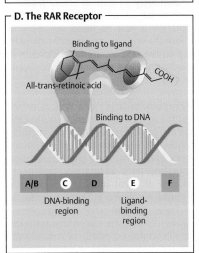

C. Marginal Vitamin A Deficiency

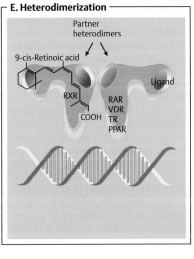

D. The RAR Receptor

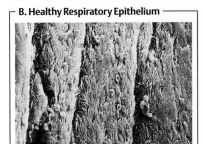

Binding to ligand

All-trans-retinoic acid

Binding to DNA

| A/B | C | D | E | F |

DNA-binding region

Ligand-binding region

E. Heterodimerization

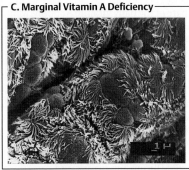

Partner heterodimers

9-cis-Retinoic acid

RXR
COOH

Ligand

RAR
VDR
TR
PPAR

Vitamin A:
Occurrence and Requirements

In a mixed diet most of the vitamin A comes from retinyl esters contained in **animal products**. The consumption of 5–10 g liver/d is enough to cover the recommended daily requirement (**A**). Eel, tuna, and herring, which contain 0.2–0.7 mg/100 g are also good vitamin A sources. Other types of fish and muscle meat contain less than 30 µg/100 g, making them insignificant as vitamin A sources. Milk and milk products, particularly cheese and eggs contribute a large share of the daily vitamin A supply. Milk and breakfast cereals are often fortified with vitamin A in the U.S. and many other countries. Vegetable oils and sugar can also be vitamin A fortified.

The **recommended intakes** are given in **retinal activity equivalents** (**RAE**) and range between 0.3 mg and 0.6 mg for children and are 0.7 mg and 0.9 mg, respectively, for females and males (1000 µg RAE ≃ 3000 IU) (see also p. 136). During pregnancy and lactation the requirements are higher since plasma values in neonates are always lower than in the mother, and vitamin A use increases significantly during pregnancy. For this reason, supplementation of 0.7 mg/d is recommended during pregnancy and 0.6 mg during lactation. Official recommendations state that **liver** should not be eaten **during pregnancy**. Depending on the feed, liver may contain up to 2500 IU vitamin A/g. With average portions of 100 g and a 45% absorption rate, such consumption could result in an uptake of more than 100 000 IU in extreme cases.

However, no teratogenic effects of eating liver have been proven with certainty. The warnings are based mostly on findings from pharmacological use of retinoic acid for therapy of severe acne. There are reports of miscarriages and malformations. Since retinoic acid cannot be metabolized to its reduced forms (retinal, retinol), it is questionable whether these results apply to vitamin A from foods. Nevertheless, to be on the safe side, women wanting to get pregnant, as well as during the first trimester, should abstain from eating liver. Outside of pregnancy, toxic effects of high doses of vitamin A from foods are not relevant. Reports of **hypervitaminosis** A are rare, and it occurs mostly in children after intake of medications. The **UL** is 3000 µg/d for adults.

Vitamin A deficiency is of much greater significance. Even though in the industrial nations, intakes tend to be above the recommendations, depletion of the liver pool may occur through disease or insufficient intakes in case of predominantly plant-based nutrition. Worldwide, vitamin A deficiency has enormous impact: the FAO assumes approximately 14 million children under five to be vitamin A deficient, up to 500 000 a year go blind, and 60% of those die within a few months thereafter. In the U.S., vitamin A deficiency is the main cause of blindness in people over 65.

Xerophthalmia (**C**) is a typical symptom of advanced deficiency, causing the cornea to become opaque and necrotic. Without treatment this leads to blindness. Early stages are characterized by impaired dark adaptation, commonly known as night blindness, caused by vitamin A deficiency. There may also be changes in skin and mucous membranes, causing increased susceptibility to infections, especially of the respiratory tract (see p. 142).

A. Occurrence and Daily Requirement

The daily requirement of 0.9 mg vitamin A (retinol) is contained in:

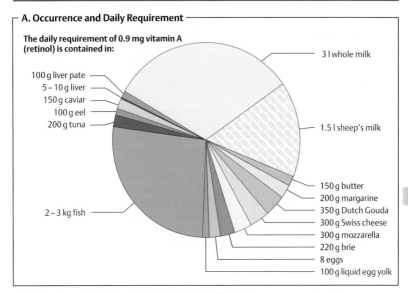

- 3 l whole milk
- 100 g liver pate
- 5 – 10 g liver
- 150 g caviar
- 100 g eel
- 200 g tuna
- 1.5 l sheep's milk
- 150 g butter
- 200 g margarine
- 350 g Dutch Gouda
- 300 g Swiss cheese
- 300 g mozzarella
- 220 g brie
- 8 eggs
- 100 g liquid egg yolk
- 2 – 3 kg fish

B. Recommended Intakes (DRI/AI*, 2000) and UL

Life Stage and Gender Group	Age	Vitamin A (µg RAE/d)	(IU)	UL (µg RAE/d)
Infants	0 – 6 mo	400*	1200	600
	7 – 12 mo	500*	1500	600
Children	1 – 3 y	300	900	600
	4 – 8 y	400	1200	900
	9 – 13 y	600	1800	1700
Males	14 – 18 y	900	2700	2800
	≥ 19 y	900	2700	3000
Females	14 – 18 y	700	2100	2800
	≥ 19 y	700	2100	3000
Pregnancy	14 – 18 y	750	2250	2800
	19 – 50 y	770	2310	3000
Lactation	14 – 18 y	1200	3600	2800
	19 – 50 y	1300	3900	3000

C. Deficiency Symptoms

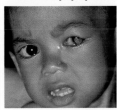

Xerophthalmia

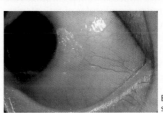

Bitot spots

β-Carotenes:
Chemistry and Metabolism

Carotenoids are always of plant origin. Chemically, they are tetraterpenes, consisting of eight symmetrically arranged isoprene units (**A**). Their behavior is determined by their long hydrocarbon chains, which contain many conjugated double bonds: they are lipophilic and colored.

Several hundred different **carotenoids** have been found in plants, but only 40 of them have provitamin A activity. Quantitatively of the greatest importance to humans are the β-carotenes, which are responsible for the red color in carrots; lycopene, which, as opposed to β-carotenes, has no aromatic components, is the main pigment in tomatoes and red bell peppers. **Xanthophylls** form through insertion of hydroxy groups into the carotenoid rings. Among others, they cause the yellow color of leaves during fall (mostly lutein, also called leaf xanthophyll). Zeaxanthin gives corn its yellow color. Egg yolk contains a mixture of several xanthophylls and β-carotenes; its color depends on the feed composition.

Since β-carotenes are fat-soluble, they are **absorbed** in the small intestine together with the other lipids (**B**). The absorption rate of β-carotenes from plant sources ranges between 10 and 50%, with large individual differences. Inside the mucosal cell, β-carotenes are split into two molecules of retinal (vitamin A) at the central double bond. The splitting enzyme, 15,15-dideoxygenase, is regulated: the better the vitamin A supply, the lower the activity of the enzyme. Asymmetrical splitting yields intermediates with uneven side chains. The longer fragments, β-apocarotinals, can be converted into vitamin A. This conversion seems to be dependent on the respective cell's vitamin A needs. Finally, it appears that β-carotene may interfere with oxidative processes as soon as it enters the mucosa cells (see p. 138).

For purposes of **transportation**, some of the β-carotenes, as well as the esterified retinol, are packaged in chylomicrons and taken to the blood via lymphatic fluid. When endothelial LPL degrades the chylomicrons, β-carotenes are taken up by the cells as well. The remnants are taken to the liver, where β-carotene is also converted to vitamin A. Excess β-carotene is packaged in LDL and VLDL and thus made available to extrahepatic tissues. Polar vitamin A metabolites such as retinoic acid can leave the mucosal cells directly with portal blood.

β-carotene is stored predominantly in fatty tissue and to a lesser extent in the liver, with concentrations in both tissues subject to large individual variations. The high **storage** capacity of fatty tissue and liver and/or the concentration-dependent absorption and concentration processes are thought to be responsible for the benign effects of high dosages of β-carotene as opposed to similar amounts of vitamin A: β-carotene is nontoxic and nonteratogenic.

A. Carotenoids

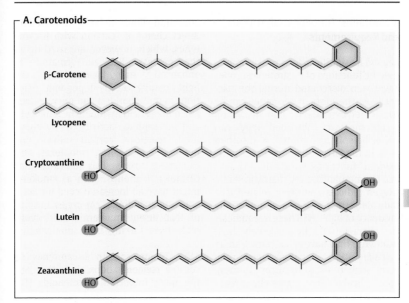

B. β-Carotene Metabolism

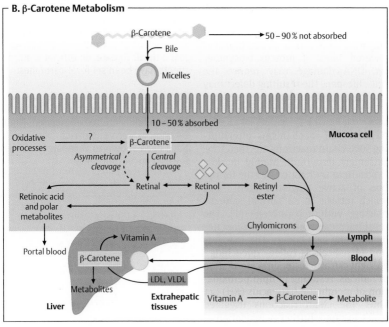

β-carotenes: Functions, Occurrence, and Requirements

Beyond its significance as provitamin A, specific functions of β-carotenes proper have been discovered during the past decades. Therefore, β-carotenes can be considered essential for humans. When β-carotenes are absorbed they can either be split into retinal or absorbed as is. In the latter case they have "**anti-oxidant**" functions in the cell.

In all human cells—particularly in skin—oxygen radicals and other related **free radicals** form continuously, under the influence of light (**A**). These free radicals are characterized by extremely high reactivity: they have an extremely short half-life (10^{-11} sec), after which they react with other substances, forming new radicals. This triggers chain reactions, which may damage essential cell components. The damage may cause acutely reduced cell function due to membrane damage, inactivation of enzymes, destruction of receptors, or lowered rates of protein biosynthesis. DNA damage may reduce the cell's lifespan. The resulting defect may also be passed on during cell division and thereby potentially affect entire tissues.

Physiological mechanisms interrupting such chain reactions are, therefore, extremely important. Mainly in skin, exposure to UV light causes the formation of active **singlet oxygen** ($^1O_2$), which returns to its normal state by reacting with a β-carotene (1). The resulting β-carotene radical regenerates by releasing heat energy. This inactivation of radicals is called "quenching." UV light can also foster direct formation of radicals, resulting in **lipid peroxidation** of membrane fatty acids (RH) (2). Thus, the chain reactions triggered result in rapid, further peroxidation of membrane lipids. It can be inhibited by direct chemical reaction with β-carotenes, which, however, are used up in the process. Radical formation is enhanced by many factors: besides UV light, mainly by O_2-dependent reactions in mitochondria and microsomes, arachidonic acid metabolism, leukocyte and macrophage activity, many enzymatic reactions, certain sulfur compounds, reduced iron complexes, and exogenous toxins. This indicates that certain risk groups, such as smokers, might have an increased need for antioxidants including β-carotenes. In spite of this, heavy smokers should avoid high doses (>10 mg) from supplements.

Most plants contain β-carotenes in varying concentrations since they are the most important carotenoids (**B**). Depending on fruit and vegetable intake, β-carotenes play a more or less important role as a source of vitamin A: in the U.S., half of the required vitamin A comes from β-carotenes, in England just a third. To date, no official requirements have been set for β-carotenes.

For an optimal antioxidant effect as well as for cancer prevention ~15–50 mg/d of carotenoids are recommended. High intakes of carotenoid-rich vegetables have been shown to correlate with the lowest cancer morbidity.

A. The Skin-Protective Effect of β-Carotenes

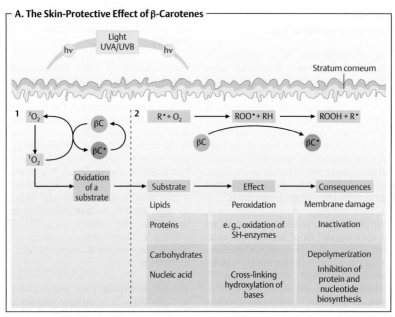

Substrate	Effect	Consequences
Lipids	Peroxidation	Membrane damage
Proteins	e. g., oxidation of SH-enzymes	Inactivation
Carbohydrates		Depolymerization
Nucleic acid	Cross-linking hydroxylation of bases	Inhibition of protein and nucleotide biosynthesis

B. Occurrence and Daily Requirement

The daily requirement of 2 –4 mg β-carotene is contained in:

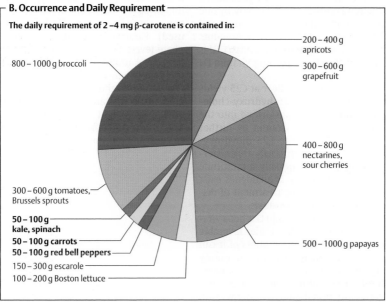

800 – 1000 g broccoli

200 – 400 g apricots

300 – 600 g grapefruit

400 – 800 g nectarines, sour cherries

500 – 1000 g papayas

300 – 600 g tomatoes, Brussels sprouts

50 – 100 g kale, spinach

50 – 100 g carrots

50 – 100 g red bell peppers

150 – 300 g escarole

100 – 200 g Boston lettuce

Vitamin D:
Chemistry and Metabolism

The characteristic bone deformities caused by vitamin D deficiency were most common in the industrial cities of the nineteenth century. In Boston, around 1900, approximately 80% of poor children suffered from bone deformities. Symptomatic treatment with cod liver oil and natural sunlight was not discovered until 1919. Another 20 years were needed until in vitro synthesis of this vitamin became possible, permitting large-scale prophylaxis.

The vitamin D family includes a number of compounds, all of which have vitamin activity. The most important compound in animals is vitamin D_3 (**cholecalciferol**) which forms from **7-dehydrocholesterol (A)** under the influence of light. Plants contain traces of the provitamin ergosterol. Its metabolite, vitamin D_2 differs from D_3 only by one double bond and one methyl group and has the same vitamin activity. Amounts are given in **international units**: 1 IU is equivalent to 0.025 µg, 1 µg vitamin D_3 or D_2 = 40 IU.

Hydroxylation in the liver at C25 yields the intermediate **25-hydroxy-cholecalciferol**. This is transformed into the active form of the vitamin by further hydroxylation at C1 to **1,25-dihydroxycholecalciferol** (1,25-$(OH)_2$-D_3), a steroid hormone. Additionally, a multitude of synthetic vitamin D analogues exist that are used for the treatment of disturbances in Ca homeostasis.

Strictly speaking, vitamin D is not a vitamin for humans since under favorable conditions sufficient amounts of it can be **endogenously synthesized** during sun exposure. The 7-dehydro-cholesterol made from cholesterol is converted to provitamin D_3 in the **skin** under UV exposure, which turns into active vitamin D_3 under the influence of heat **(B)**.

Since vitamin D from foods is fat-soluble, it is transported to the liver in chylomicrons. All free vitamin D metabolites are **transported** in the blood, as well as in the liver, by a specific, vitamin D-binding protein (DBP).

In the mitochondria of the **renal** proximal tubular cells, 1,25-$(OH)_2$-D is hydroxylated a second time, this time at C24, by another enzyme. In case of oversupply of 1,25-$(OH)_2$-D this pathway is favored, leading to inactivation of the hormone. The active 1,25-$(OH)_2$-D reaches its target organs through the bloodstream where it circulates bound to proteins.

The last metabolic step, hydroxylation to 1,25-$(OH)_2$-D, is **strictly regulated**: the presence of 1,25-$(OH)_2$-D provides inhibiting feedback control (an alternative pathway to inactive 1,24-$[OH]_2$-D is used). Parathormone and low phosphate levels activate the hydroxylating enzyme. A multitude of additional factors exert their influence mostly indirectly via parathormone: Ca, estrogen, glucocorticoids, and calcitonin among others. This tight regulation permits short-term adjustment depending on calcium and phosphate needs.

A. Chemistry

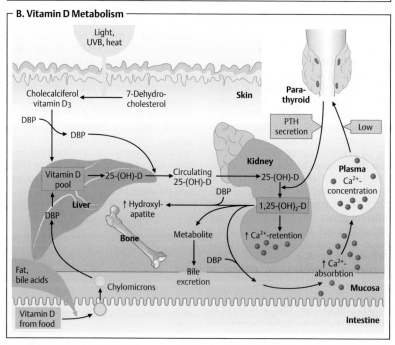

B. Vitamin D Metabolism

Vitamin D: Functions

The classic vitamin D function is to maintain **calcium (Ca)** and **phosphate (P) homeostasis**. Its cellular effects on **intestinal Ca transport** are best understood **(A)**. In the cytosol, 1,25-$(OH)_2$-D is probably bound to a cytosol receptor before being transferred to a DNA-associated nuclear receptor. This process induces the synthesis of several proteins, such as calcium-binding protein (CaBP), an ATPase, alkaline phosphatase, phytase, etc. At the same time, lipid synthesis is increased, altering membrane lipids. The subsequent step, Ca transport from the brush border membrane to the basal membrane is not yet understood. It cannot be CaBP synthesis, which was once thought to be responsible since it is too slow to provide a sufficient explanation for a Ca transport that can be triggered within a few minutes.

Bones and kidneys are other classic target organs of vitamin D **(B)**. In **bones**, the activity of osteoclasts and osteoblasts maintains homeostasis between demineralization, i.e., the release of Ca and P, and mineralization. Because of its significance for Ca homeostasis (making Ca available to the organism), vitamin D is responsible for demineralization. Increased absorption of Ca out of the bones under the influence of 1,25-$(OH)_2$-D is due to two factors: increased differentiation of macrophages into osteoclasts, on the one hand; and a much more rapidly occurring process, on the other hand, in which 1,25-$(OH)_2$-D triggers osteoblasts to release an osteoclast-stimulating factor.

Vitamin D's **renal** effects are not fully understood to date. They also serve Ca homeostasis, enhancing Ca reabsorption and P excretion in the distal renal tubules.

During recent years, further tissues and cells have been found to be responsive to 1,25-$(OH)_2$-D **(B)**. The present discussion centers on cellular mechanisms like the above-mentioned induction of protein synthesis, or activation of various phospholipases (C, A_2, D) with subsequent second messenger formation. A 1,25-$(OH)_2$-D-specific membrane receptor is also under consideration. Many cells respond to 1,25-$(OH)_2$-D by **releasing Ca from the intracellular pool**. To what extent this constitutes a contribution to Ca homeostasis is unknown; it may simply be an intracellular signal. It has been observed that vitamin D deficiency and bone diseases are often accompanied by weakness of skeletal or cardiac muscle, leading to the conclusion that vitamin D may have a **function in muscle cells**. Today, it is assumed that 1,25-$(OH)_2$-D activates voltage-dependent Ca channels in muscle cell membranes and is thus involved in the regulation of cross-membrane Ca transport. In the **pancreas**, insulin secretion is influenced by 1,25-$(OH)_2$-D; in **skin**, the hormone influences growth and cell differentiation. There are also receptors for it in **immune system cells**, as well as various tumor cells, where 1,25-$(OH)_2$-D usually inhibits cell proliferation.

A. Induction of Ca Absorption

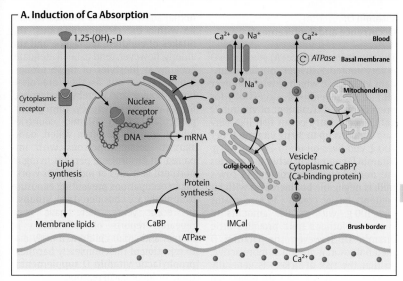

B. Classic and Recently Discovered Vitamin D Target Organs

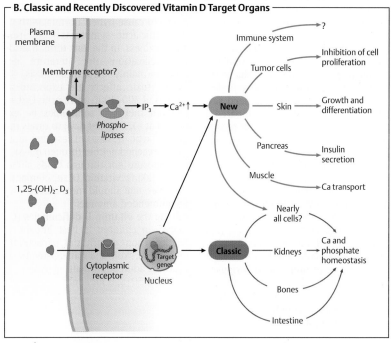

Vitamin D:
Occurrence and Requirements

The natural **occurrence (A)** of vitamin D is very limited. Fish liver contains abundant vitamin D, which is why fish liver oil has long been used successfully for prevention and treatment of vitamin D deficiencies. Fatty ocean fish like herring contains up to 30 µg vitamin D per 100 g, cod liver oil up to 200 µg/100 g. Vitamin D contents of other fish species are much lower. The content in cow's milk is negligible but increases with fat content: heavy cream (30%) contains 1 µg/100 g, with similar amounts in cheeses. Mother's milk provides little vitamin D; however, the vitamin D metabolites in it are much more active, so that the risk of rickets is generally very low in infants who are breast-fed exclusively.

The **requirements (B)** for exogenous vitamin D depend largely on the duration and intensity of UV exposure and the resulting endogenous vitamin D synthesis and skin tone. To achieve the same rate of vitamin D synthesis in skin, a dark-skinned person may need several times longer exposure compared to a light-skinned person. Current recommendations of 5 µg/d for children and adults are based on an assumption of insufficient skin synthesis. In the U.S., fortified foods are the major source of dietary vitamin D. Milk is fortified with 10 µg/l vitamin D_3. All industrially produced infant formulas are enriched with 400 IU (= 10 µg) vitamin D_3/l. Unless fortified milk products are used, an additional daily supply of 400 IU in tablet form is recommended during the first year of life. Health Canada recommends infant supplementation of 10 µg (400 IU) during summer and 20 µg (800 IU) during winter.

Actual adult vitamin D **intakes** usually lie within the recommendations; the intakes of children, teenagers, and the elderly, however, tend to be inadequate. Looking at lifestyles of these groups, seniors stand out as they are often house-bound, and thereby predestined for vitamin D deficiency. Immigrants, particularly from Islamic countries where women are often veiled, dark-skinned persons, persons with impaired fat absorption, persons living in northern latitudes or individuals working in occupations preventing exposure to sunlight are considered risk groups.

In recent years, there have been repeated reports of deficiencies in infants and small children, mostly due to rejection of the completely harmless **prophylactic vitamin D supplementation**, for ideological reasons.

Vitamin D has to be massively **overdosed** to cause hypercalcemia, with its unspecific acute symptoms of vomiting and dizziness. In the long term, it leads to calcifications—the literature describes mainly nephrocalcinosis. In adults, toxic effects are expected at intakes of 500–1000 µg vitamin D/d, in children they can sometimes be expected at >150 µg per day (10 times the prophylactic dosage). These amounts can be reached neither through massive UV exposure nor through foods alone. When taking vitamin D supplements, however, one should not exceed the recommended amounts.

Among the **vitamin D deficiencies (C)**, rickets in children is best known. It results in bone deformities, particularly of sternum, skull, and spine. Osteomalacia is the adult equivalent.

The **UL** is 50 µg/d for adults.

A. Occurrence and Daily Requirement

The daily requirement of 5 µg vitamin D is contained in:

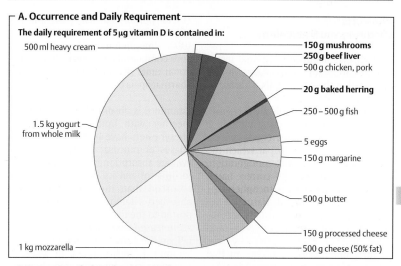

500 ml heavy cream

150 g mushrooms
250 g beef liver
500 g chicken, pork

20 g baked herring

250 – 500 g fish

5 eggs

150 g margarine

1.5 kg yogurt
from whole milk

500 g butter

150 g processed cheese
500 g cheese (50% fat)

1 kg mozzarella

B. Recommended Intakes (AI, 1999)

Life Stage and Gender Group	Age	Vitamin D		UL
		(µg/d)	(IU)	
Infants	0 – 12 mo	5.0	200	25
Children	1 – 8 y	5.0	200	50
Males and females	9 – 50 y	5.0	200	50
	51 – 70 y	10.0	400	50
	> 70 y	15.0	600	50
Pregnancy	18 – 50 y	5.0	200	50
Lactation	18 – 50 y	5.0	200	50

C. Deficiency Symptoms

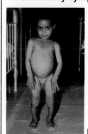

Rickets

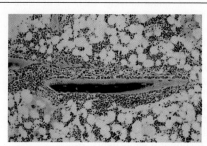

Uncalcified bone matrix (blue)

Vitamin E:
Chemistry and Metabolism

First reports about a nutritional factor required to maintain pregnancy in rats appeared in the early 1920s. This factor was named vitamin E.

α-tocopherol is the naturally occurring compound with the highest vitamin E activity (**A**). It has three chiral centers (at 2′, 4′, 8′ in the figure) at which the methyl groups are in R-configuration. According to IUPAC, the correct name is therefore 2R,4R,8R-α-tocopherol or short RRR-α-tocopherol. Naturally occurring α-tocopherol is usually accompanied by small amounts of β-, γ-, and δ-tocopherol, which differ by the number and positions of the methyl groups attached to the ring. Additionally, there are naturally occurring tocotrienoles with three additional double bonds in the side chain. Lastly, various synthetic or half-synthetic α-tocopherols are always mixtures of various stereoisomers. The most common form of synthetic vitamin E consists of eight stereoisomers, and has a 12.5% RRR-α-tocopherol content. The mixture is called all-rac-α-tocopherol. IUPAC recommends the use of the biochemical nomenclature (in analogy to vitamin A): vitamin E comprises all tocopherols and tocotrienoles that have the same qualitative biological activity as RRR-α-tocopherol. However, quantitatively, their biological effects vary greatly. All naturally occurring tocopherols/tocotrienoles exhibit less than 50% of the activity of RRR-α-tocopherol (= 100%), all-rac-α-tocopherol 74%, and all-rac-α-tocopherol acetate, which is frequently used in medications and is esterified for increased stability, 67%. In order to account for these various degrees of vitamin E activity, nutrient tables use the term **α-tocopherol equivalents** (α-TE), for purposes of which the effect of RRR-α-tocopherol is equivalent to 100%. Vitamin E in medications and in pure compounds is counted in international units (IU) or USP (United States Pharmacopeia).

Vitamin E is **absorbed** in the intestine together with lipids after any tocopheryl esters have been hydrolyzed by lipases or mucosal esterases (**B**). The average absorption rate is 30%, with α-tocopherol and its esters being better absorbed than the other forms. The absorbed vitamin E is rapidly transported to the liver; only small amounts are released from the chylomicrons by LPL on the surface of endothelial cells. Vitamin E incorporated in VLDL is released back into the bloodstream. There, a dynamic equilibrium exists between all lipoprotein fractions due to a rapid interchange. **Uptake into the target cells** occurs either through release by endothelium-based LPL or via receptor-mediated LDL endocytosis.

Vitamin E is stored in fatty tissue and muscle, preferentially as RRR-α-tocopherol. Recently, an explanation for this was found in a cloned human gene that encodes for a hepatic α-tocopherol transfer protein. It causes RRR-α-tocopherol to be preferentially incorporated into VLDL, while other forms of vitamin E are quickly excreted via bile fluid.

A. Chemistry and Biological Activity

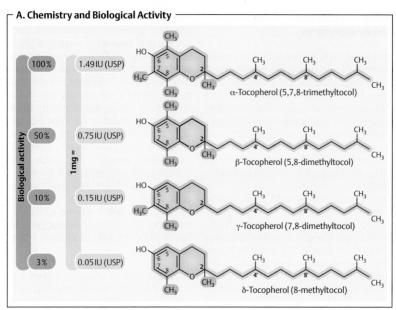

B. Vitamin E Metabolism

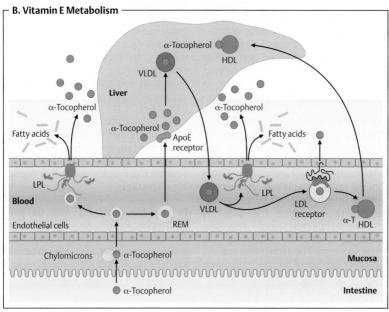

Vitamin E: Functions, Occurrence, and Requirements

In animal cells, α-tocopherol is a component of all biological membranes. According to the current state of knowledge, its most important function is to protect membrane lipids and stored lipids from being degraded by lipid peroxidation. The food industry has long used the common knowledge about this **antioxidant** effect by enriching fats and oils with vitamin E to prevent peroxidation.

Due to exposure to light, heat, and/or chemicals, as well as through many metabolic processes, **free radicals (A)** form in the body. If a polyunsaturated fatty acid is attacked by a radical X, one of the two H atoms is removed from the methylene group between the two double bonds, resulting in a highly reactive lipid radical (missing electron). When the latter bonds with O_2, a highly reactive lipid peroxide radical is formed. The latter will either react with another fatty acid to form a stable, nonphysiological but cytotoxic **lipid peroxide** or "fuse with" another peroxide molecule. During the transfer of the H atom, an additional lipid radical is formed, triggering an autocatalytic chain reaction. Uninterrupted, this process can quickly destroy the affected biological membrane's function. Vitamin E has a very strong affinity for lipid peroxide radicals: transfer of an H atom from vitamin E to the lipid peroxide radical results in a stable lipid hydroperoxide and a vitamin E radical. Since the latter is resonance-stabilized and therefore extremely inert, this interrupts the chain reaction. The tocopherol radical, which is anchored in the cell membrane, is probably reconverted to vitamin E by ascorbic acid (vitamin C) inside the watery cytosol (see p. 206).

Plant germs and seeds, as well as their oils, and products derived from them are the best **sources** of vitamin E **(B)**. In wheat germ, sunflower seeds, cottonseed, and olive oil, RRR-α-tocopherol makes up most (50–100%) of the vitamin E, while γ-tocopherol, which has only 10% of the biological activity, dominates in soy and corn oil. Most oils sold as "vegetable oil" contain various amounts of soy, corn and cottonseed oil, margarines mostly soy, corn, and sunflower oil. Their natural vitamin E activity depends on their sunflower or cottonseed components, otherwise, synthetic vitamin E may be added as a stabilizer. Cold-pressed wheat germ oil has the highest natural vitamin E content.

Estimates of adequate vitamin E intakes (C) depend on the intake of polyunsaturated fatty acids: 0.5 mg RRR-α-tocopherol should be supplied for every gram of diene fatty acids; even many plant oils do not contain these amounts (e.g., soy oil, approximately 0.3 mg). An intake of 24 g of diene equivalents (18 g linoleic acid, 3 g linolenic acid) would, therefore, mean a calculated requirement of 12 mg α-TE per day. People in the U.S. generally achieve these approximate intakes, but higher intakes may well be desirable for optimal protection from peroxidation. People on low fat diets may be at risk of vitamin E deficiency due to low vegetable oil intakes.

In preemies, patients with fat malabsorption, various diseases like cystic fibrosis or coronary artery disease, vitamin E supplements have proven beneficial. The **UL** is 1000 mg of supplemental α-tocopherol (1500 IU vitamin E).

A. Protective Effects of Vitamin E

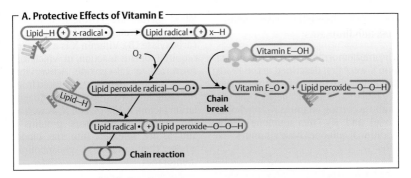

B. Occurrence and Daily Requirement

The daily requirement of 12 mg vitamin E is contained in:

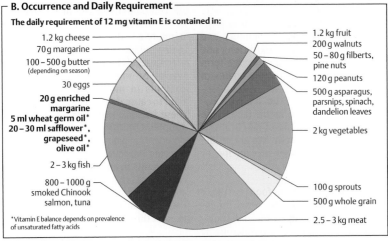

- 1.2 kg cheese
- 70 g margarine
- 100 – 500 g butter (depending on season)
- 30 eggs
- **20 g enriched margarine**
- **5 ml wheat germ oil***
- **20 – 30 ml safflower*, grapeseed*, olive oil***
- 2 – 3 kg fish
- 800 – 1000 g smoked Chinook salmon, tuna

- 1.2 kg fruit
- 200 g walnuts
- 50 – 80 g filberts, pine nuts
- 120 g peanuts
- 500 g asparagus, parsnips, spinach, dandelion leaves
- 2 kg vegetables
- 100 g sprouts
- 500 g whole grain
- 2.5 – 3 kg meat

*Vitamin E balance depends on prevalence of unsaturated fatty acids

C. Recommended Intakes (AI*, DRI, 2000)

Life Stage and Gender Group	Age	Vitamin E			UL	
		(mg/d)	(µmol)	(mg/kg)	(mg/d)	(µmol/d)
Infants	0 – 6 mo	4*	9.3	~ 0.6*	No supplements	
	7 – 12 mo	5*	11.6	~ 0.6*		
Children	1 – 3 y	6	13.9		200	465
	4 – 8 y	7	16.3		300	698
Adolescents	9 – 13 y	11	25.6		600	1395
Adults	14 – 18 y	15	34.9		800	1860
	≥ 19 y	15	34.9		1000	2326
Pregnancy	14 – 18 y	15	34.9		800	1860
	19 – 50 y	15	34.9		1000	2326
Lactation	14 – 18 y	15	34.9		800	1860
	19 – 50 y	19	44.2		1000	2326

Vitamin K: Chemistry, Metabolism, and Functions

The antihemorrhagic properties of vitamin K were first described in the 1930s; the newly discovered factor was called "coagulation vitamin." Besides the naturally occurring vitamins K_1 (phylloquinone) and K_2 (menaquinone), some additional quinones have vitamin K-like effects.

The **basic structure** of vitamin K (**A**) is 1,4-naphtoquinone. Its vitamin activity depends on the methyl group in position two, while its fat solubility and other properties are due to the long side chains. Vitamin K_2 is a collective term for menaquinones with side chains of different lengths—always with an isoprene unit attached. From a pharmacological perspective, only the fat-soluble vitamins K_1 and K_2 are of practical significance. The synthetic, water-soluble K_3 and its derivatives are no longer used.

Vitamin K supplied with **food** is actively absorbed in the proximal small intestine during lipid digestion and transported to the liver in chylomicrons. It also circulates in all other lipoprotein fractions (particularly VLDL). Its **absorption rate** is 20–70 %. Vitamin K_2 is also synthesized by intestinal bacteria in the distal small intestine and colon. In that part of the digestive tract, however, the concentration of bile acids is so low that the absorption of fat-soluble K_2 from intestinal bacteria is of no great significance.

The first function of vitamin K to be discovered was its role in **blood coagulation**, and it has been used for therapeutic purposes in this context for a long time. Inactive precursors of the coagulation factors are synthesized in the liver and activated there by γ-glutamyl carboxylase (**B**). Vitamin K is a cofactor required for this reaction, in which it is converted to 2,3-epoxide. Active vitamin K is subsequently regenerated from the latter in a two-step reaction. Coagulation factors II, VII, IX, and X, as well as the coagulation inhibitors, proteins C and S, are released into the blood, where they attach to phospholipid membranes.

All components of the blood coagulation system are present in the normal **neonate's** body; however, the vitamin K-dependent factors will not reach the activity levels found in adults for several weeks or months. Additionally, low contents in mother's and cow's milk tend to cause deficiencies in infants. For these reasons, **prophylactic vitamin K supplementation** has been common practice for a long time. Vitamin K is injected IM right after birth or administered orally in an oily solution.
Antagonists that block vitamin K effects also have a long history of therapeutic use: coumarin derivatives are widely used in thrombosis prevention.

In the past decades, additional vitamin K effects have been discovered. It is involved in the formation (carboxylation) of osteocalcin, a bone protein that inhibits Ca^{2+} mobilization from bone during postmenopause. **Matrix Gla-proteins** (MGP), which have been found in bone, kidneys, lungs, and heart among others, are also vitamin K dependent.

A. Chemistry

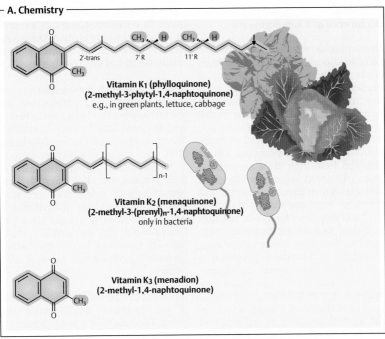

Vitamin K₁ (phylloquinone)
(2-methyl-3-phytyl-1,4-naphtoquinone)
e.g., in green plants, lettuce, cabbage

Vitamin K₂ (menaquinone)
(2-methyl-3-(prenyl)ₙ-1,4-naphtoquinone)
only in bacteria

Vitamin K₃ (menadion)
(2-methyl-1,4-naphtoquinone)

B. Effects of Vitamin K

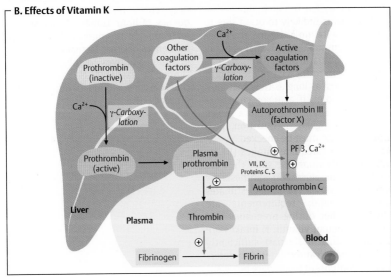

Vitamin K:
Occurrence and Requirements

Phylloquinone (vitamin K_1) is present in variable concentrations in the chloroplasts of green plants, where it is needed for photosynthesis. Gram-positive bacteria, like certain strains of *Escherichia coli* and *Bacteroides fragilis* produce menaquinones (vitamin K_2), which animals obtain from plant foods, together with K_1. So vitamin K can be obtained from both plant and animal **foods (A)**. Green vegetables like green cabbages, green lettuces, broccoli, and chives are excellent sources of vitamin K. This is why older textbooks still suggest that patients on coumarin drugs avoid eating cabbage. When using anticoagulants as **thrombosis prophylaxis**, a balance between the agonist vitamin K and the coumarin antagonist has to be maintained. With larger amounts of vitamin K, the balance shifts in favor of the agonist, resulting in an increased tendency towards coagulation. However, more recent research shows that such a shift is unlikely to occur due to nutritional vitamin K. Hence, the more recent recommendation is that patients receiving coumarin drugs do not have to pay attention to the vitamin K content of their foods, as long as they maintain their usual diet. If a major change is made, such as a change from a mixed to a strict vegetarian nutrition, prothrombin time must be checked.

Estimates of Adequate Intakes (B) for vitamin K are imprecise since they are based on the uncertain synthesis by intestinal bacteria. For adults, estimates are 65–80 µg/d; requirements are slightly higher during pregnancy and lactation. Actual vitamin K intakes are unknown since, in the past, sufficiently reliable analytical techniques to determine K contents of foods were not available. It can be assumed, however, that more than sufficient amounts are supplied with a mixed nutrition. There is no known toxicity from vitamin K from foods. No **UL** has been established.

Classic **vitamin K deficiencies (C)** are usually found only in infants who are exclusively breast-fed. It causes bleeding, the most feared variant of which is bleeding into the ventricles of the brain. This can cause irreversible damage including death; prophylaxis is, therefore justified, even if without it, there would only be a few cases per year. One mg intramuscular (IM) vitamin K or 2 mg orally on the 1st and 5th day of the neonate's life, repeated during the 4th–6th week, can prevent most cases of bleeding caused by vitamin K deficiency.

Until 1991, IM administration of vitamin K was practiced almost exclusively. Then, a scandal hit the press: Scandinavian research showed a correlation between IM prophylaxis and the frequency of brain tumors. Other studies were unable to confirm this; further, influences of other factors like solvents or other additives to the IM solution cannot be excluded. No such correlations have been found for oral vitamin K prophylaxis.

A. Occurrence and Daily Requirement

The daily requirement of 65 µg vitamin K is contained in:

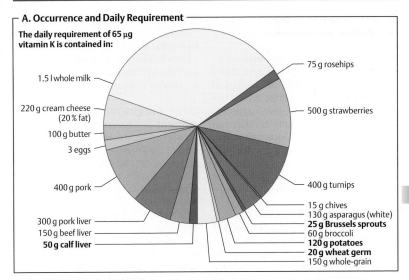

- 1.5 l whole milk
- 220 g cream cheese (20 % fat)
- 100 g butter
- 3 eggs
- 400 g pork
- 300 g pork liver
- 150 g beef liver
- **50 g calf liver**

- 75 g rosehips
- 500 g strawberries
- 400 g turnips
- 15 g chives
- 130 g asparagus (white)
- **25 g Brussels sprouts**
- 60 g broccoli
- **120 g potatoes**
- **20 g wheat germ**
- 150 g whole-grain

B. Adequate Intakes (AI, 2002)

Life Stage and Gender Group	Age	Vitamin K (µg/d)
Infants	0 – 6 mo	2.0
	7 – 12 mo	2.5
Children	1 – 3 y	30
	4 – 8 y	55
Adolescents	9 – 13 y	60
	14 – 18 y	75
Males	≥ 19 y	120
Females	≥ 19 y	90
Pregnancy and Lactation	14 – 18 y	75
	19 – 50 y	90

C. Typical Extensive Hemorrhages Caused by Vitamin K Deficiency

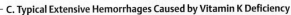

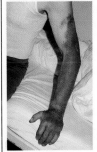

Subcutaneous

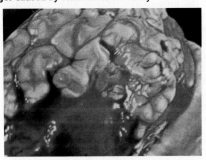

Cerebral

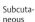

Ascorbic Acid: Chemistry, Metabolism, and Functions

The term "vitamin C" encompasses L-[+]-ascorbic acid and its derivatives with identical levels of biological effects. **Chemically**, ascorbic acid is the enolic form of 3-oxo-L-gulofuranolactone (**A**). Plants and many animals can synthesize it from glucuronic acid. Since humans, apes, and guinea pigs lack the last enzyme in the enzyme pathway, L-gulonolactone oxidase, the vitamin is essential for them.

Vitamin C **absorption** begins at the buccal mucosa, but most of it is absorbed in the proximal small intestine. There are probably several active transport mechanisms. Passive diffusion requires very high concentrations in the intestinal lumen. The absorption rate at physiological doses is ~80 %. With megadoses it may drop to 15 %. In plasma, about three-fourths is found as free ascorbic acid, the remaining one-fourth is protein bound. Optimal plasma concentrations are estimated to be around 1 mg/l; classic deficiency symptoms occur around 0.2 mg/l.

The kidneys are the **main excretory organ**, whereas after megadose supplementation (>3 g) increasingly large amounts are excreted through feces.

Some of the **biological effects** of vitamin C can be explained by L-ascorbic acid's **reductant** properties. When L-ascorbic acid is oxidized to dehydroascorbic acid, the extremely reactive intermediate semidehydro-L-ascorbate is formed. These three forms of vitamin C represent a reversible redox system. The oxidized form can be reduced to ascorbate by a reductase. Other redox systems like glutathione or tocopherol are involved in the latter enzyme's function. This allows ascorbic acid to play a hydrogen donor role in hydroxylation reactions, as, for instance, during biosynthesis of the **catecholamines**, noradrenaline, and adrenaline, where ascorbic acid functions as a cofactor for dopamine-β-mono oxygenase.

Other biological effects are based on different mechanisms, some of which are still unknown. For instance, ascorbic acid is involved in collagen biosynthesis. However, even though intracellular protein modification of pre-collagen occurs through hydroxylation of proline and lysine, ascorbic acid is not involved as a hydrogen donor here. Also, during **degradation of tyrosine**, activation of one of the enzymes occurs without involvement of the ascorbic acid/dehydroascorbate redox system. Ascorbic acid is involved in the **synthesis of bile acids** from cholesterol and the **synthesis of carnitine** from the amino acids lysine and methionine.

Neuroendocrine hormones such as gastrin, bombesin, CRH, and TRH are activated by ascorbic acid-dependent amidation. The synthesis of cytochrome P_{450} in liver microsomes, required for detoxification reactions, is stimulated by ascorbic acid. Its iron absorption enhancing function has been known for a long time just like its role as inhibitor of nitrosamine formation from nitrite and amines in the stomach. The competitive inhibition that vitamin C exerts on protein glycosylation may be particularly important for long-term prognosis for diabetics. For its antioxidant effects see p. 206.

A. Chemistry and Function

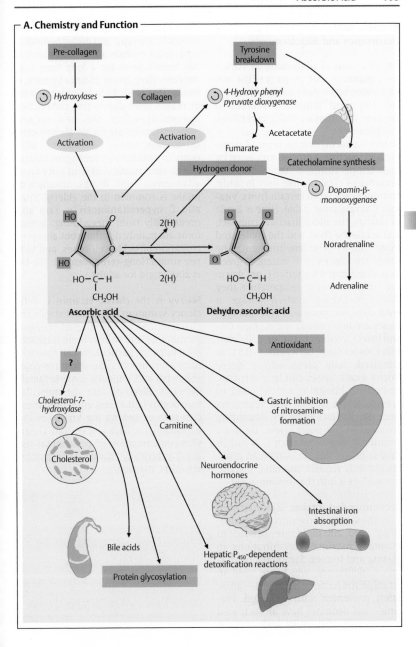

Ascorbic Acid:
Occurrence and Requirements

Ascorbic acid is ubiquitous in nature since plants, as well as many of the animals eaten by humans, can synthesize it (**A**). The most important **sources** in Western nutrition are fruits, vegetables, and potatoes.

Oxidation during storage renders ascorbic acid inactive, a process enhanced by high temperatures, as well as by the presence of catalysts like iron. In acidic environments, as in certain fruits, vitamin C is relatively stable. Here is a rule of thumb: the more inactive, compact, and acidic the food, and the colder and more humid the environment, the lower the **losses**. For instance, green peas lose about 4% vitamin C per day in the fridge; at room temperature they lose 12%. During modern storage at controlled temperatures (CA storage), losses are minimized: at 3° C, high CO_2 and low O_2 content in the air, daily vitamin C losses range between 0.1–0.3%. In sterilized, fully preserved, or deep-frozen foods, losses can be enormous. Immediate blanching can be used to prevent losses in fruit and vegetables since this inhibits vitamin C-destroying enzymes in the outer layers. Up to an additional 50% of vitamin C is lost in further processing; in particular, cooking not only renders vitamin C inactive but leaches it into the cooking water.

Recommended intakes (**B**) for vitamin C are the subject of considerable controversy; 100–200 mg/d are needed to maintain maximal concentrations in plasma and tissues. Symptoms of vitamin C deficiency—which are used to establish the recommendations—can be safely prevented with 100 mg/d. Preemies and neonates have an increased requirement of 6 mg/kg body weight.

During pregnancy and lactation, during antibiotic therapy, and under hemodialysis, requirements are also elevated. It has been known for a long time that smokers have lower plasma vitamin C levels. This is likely to be caused by an increased need due to free radical formation. Therefore, the new recommended intakes are higher for smokers. On average, vitamin C intake is adequate in children and teenagers, largely due to consumption of fruit juices and vitaminized fruit drinks. Insufficient intake is common in the elderly. Vitamin C **hypervitaminosis** is rare and occurs only from megadosing. Symptoms are mainly diarrhea, but also precipitation of sickle-cell crises, and kidney stones (long-term overuse). The **UL** is 2000 mg/d for adults.

Scurvy is the classic **vitamin C deficiency symptom** (**C**). Earliest stages are characterized by bleeding of mucosal membranes and pain in more intensely used muscles, particularly calf muscles. After a few months, the skin turns pale-yellowish and follicular hyperkeratosis develops. Bleeding into the musculature begins in the frequently used muscles such as behind the knees—in the bedridden, the back and bottom. Gingivitis (inflammation of periodontal tissues) practically always accompanies vitamin C deficiency.

A. Occurrence and Daily Requirement

The daily requirement of 100 mg vitamin C is contained in:

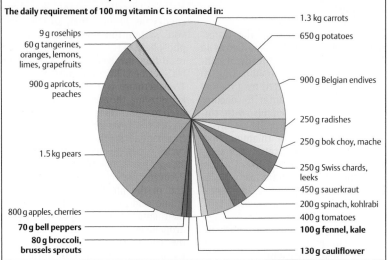

- 9 g rosehips
- 60 g tangerines, oranges, lemons, limes, grapefruits
- 900 g apricots, peaches
- 1.5 kg pears
- 800 g apples, cherries
- **70 g bell peppers**
- **80 g broccoli, brussels sprouts**

- 1.3 kg carrots
- 650 g potatoes
- 900 g Belgian endives
- 250 g radishes
- 250 g bok choy, mache
- 250 g Swiss chards, leeks
- 450 g sauerkraut
- 200 g spinach, kohlrabi
- 400 g tomatoes
- **100 g fennel, kale**
- **130 g cauliflower**

B. Recommended Intakes (DRI/AI*, 2000) and UL

Life Stage and Gender Group	Age	Vitamin C (mg/d)	(µmol)	(mg/kg)	UL (mg/d)
Infants	0 – 6 mo	40*	227	~ 6*	No supplements
	7 – 12 mo	50*	256	~ 6*	
Children	1 – 3 y	15	85		400
	3 – 8 y	25	142		650
Adolescents	9 – 13 y	45	256		1200
Adolescent males	14 – 18 y	75	426		1800
Adolescent females	14 – 18 y	65	370		1800
Men	≥ 19 y	90	511		2000
Women	≥ 19 y	75	426		2000
Pregnancy	14 – 18 y	80	454		1800
	19 – 50 y	85	483		2000
Lactation	14 – 18 y	115	568		1800
	19 – 50 y	120	682		2000

C. Deficiency Symptoms

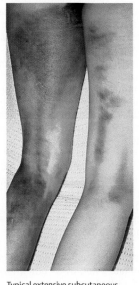

Typical extensive subcutaneous hemorrhage caused by vitamin C deficiency

Thiamin: Chemistry, Metabolism, and Functions

Thiamin was the first of the water-soluble B vitamins to be identified as an essential nutrient. **Chemically**, it consists of a substituted pyrimidine ring (**A**) and a thiazole, connected by a methyl group. The term vitamin B_1 encompasses several compounds with thiamin-like effects. Naturally occurring B_1 consists mostly of thiamin phosphates. In pharmaceuticals, water-soluble thiamin derivatives like thiamin hydrochloride or nitrate as well as lipophilic thiamin analogues like benfotiamine or fursultiamine are used.

Absorption of thiamin occurs predominantly in the jejunum after its release in the intestinal lumen during digestion. The active transport mechanism for water-soluble thiamin is saturable and rate-limiting. At higher luminal concentrations, some minor passive diffusion occurs. Overall, absorption at physiological doses is near 100%, while it drops to ~25% at pharmacological dosages. Lipophilic thiamin analogues pass through cell membranes more easily and are, therefore, absorbed in amounts corresponding to intakes. In the intestinal mucosa, free thiamin is converted to active thiamin diphosphate (TDP)—a process that consumes ATP—released into the bloodstream, bound to albumin, and transported to the target cells. The entire body contains ~30 mg thiamin, 40% of which is found in the musculature. Since its storage is so limited and because of its short half-life, daily exogenous supply is required. Excretion is mainly renal, either as thiamin, as its sulfate ester, or as other, hitherto unidentified, metabolites.

The **biochemical functions** of thiamin are based mostly on its role as the TDP **coenzyme**. Beyond that, specific nervous system functions of thiamin triphosphate (TTP) are under discussion regarding involvement of TTP in the Na^+-permeability of membranes.

Transketolase is a thiamin-dependent key enzyme, the activity of which is also used to assess thiamin status (**B**). It catalyzes the reversible transfer of a C2 fragment during the pentose phosphate cycle, thereby converting various aldoses into ketoses and vice versa.

Pyruvate, the end product of glycolysis and of the breakdown of glucogenic amino acids, is converted to acetyl by the thiamin-dependent **pyruvate dehydrogenase** (**C**) after which it can enter the citrate cycle as acetyl-CoA. The formation of succinyl-CoA during the citrate cycle requires the enzyme **α-ketoglutarate dehydrogenase**, which also depends on a thiamin cofactor.

Generally, thiamin is involved in reactions (**D**) that lead either to decarboxylation of α-keto acids (1), formation of α-hydroxy ketones (2), or transfer of an α-keto R-group (3,4). During an intermediate stage (5), a negatively charged C atom is formed, the charge of which is stabilized by TDP, making it available for further reactions at the enzyme complex.

A. Chemistry

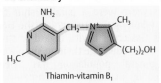

Thiamin-vitamin B$_1$

B. Coenzyme Function

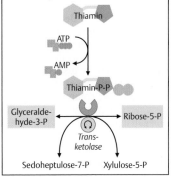

Thiamin

ATP → AMP

Thiamin-P-P

Glyceralde-hyde-3-P ↔ Ribose-5-P

Transketolase

Sedoheptulose-7-P ↔ Xylulose-5-P

C. Thiamin in the Citrate Cycle

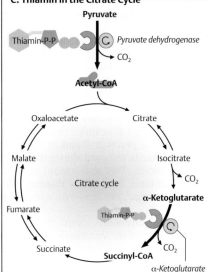

Pyruvate

Thiamin-P-P — Pyruvate dehydrogenase → CO$_2$

Acetyl-CoA

Oxaloacetate — Citrate

Malate — Isocitrate → CO$_2$

Fumarate — Citrate cycle — **α-Ketoglutarate**

Succinate — Thiamin-P-P → CO$_2$

Succinyl-CoA

α-Ketoglutarate dehydrogenase

D. Effects of Thiamin

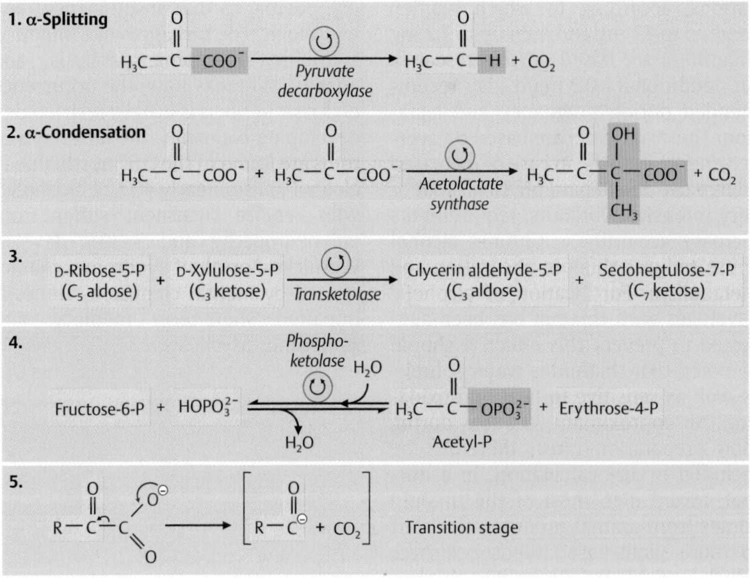

1. α-Splitting

$$H_3C-\overset{O}{\overset{\|}{C}}-COO^- \xrightarrow{\text{Pyruvate decarboxylase}} H_3C-\overset{O}{\overset{\|}{C}}-H + CO_2$$

2. α-Condensation

$$H_3C-\overset{O}{\overset{\|}{C}}-COO^- + H_3C-\overset{O}{\overset{\|}{C}}-COO^- \xrightarrow{\text{Acetolactate synthase}} H_3C-\overset{O}{\overset{\|}{C}}-\overset{OH}{\underset{CH_3}{C}}-COO^- + CO_2$$

3.

D-Ribose-5-P (C$_5$ aldose) + D-Xylulose-5-P (C$_3$ ketose) $\xrightarrow{\text{Transketolase}}$ Glycerin aldehyde-5-P (C$_3$ aldose) + Sedoheptulose-7-P (C$_7$ ketose)

4.

Fructose-6-P + HOPO$_3^{2-}$ $\xleftarrow[\text{Phospho-ketolase}]{H_2O}$ $H_3C-\overset{O}{\overset{\|}{C}}-OPO_3^{2-}$ + Erythrose-4-P

Acetyl-P

5.

$$R-\overset{O}{\overset{\|}{C}}-\overset{O^{\ominus}}{\underset{O}{C}} \longrightarrow \left[R-\overset{O}{\overset{\|}{C}}^{\ominus} + CO_2 \right]$$ Transition stage

Thiamin:
Occurrence and Requirements

Thiamin is found in all animal **foods (A)**. Good sources are several species of fish (e. g., farmed catfish, sole, Florida pompano) as well as liver and muscle, especially porcine (e. g., ham), and egg yolk. Good plant sources are whole grains, potatoes, legumes, soy milk, and acorn squash. Like most B vitamins, most of the thiamin in grains is found in the seed coat that is removed during the refining process. This also applies to rice, which loses most of its thiamin during polishing.

Thiamin requirements vary with energy expenditure. Vitamin balance research shows that ~0.5 mg of thiamin per 1000 kcal (4.2 MJ) used is needed daily to maintain erythrocyte transketolase activity as well as sufficient tissue thiamin levels. Current recommendations, according to which women need up to 1.1 mg and men up to 1.2 mg thiamin/d, are based on this research. An additional 0.3 mg/d is recommended during pregnancy and lactation. These amounts are based on average energy intakes; in case of increased energy use due to hard physical labor or very intensive workouts, requirements increase accordingly. Chronic alcohol abuse reduces thiamin absorption and metabolism. Fortification of alcoholic beverages with thiamin has been suggested to prevent this effect. It should be noted that thiamin is water soluble, as well as sensitive to heat and oxidation. An approximate 30 % loss during food preparation must, therefore, be included in any calculation. In a normal, mixed diet, most of the thiamin comes from animal products. If a shift to more plant-based foods occurred, which would be desirable, thiamin intakes might become problematic unless there were a parallel shift to more whole-grain products. In the U.S. this is less crucial with regard to thiamin, since adequate thiamin supply of the general population has been insured by mandatory enrichment of refined flour. No **UL** has been established.

The classic **vitamin B$_1$ deficiency syndrome (C)** is **beriberi**. The wet form causes generalized edema; in the dry form, nerve lesions dominate; in breast-fed children it may be associated with carbohydrate intolerance (infantile beriberi). Beriberi was common in the U.S. before government-mandated enrichment began in the 1940s. In 1932 alone, there were nearly 50 000 cases of beriberi. Based on thiamin's biochemical functions, there are two main categories of symptoms: cardiovascular disturbances, with insufficient blood supply, edema, cardiac insufficiency; neurological disturbances like impaired sensibility, cramping, paralysis, and anxiety. Whereas now, the occurrence of classic beriberi is usually restricted to developing countries, the latter symptoms are found in the U.S. mostly due to alcohol abuse: nearly 40 % of alcoholics who require treatment suffer from polyneuropathy and 3–10 % develop Wernicke-Korsakoff syndrome, characterized by mental confusion, amnesia, impaired short-term memory, and sometimes psychosis.

A. Occurrence and Daily Requirement

The daily requirement of 1 mg vitamin B₁ is contained in:

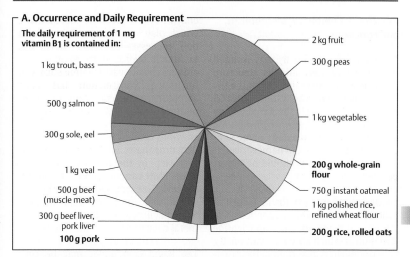

- 1 kg trout, bass
- 500 g salmon
- 300 g sole, eel
- 1 kg veal
- 500 g beef (muscle meat)
- 300 g beef liver, pork liver
- **100 g pork**
- 2 kg fruit
- 300 g peas
- 1 kg vegetables
- **200 g whole-grain flour**
- 750 g instant oatmeal
- 1 kg polished rice, refined wheat flour
- **200 g rice, rolled oats**

B. Recommended Intakes (DRI/AI*, 2000)

Life Stage and Gender Group	Age	Thiamin (mg/d)	Thiamin (mg/kg)
Infants	0 – 6 mo	0.2*	~ 0.3*
	7 – 12 mo	0.3*	~ 0.3*
Children	1 – 3 y	0.5	
	3 – 8 y	0.6	
Boys and girls	19 – 13 y	0.9	
Boys	14 – 18 y	1.2	
Girls	14 – 18 y	1.0	
Men	>19 y	1.2	
Women	>19 y	1.1	
Pregnancy and lactation	14 – 50 y	1.4	

C. Deficiency Symptoms

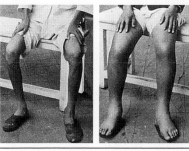

Atrophic (dry) beriberi

Exudative (moist) beriberi

Riboflavin: Chemistry, Metabolism, and Functions

Riboflavin or vitamin B_2 was isolated from yeast in 1932 and its **structure** described soon thereafter (**A**): it is a tricyclic nitrogenous ring system with a C5 side chain, in which the last hydroxy group can be esterified with phosphoric acid. Riboflavin is the short name suggested by IUPAC; the old names "ovoflavin" and "lactoflavin" should no longer be used.

Foods contain free riboflavin as well as protein-bound flavin mononucleotide (**FMN**) and flavin adenine dinucleotide (**FAD**), all of which are called vitamin B_2. Free riboflavin is **absorbed** in the proximal small intestine after dephosphorylation. Inside the mucosa cells, the enzyme riboflavin kinase phosphorylates it back to FMN. Absorption in the intestine is active and subject to saturation kinetics. At higher concentrations, however, passive diffusion may occur. In the blood, free riboflavin, FMN, and FAD are bound to albumin or to riboflavin-binding proteins (RFBPs). Storage capacity for riboflavin depends largely on the available amount of apoprotein. Maximal reserves last 2–6 weeks, much less in case of protein deficiency. Vitamin B_2 is excreted through active secretion into the renal tubules either as riboflavin or as metabolites like 7-α-hydroxy riboflavin. Its concentration in urine can be used as an indicator of B_2 status: <40 µg riboflavin/g creatinine indicates **riboflavin deficiency**.

Riboflavin's **biochemical functions** are based on the **oxidoreductase** effects of FMN and FAD as **coenzymes** or **prosthetic groups** of enzymes (**B**). Because of the yellow color of the coenzyme they are called flavoproteins or flavin enzymes. To date, more than 60 such enzymes have been found, many of which play key roles in various metabolic processes. FMN and FAD are able to attach hydrogen to riboflavin's N atoms in positions 1 and 5 and can thus function as hydrogen donors. Hydrogen acceptors can be ubiquinone in the respiratory chain, NAD^+, or even oxygen (formation of H_2O_2). Most flavin enzymes contain FAD, such as acyl-CoA dehydrogenase, which catalyzes the first step in the β-oxidation of fatty acids. FMN can be found, for instance, in NADH-dehydrogenase (respiratory chain) and in amino acid oxidases. Some flavin enzymes contain additional metal cofactors like Fe, Cu, Mn, or Mo.

The flavin component may be covalently attached to the apoprotein, as in the mitochondrial enzymes of the respiratory chain, in succinate dehydrogenase (SuccDH), or in the monoamine oxidases (MAO). Lastly, prosthetic groups may be loosely and reversibly attached to the protein, as for instance in xanthine oxidase or glutathione reductase.

FMN and FAD (**C**) form predominantly in the liver, kidneys, and heart under hormonal control (e. g., T_3). Their synthesis requires ATP.

A. Chemistry

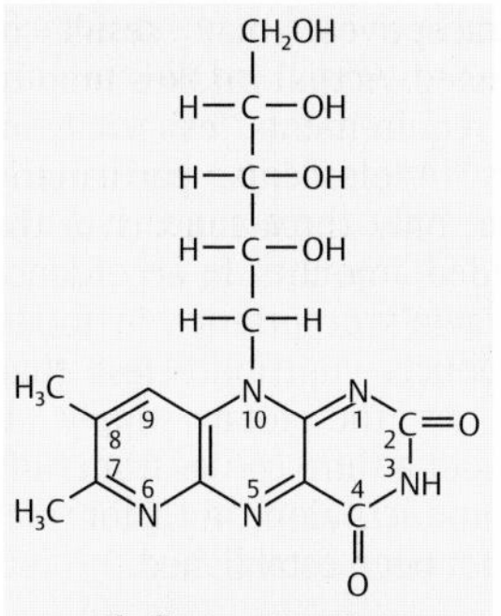

CH$_2$OH
H—C—OH
H—C—OH
H—C—OH
H—C—H

Riboflavin – vitamin B$_2$

B. Cellular Metabolism

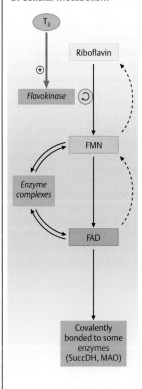

T$_3$

Riboflavin

$\oplus$

Flavokinase

FMN

Enzyme complexes

FAD

Covalently bonded to some enzymes (SuccDH, MAO)

C. Biosynthesis of FMN and FAD

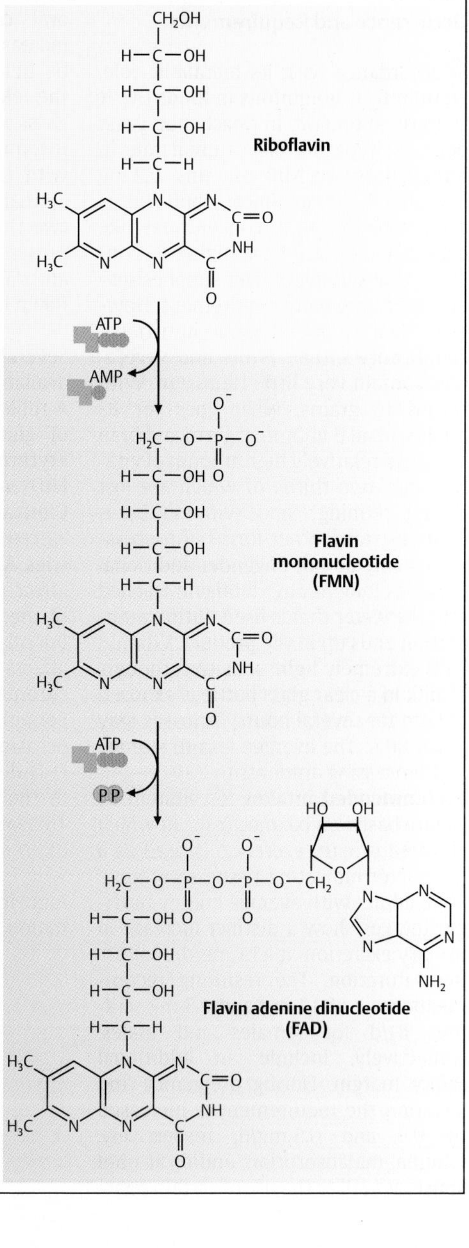

CH$_2$OH
H—C—OH
H—C—OH
H—C—OH
H—C—H

Riboflavin

ATP

AMP

H$_2$C—O—P
H—C—OH
H—C—OH
H—C—H

Flavin mononucleotide (FMN)

ATP

PP

H$_2$C—O—P—O—P—O—CH$_2$
H—C—OH
H—C—OH
H—C—OH
H—C—H

NH$_2$

Flavin adenine dinucleotide (FAD)

Riboflavin:
Occurrence and Requirements

In accordance with its metabolic role, vitamin B_2 is ubiquitous in **foods (A)**. It is most abundant in yeast, but yeast does not typically play a great role in human nutrition. Milk contains ~0.2 mg vitamin B_2/100 g. Since riboflavin is protein bound, milk concentrates like cheese and ricotta have higher B_2 contents. One serving of liver supplies several times the daily requirement. However, liver is not of great nutritional significance either. Fruits and vegetables contain very little riboflavin. With regard to grains, what goes for B_2 applies to all B vitamins: germ and bran contain a relatively high amount of vitamin B_2, ~two-thirds of which are lost during refining. Since vitamin B_2 is **heat-resistant**, other forms of processing usually do not engender additional losses as long as any riboflavin leached into the water that is used during preparation ends up in the product. Vitamin B_2 is extremely **light-sensitive**, though. If milk in a clear glass bottle is exposed to light for several hours, B_2 losses may reach 80%. The average loss to storage and processing amounts to 20%.

Recommended intakes for vitamin B_2 **(B)** are based on balance tests, in which elevated urinary excretion is used as a parameter indicating tissue saturation. Male adults with average energy nutrient intakes show a distinct increase in urinary excretion at ≥1.1 mg/d, indicating saturation. The resulting recommendations of 1.1 mg and 1.3 mg vitamin B_2/d for females and males, respectively, include an additional safety margin. During pregnancy and lactation the requirement is increased by 0.3 and 0.5 mg/d, respectively. Trauma, malabsorption, and/or alcohol abuse, as well as the use of certain phar-

maceuticals (antidepressants, some oral contraceptives) may result in increased need. **Actual intakes** tend to be below requirements, especially in the elderly. Adolescents, particularly girls, obtain only three-fourths of the recommended amounts. In accordance with riboflavin's occurrence in foods, animal products contribute less than two-thirds of the total supply at present; about a third comes from milk and dairy products alone. A **UL** for riboflavin has not been established.

Several possible test parameters are available to determine B_2 deficiency **(C)**. A reliable method is the measurement of glutathione reductase activity (in erythrocytes) after stimulation with FAD (α-EGR-method).

Clinical deficiency symptoms are extremely rare in industrialized countries. At first, they are unspecific **(D)** and affect mainly the mucous membranes of the head (e.g., stomatitis, inflamed buccal mucosa). B_2 deficiency also affects Fe metabolism, causing hypochromic anemia in advanced stages. Sometimes there is also dermatitis, occasionally generalized. FMN- and FAD-dependent enzymes also play roles in the metabolism of other vitamins. This fact, and the fact that the vitamins often occur in foods together, explains why isolated B_2 deficiency is uncommon. Instead it usually occurs in combination with other vitamin deficiencies.

A. Occurrence and Daily Requirement

The daily requirement of 1.5 mg vitamin B₂ is contained in:

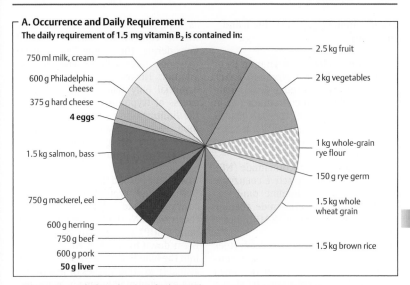

- 750 ml milk, cream
- 600 g Philadelphia cheese
- 375 g hard cheese
- **4 eggs**
- 1.5 kg salmon, bass
- 750 g mackerel, eel
- 600 g herring
- 750 g beef
- 600 g pork
- **50 g liver**

- 2.5 kg fruit
- 2 kg vegetables
- 1 kg whole-grain rye flour
- 150 g rye germ
- 1.5 kg whole wheat grain
- 1.5 kg brown rice

B. Recommended Intakes (DRI/AI*, 2000)

Life Stage and Gender Group	Age	Riboflavin (mg/d)	Riboflavin (mg/kg)
Infants	0 – 6 mo	0.3*	~ 0.4*
	7 – 12 mo	0.4*	~ 0.4*
Children	1 – 3 y	0.5	
	4 – 8 y	0.6	
Boys	9 – 13 y	0.9	
	14 – 18 y	1.3	
Girls	9 – 13 y	0.9	
	14 – 18 y	1.0	
Men	>19 y	1.3	
Women	>19 y	1.1	
Pregnancy	14 – 50 y	1.4	
Lactation	14 – 50 y	1.6	

C. Deficiency

Test parameters	Normal	Marginal deficiency	Severe deficiency
Riboflavin in urine (μg/g creatine)	>80	27 – 79	<27
Riboflavin in erythrocytes (μg/g hemoglobin)	>0.45		
Erythrocyte glutathion reductase activation coefficient	<1.2	1.2 – 1.4	>1.4

D. Cheilosis

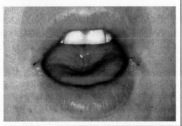

Niacin: Chemistry, Metabolism, and Functions

Niacin used to be called vitamin B_3 or vitamin PP (pellagra preventive). Today, the term "niacin" is used to denominate **nicotinic acid** and **nicotinamide** (**A**). In their biological activity they are quantitative and qualitative equivalents since the body can convert them into one another (**B**).

Nicotinic acid (NA), nicotinamide (NE), and the metabolically active coenzyme form nicotinamide adenine dinucleotide (**NAD**), and nicotinamide adenine dinucleotide phosphate (**NADP**), occur in foods.

In order to be absorbed, the coenzymes have to be split and NE partially converted to NA by bacteria of the small intestine. Mucosa cells absorb NA and some NE actively, at higher concentrations also by passive diffusion (**C**). At low dosages, nearly all niacin is immediately converted to NAD in the liver (first-pass effect, i.e., quantitative conversion during the initial passage through the liver).

There are three pathways for **NAD synthesis**. The first one uses NA as a precursor and requires 5-phospho ribosyl-1-diphosphate (PRPP), glutamine, and ATP. If NE is used as a precursor, only PRPP and ATP are needed. The third pathway is independent of niacin. In an alternative pathway for the breakdown of tryptophan, nicotinic acid mononucleotide (NMN) is made via the intermediates kynurenine and quinolinic acid. NMN can be converted to NAD with glutamate and ATP as above. This pathway is important only in the liver and kidneys, whereas peripheral organs preferentially use NE for the synthesis. On average, 60 mg L-tryptophan can be converted to the same amount of NAD as 1 mg NE. For this reason, the term **niacin equivalents** was introduced. Considering this equivalency, niacin may not necessarily be considered a vitamin. However, it becomes non-essential only when there is a large excess of tryptophan. If tryptophan is the limiting amino acid or, as is common with adequate protein supply, there is just enough of it, it is used exclusively for protein synthesis.

In the liver, beyond the synthesis of NAD from NA and tryptophan, there is also constant breakdown to NE and resynthesis of NMN. The liver regulates NAD (and NADP) metabolism by breaking them down to NE. And NE is secreted into the bloodstream and thereby made available to other tissues or inactivated and excreted mainly renally as methyl-NE. Humans can store a niacin supply sufficient for up to 2–6 weeks.

The **biochemical functions** of niacin are based on its role as a **coenzyme** of various **dehydrogenases**. The active form is NAD and/or NADP, into which NAD is converted by phosphorylation, using ATP. Both play a role in hydrogen transfer. For this, one H out of H_2 attaches to the niacinamide ring bringing with it its pair of electrons (NADH, NADPH) and leaving behind a proton (H^+). NAD-dependent dehydrogenases are found mostly in the mitochondria while NADP is predominantly involved in cytosolic synthesis pathways (e.g., fatty acid synthesis).

A. Chemistry

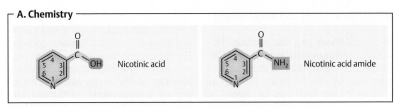

Nicotinic acid

Nicotinic acid amide

B. Nicotinic Acid Amide Synthesis

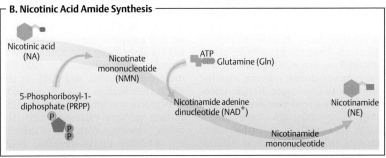

Nicotinic acid (NA)

5-Phosphoribosyl-1-diphosphate (PRPP)

Nicotinate mononucleotide (NMN)

ATP   Glutamine (Gln)

Nicotinamide adenine dinucleotide (NAD$^+$)

Nicotinamide mononucleotide

Nicotinamide (NE)

C. Niacin Metabolism

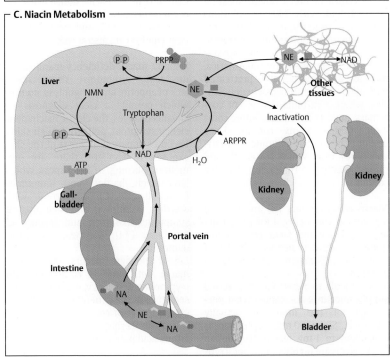

Niacin: Occurrence and Requirements

In animal **foods (A)**, niacinamide (NE) occurs predominantly as NAD or NADP. In the U.S., nearly half of the niacin is supplied by beef, pork, turkey, or chicken. Some NAD can be stored in liver, making calf, beef, and pig liver good sources of niacin that contain ~15 mg/100 g. Lean muscle meat—particularly heart muscle—is rich in niacin (5–7 mg/100 g). Whole grains contain 5 mg niacin/100 g, but most of it is removed during refining, together with the aleuron layer. Hence, unenriched white bread contains less than 1 mg niacin/100 g. In some grains, niacin is bound to a carbohydrate complex (niacytin), which is difficult for enzymes to break down. Roasting or treatment with alkaline solutions releases NA from these complexes. This is particularly important in countries in which corn and sorghum/millet are staple foods. In South and Central America, tortillas are traditionally pretreated with alkali, preventing niacin deficiencies, whereas in India that is not customary, making deficiencies more common. Coffee beans contain large amounts of methyl-nicotinic acid (trigonelline), from which NA is released during roasting so that a cup of coffee contains 1–2 mg niacin.

Niacin requirements (B) are 14 mg/d for women and 16 mg/d for men. During pregnancy and lactation an additional 3–4 mg/d is needed. The **UL** of supplemental niacin for adults is 35 mg/d.

It is difficult to determine the **actual supply** since it is not known what percentage of the intake is actually absorbed. Since 60 mg tryptophan is equivalent to 1 mg niacin, tryptophan intake levels are highly significant. Tryptophan in corn constitutes ~0.6%, in cereals, vegetables, etc. ~1%, and in animal products >1.1% of protein content. The 60 g recommended minimum protein intake of a 2000 calorie diet alone provides nearly 10 mg niacin. With an average protein intake >200 g per person/d in the U.S., adequate niacin intake is amply assured in most people. This was not always so: in the 1900s, corn became a staple in the southeastern U.S. In 1915 alone, more than 10 000 Americans died from pellagra, and ~200 000 more between 1918 and 1945. In the 1940s, fortification of grain products with niacin was introduced in the U.S., making pellagra extremely rare (see below). However, with 40% of the elderly admitted to U.S. hospitals being malnourished, niacin deficiencies do occur, especially due to protein energy malnutrition (PEM) and alcohol abuse. Poor children are also at risk.

Initially, **niacin deficiency** manifests as unspecific symptoms: sleeplessness, lack of appetite and weight loss, none of which permits a clear diagnosis. In advanced stages, the classic niacin deficiency symptom, **pellagra** (rough skin), becomes apparent. In areas of the skin exposed to sunlight, there are pigmented, burning, or itchy spots, which later swell, harden, and sometimes form blisters (**C**), concurrent with diarrhea, vomiting, and neurological symptoms like pain and feelings of numbness (3 D: diarrhea, dermatitis, dementia).

Classic pellagra occurs only when niacin deficiency is combined with tryptophan deficiency, mainly as a consequence of the general PEM. Exclusive consumption of corn (e.g., in parts of Africa) exacerbates this, due to the amino acid pattern of corn.

A. Occurrence and Daily Requirement

The daily requirement of 15 mg niacin is contained in:

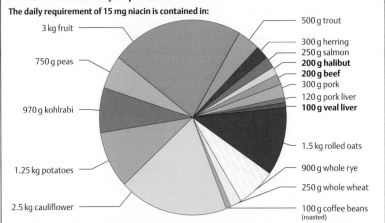

- 3 kg fruit
- 750 g peas
- 970 g kohlrabi
- 1.25 kg potatoes
- 2.5 kg cauliflower
- 500 g trout
- 300 g herring
- 250 g salmon
- **200 g halibut**
- **200 g beef**
- 300 g pork
- 120 g pork liver
- **100 g veal liver**
- 1.5 kg rolled oats
- 900 g whole rye
- 250 g whole wheat
- 100 g coffee beans (roasted)

B. Recommended Intakes (DRI/AI*, 2000) and UL

Life Stage and Gender Group	Age	Niacin Equivalents (mg/d)	(mg/kg)	UL (mg/d)
Infants	0 – 6 mo	2* (preformed)	~ 0.2*	No supplements
	7 – 12 mo	4*	~ 0.4*	
Children	1 – 3 y	6		10
	4 – 8 y	8		15
Boys	9 – 13 y	12		20
	14 – 18 y	16		30
Girls	9 – 13 y	12		20
	14 – 18 y	14		30
Men	≥ 19 y	16		35
Women	≥ 19 y	14		35
Pregnancy	14 – 18 y	18		30
	19 – 50 y	18		35
Lactation	14 – 18 y	17		30
	19 – 50 y	17		35

C. Pellagra

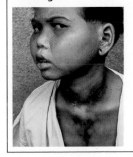
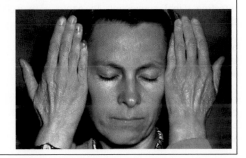

Pantothenic Acid: Chemistry, Metabolism, and Functions

Pantothenic acid, also known as vitamin B_5, was first discovered as an essential growth factor for yeast cells. After it was found to have a similar function in lactic acid bacteria, chicks, and rats, the substance was called pantothenic acid (Greek pantothen = everywhere) in reference to its ubiquitous occurrence.

Chemically, the pantothenic acid molecule consists of pantoic acid and β-alanine (**A**). The alcohol (R)-panthenol, also known as D-panthenol, is also biologically active. The pantothenic acid molecule has a chiral center. Only the D(+) form occurs naturally. Since this is also its only active form, and synthetic mixtures contain the S-enantiomer and other inactive derivatives as well, the term **pantothenic acid activity** is used. Since the acid is relatively unstable, synthetic forms usually contain Na^+ or Ca^{2+} salts of the acid or the alcohol (panthenol).

Pantothenic acid in **foods** occurs mostly in the form of its active coenzymes, CoA and fatty acid synthase, of which it is a constituent. In the stomach and intestines, they are broken down into the intermediate pantetheine and pantothenic acid, both of which are passively absorbed in all segments of the small intestine. Final conversion to pantothenic acid occurs inside the intestinal mucosa. Panthenol, applied to the skin or supplied orally, is also absorbed passively and converted to pantothenic acid by enzymatic oxidation. In blood, pantothenic acid is protein-bound and thus transported directly to the target cells. There are no specific storage organs. Pantothenic acid is excreted as such via the urine.

In tissues, pantothenic acid is used for synthesis of **coenzyme** A (CoA) (**B**). For this, it is first phosphorylated with ATP, then amidated with cysteine, and decarboxylated to pantetheine. This introduces the HS-group, which is so important for the function of CoA (in A on the right side of the molecule). Transfer of the nucleotide R-group results in the finished CoA, which can be used for metabolism or further converted to fatty acid synthase.

The **biological effects** of pantothenic acid are ubiquitous since CoA (and CoASH) participate in numerous reactions. This applies to many metabolic pathways, such as the energy and lipid metabolism (**C**), which will serve as an example: CoA is involved in the release and transfer of fatty acids for β-oxidation in mitochondria (1) as well as in triglyceride and phospholipid synthesis (2). For the synthesis of fatty acids (3), C2 building blocks in the form of acetyl-CoA from the mitochondria are bonded together inside the cytosol, using CoA-intermediates. The fatty acid synthase complex is also involved in this process. In its large carrier protein, the HS-group of the pantetheine group serves as an anchor for the fatty acid as it undergoes elongation. In these reactions, CoA functions as transfer agent for activated (i.e., raised to a higher energy level) acyl or acetyl groups.

A. Chemistry

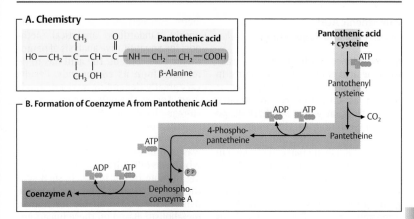

Pantothenic acid

$$HO-CH_2-\underset{\underset{CH_3}{|}}{\overset{\overset{CH_3}{|}}{C}}-\underset{\underset{OH}{|}}{CH}-\overset{\overset{O}{||}}{C}-NH-CH_2-CH_2-COOH$$

β-Alanine

B. Formation of Coenzyme A from Pantothenic Acid

Pantothenic acid + cysteine

ATP

Pantothenyl cysteine

CO$_2$

Pantetheine

ADP + ATP

4-Phospho-pantetheine

ATP

PP

Dephospho-coenzyme A

ADP + ATP

Coenzyme A

C. Pantothenic Acid in Intermediate Metabolism

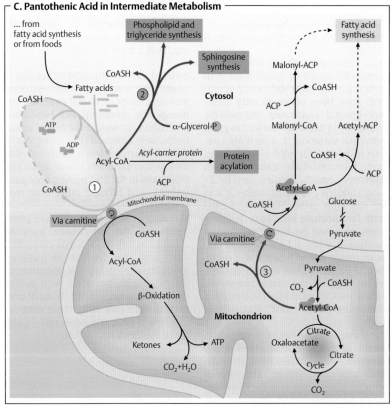

... from fatty acid synthesis or from foods

Phospholipid and triglyceride synthesis

Fatty acid synthesis

Cytosol

Malonyl-ACP

CoASH ②

Sphingosine synthesis

ACP

CoASH

Fatty acids

Malonyl-CoA

Acetyl-ACP

α-Glycerol-P

ATP

CoASH

ACP

ADP

Acetyl-ACP

CoASH

ACP

Acyl-CoA

Acyl-carrier protein

Protein acylation

ACP

Acetyl-CoA

CoASH

CoASH ①

Glucose

Via carnitine

Mitochondrial membrane

Via carnitine C

Pyruvate

CoASH

Acyl-CoA

CoASH

β-Oxidation

③

Pyruvate

CO$_2$

CoASH

Acetyl-CoA

Ketones

ATP

Mitochondrion

Citrate

Oxaloacetate

Citrate

CO$_2$+H$_2$O

Cycle

CO$_2$

Pantothenic Acid:
Occurrence and Requirements

In accordance with its name, pantothenic acid is ubiquitous in **foods**. In plant and animal tissues 50–95 % is present as CoA and as pantetheine, mostly from fatty acid synthase. Royal jelly, a secretion of the pharyngeal glands of the honeybee, and the ovaries of dried cod fish are particularly high in pantothenic acid. Among those foods important for human nutrition, sunflower seeds, liver, eggs, and wholegrain products stand out (**A**). More important, though, is its ubiquitous occurrence: practically all foods provide pantothenic acid, so that even low contents add up to considerable overall amounts.

Exact human **pantothenic acid requirements (B)** cannot be established with certainty since clear deficiency symptoms have been observed only under experimental conditions. Pantothenic acid levels in blood are subject to great individual variation: 1–4 mg/l are considered normal for adults. Daily losses through excretion are also only rough estimates: healthy adults excrete 2–7 mg, children 2–3 mg pantothenic acid per day with urine. The 6 mg/d **estimate for adequate intakes** is therefore based on actual intakes. Older studies mention a daily intake of 7–10 mg; more recent research found 4–6 mg/d. Even at intakes as low as 1 mg/d, there are normally no deficiency symptoms. Deficiencies are most likely in teenagers consuming mostly "fast" and refined foods.

There are several reasons why pantothenic acid has not received much attention from researchers to date. Studies on actual intakes and vitamin content tables often lack data pertaining to pantothenic acid. One causative factor can certainly be found in the poorly standardized analytical methods: for a quantitative analysis of pantothenic acid content, the acid has to be released from its compounds. Results vary greatly, depending on the methods used. Losses through preparation and storage have not been determined exactly, but are estimated at ~30 %. At one point, it was assumed that there was synthesis by intestinal bacteria, which was difficult to calculate. According to more recent research, such synthesis, if it occurs, does not produce pantothenic acid available for human metabolism. Based on these uncertainties, many countries have not established requirements for pantothenic acid. In the U.S., **adequate intakes (AI)** are set at 5 mg/d for adults.

Isolated pantothenic acid deficiency is practically unknown. With extreme malnutrition or in animal experiments, nonspecific symptoms like headaches and fatigue, as well as the loss of visual fields, were observed (**C**). During World War II, "burning feet syndrome" was observed in prisoners of war in Burma, Japan, and in the Philippines; only pantothenic acid brought relief from that syndrome.

The alcohol of pantothenic acid (dexpanthenol) has long been used in creams and lotions for burns, conjunctivitis, and anal fissures. In patients receiving total parenteral nutrition or dialysis, supplementation with pantothenic acid is important. Hypervitaminosis is not a risk, since there were no side effects even at dosages up to 5 g/d. No **UL** has been established.

A. Occurrence and Daily Requirement

The daily requirement of 6 mg pantothenic acid is contained in:

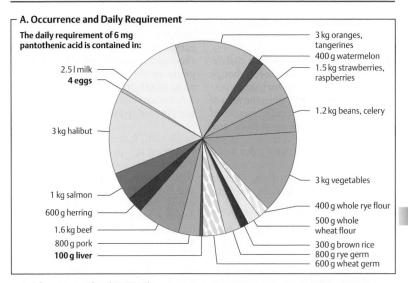

- 2.5 l milk
- **4 eggs**
- 3 kg halibut
- 1 kg salmon
- 600 g herring
- 1.6 kg beef
- 800 g pork
- **100 g liver**

- 3 kg oranges, tangerines
- 400 g watermelon
- 1.5 kg strawberries, raspberries
- 1.2 kg beans, celery
- 3 kg vegetables
- 400 g whole rye flour
- 500 g whole wheat flour
- 300 g brown rice
- 800 g rye germ
- 600 g wheat germ

B. Adequate Intakes (AI, 2000)

Life Stage and Gender Group	Age	Pantothenic acid (mg/d)	Pantothenic acid (mg/kg)
Infants	0 – 6 mo	1.7	~ 0.2
	7 – 12 mo	1.8	~ 0.2
Children	1 – 3 y	2	
	4 – 8 y	3	
Males and females	9 – 13 y	4	
	>14 y	5	
Pregnancy	14 – 50 y	6	
Lactation	14 – 50 y	7	

C. Deficiency Symptoms

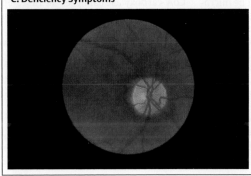

Atrophy of the optical nerve: preceded by reduced visual acuity through loss of central vision

Biotin: Chemistry, Metabolism, and Functions

The **structure** of biotin (**A**) was discovered as late as the 1940s, even though the factor had been known from experiments with yeast cells since the turn of the century. The molecule consists of two ring systems with a valerianic acid side chain. Biotin contains three asymmetrical C atoms, allowing for eight stereoisomers. However, only D-biotin is active and occurs naturally. The old name vitamin H, which is obsolete, should no longer be used.

Biotin in foods occurs partially in free-form, and is also protein-bound, particularly in animal foods. The latter is digested to biocytin in the digestive tract. Before **absorption,** biocytin has to be hydrolyzed by the enzyme biotinidase. Free biotin is actively absorbed in the proximal small intestine. At high concentrations, passive diffusion takes place as well. Not much is known about its further **metabolism.** In blood, biotin occurs in variable concentrations (200–1200 µg/L); mostly free-form, ~10% is found in erythrocytes. Excretion of the free-form or of unknown metabolites occurs via urine. Since biotin amounts found in fecal matter are higher than ingested amounts, there must be microbial synthesis. Estimates of the quantitative contribution of this bacterial synthesis differ. Children with congenital biotinidase deficiency are unable to use protein-bound biotin in foods. Without supplementation, biotin levels in plasma drop rapidly. It can be concluded from this that the available contribution from microbial synthesis in the intestine—at least as free biotin—cannot be significant.

The **biochemical effects** of biotin are based on its function as a **coenzyme** of **carboxylases.** For this, biotin's side chain is covalently bonded to a lysine R-group of the enzyme (**B**). Biotin first picks up CO_2 from bicarbonate, forming 1-N-carboxybiotin, which then carboxylates the substrate.

In humans, four such carboxylases are important (**C**): **pyruvate carboxylase** is a key enzyme in gluconeogenesis. In the mitochondria, particularly of hepatic and renal cells, it catalyzes the conversion of pyruvate to oxaloacetate, which can be converted to glucose after passing into the cytosol. Pyruvate carboxylase also plays an important role in fatty tissue since it is needed to transfer acetyl-CoA out of the mitochondria for purposes of lipogenesis.

During breakdown of various amino acids, odd-chain fatty acids, and cholesterol, the 3C compound propionic acid is synthesized. Propionic acid is converted into citrate cycle intermediates. This reaction requires the enzyme **propionyl-CoA carboxylase**, which catalyzes conversion from an odd- to an even-chain compound.

Breakdown of the amino acid leucine requires, among others, **3-methyl crotonyl-CoA-carboxylase**, whereas **acetyl-CoA-carboxylase** catalyzes the first step in fatty acid synthesis, the formation of malonyl-CoA from acetyl-CoA.

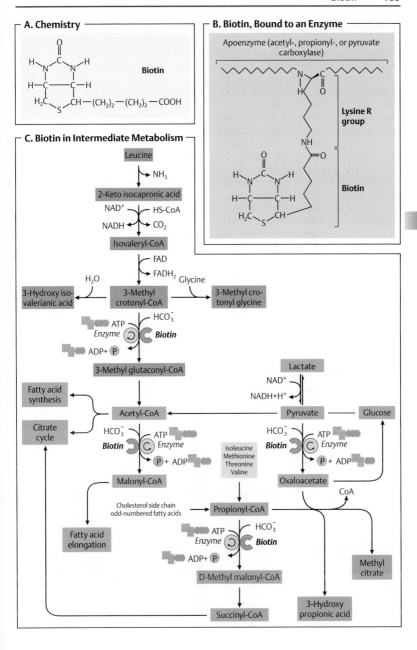

A. Chemistry

Biotin

B. Biotin, Bound to an Enzyme

Apoenzyme (acetyl-, propionyl-, or pyruvate carboxylase)

Lysine R group

Biotin

C. Biotin in Intermediate Metabolism

Leucine
→ NH_3
2-Keto isocapronic acid
NAD^+ HS-CoA
NADH CO_2
Isovaleryl-CoA
FAD
$FADH_2$ Glycine
H_2O 3-Methyl crotonyl-CoA   3-Methyl crotonyl glycine
3-Hydroxy iso-valerianic acid
ATP HCO_3^-
Enzyme   Biotin
ADP + P
3-Methyl glutaconyl-CoA

Lactate
NAD^+
$NADH + H^+$

Fatty acid synthesis
Citrate cycle
Acetyl-CoA   Pyruvate   Glucose
HCO_3^- ATP
Biotin   Enzyme
P + ADP

Isoleucine Methionine Threonine Valine

HCO_3^- ATP
Biotin   Enzyme
P + ADP
Malonyl-CoA   Oxaloacetate
CoA

Cholesterol side chain odd-numbered fatty acids   Propionyl-CoA
Methyl citrate

Fatty acid elongation
ATP HCO_3^-
Enzyme   Biotin
ADP + P
D-Methyl malonyl-CoA
3-Hydroxy propionic acid
Succinyl-CoA

Biotin: Occurrence and Requirements

Biotin is present in most **foods**, though often in low concentrations (**A**). Liver and microorganisms like yeasts are very biotin-rich, but do not play an important role in everyday nutrition. The most important sources are milk and dairy products, eggs, whole-grain products, and legumes. Some vegetables, like cauliflower or green beans, also contain fair amounts of biotin. Biotin availability from various sources differs greatly, depending on whether it is protein-bound or free-form. Feeding experiments showed that only 5 % of the total biotin contained in wheat was available to the body, whereas biotin from beet seed was 62 % available.

The determination of **biotin requirements** is subject to a host of difficulties: there is no reliable analytical method; enteral synthesis cannot be calculated; variable biological availability and late appearance of deficiency symptoms make prevention of suboptimal intakes difficult. Since it is impossible, under these conditions, to even establish **Estimated Average Requirements** (EAR), **Average Intakes** (AI) for biotin in the U.S. (30 µg/d for adults) were extrapolated based on biotin intakes of infants who were breast-fed exclusively. According to some estimates, actual average intakes from normal nutrition range between 50 and 100 µg/d. Therefore, nutrition-related deficiencies are uncommon. Since mother's milk contains only about 6–10 µg/l biotin, possible in-creased needs during pregnancy and/or lactation may not be significant. However, the recommendations suggest an additional 5 µg/d during lactation.

Earliest observations of **biotin deficiency** symptoms were made after feeding raw egg whites to rats: the characteristic skin changes and hair loss were termed "egg white injury." Egg whites contain the glycoprotein **avidin**, each molecule of which binds four biotin molecules. This avidin-biotin complex cannot be enzymatically separated and, therefore, removes large amounts of biotin from a mixed diet. Cooking denatures the avidin, so that biotin is released. In 1942, transferability of the results from animal experiments to people was tested on four volunteers. After four weeks of being fed raw egg whites, a fine, scaly skin rash developed, followed by other forms of dermatitis and cheilosis (**C**). After ten weeks, neurological symptoms (e. g., depression), muscle pain, paresthesia, etc., set in. These nonspecific symptoms, however, have rarely been described—and only after excessive consumption of raw egg whites. Some children fed a biotin-free formula parenterally had similar symptoms. Hereditary biotinidase deficiency prevents not only the absorption of protein-bound biotin, but also endogenous recycling of biotin from degraded enzymes, which appears to be of even greater importance.

There are some reports of successful biotin supplementation for various forms of dermatitis in infants that might indicate marginal biotin status of their mothers. Breaking fingernails, often used as a sales argument for biotin supplements, are not a scientifically proven deficiency symptom and the argument is therefore dubious.

Symptoms of biotin **hypervitaminosis** have never been observed in humans; supplements commonly contain 300 µg of biotin, multiples of which can be consumed without side effects. No **UL** has been established.

A. Occurrence and Daily Requirement

The daily requirement of ~50 μg biotin is contained in:

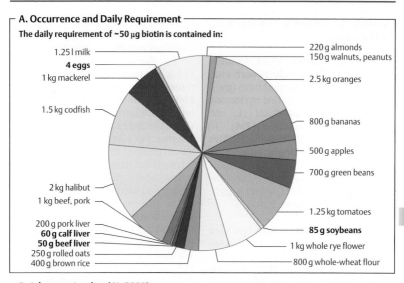

- 1.25 l milk
- **4 eggs**
- 1 kg mackerel
- 1.5 kg codfish
- 2 kg halibut
- 1 kg beef, pork
- 200 g pork liver
- **60 g calf liver**
- **50 g beef liver**
- 250 g rolled oats
- 400 g brown rice
- 220 g almonds
- 150 g walnuts, peanuts
- 2.5 kg oranges
- 800 g bananas
- 500 g apples
- 700 g green beans
- 1.25 kg tomatoes
- **85 g soybeans**
- 1 kg whole rye flower
- 800 g whole-wheat flour

B. Adequate Intakes (AI, 2000)

Life Stage and Gender Group	Age	Biotin (μg/d)	Biotin (μg/kg)
Infants	0 – 6 mo	5	~ 0.7
	7 – 12 mo	6	~ 0.7
Children	1 – 3 y	8	
	4 – 8 y	12	
Boys and girls	9 – 13 y	20	
	14 – 18 y	25	
Men and women	> 19 y	30	
Pregnancy	14 – 50 y	30	
Lactation	14 – 50 y	35	

C. Deficiency Symptoms

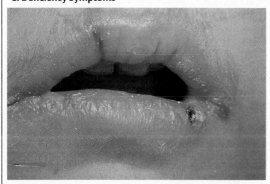

Cheilosis

Pyridoxine: Chemistry, Metabolism, and Functions

Vitamin B_6 is a collective term for all 3-hydroxy-2-methyl-pyridines with vitamin effects (**A**): the alcohol form (pyridoxol), which is also called pyridoxine (PN), the aldehyde pyridoxal (PL), and the amine pyridoxamine (PM). To denote phosphorylation of metabolites in position 5, a P is simply attached to the name (PNP, PLP, and PMP, respectively). These six substances all have the same vitamin B_6 effects, whereas pyridoxic acid has no known function.

PN, PL, and PM ingested with foods are absorbed throughout the entire small intestine by passive diffusion (**B**). The phosphates, particularly PNP, have to be hydrolyzed by membrane-bound alkaline phosphatase in order to be **absorbed**. Inside the mucosa cells, the compound is rephosphorylated, only to be again dephosphorylated on the serosal side, after which it can pass into the blood. PN, PL, and PM are transported through the blood to hepatic and peripheral tissues, where they are phosphorylated by PL-kinase. An oxidase converts PNP to its active form PLP. PLP and PNP are reversibly converted into one another by a multitude of transaminases. PLP may again be dephosphorylated to PL. Both (PLP and PL) are released into the bloodstream. PLP circulates in blood albumin-bound; in this form, it has a very low turnover rate, indicating that the PLP-albumin complex may represent some sort of pool. To be released from the complex, PLP has to be hydrolyzed in plasma by alkaline phosphatase. PL can cross the cell membrane and is again phosphorylated inside the cell. The intracellular vitamin B_6 pool, consisting of protein-bound PLP or PNP, is very small (<100 mg).

Excretion occurs mostly as pyridoxic acid; additionally, small amounts of PN and other metabolites occur in urine.

PLP is a **coenzyme for many enzymes**, mostly of the amino acid metabolism. PMP also has coenzyme function, but only for transaminases. As a coenzyme, PLP is bonded to a lysine R-group of the enzyme. PLP's aldehyde group and the amino group of the amino acids react to form a Schiff base, causing a shift of the amino acid's charges. This activated amino acid can now be decarboxylated or the side chain eliminated. Glycogen phosphorylase, which is needed to metabolize muscle glycogen, contains PLP, but it is unclear how it functions. Via the above-mentioned Schiff base, PLP can also react with other proteins, sometimes causing conformational changes. For instance, high PL concentrations in erythrocytes increase hemoglobin's affinity for O_2. A modulator effect on steroid hormone receptors is also being discussed.

Since the bonding to proteins can have relatively unspecific effects, therapeutic use of vitamin B_6 has been suggested for a large number of diseases. However, most indications for vitamin B_6 lack final scientific proof.

A. Chemistry

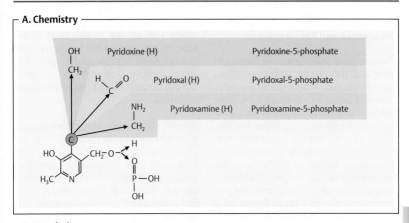

B. Metabolism

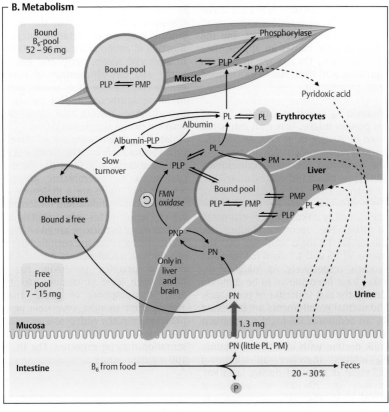

Pyridoxine:
Occurrence and Requirements

Vitamin B$_6$ is widespread in **foods (A)**. Meat and fish are good sources, so are vegetables and whole-grain products. Contents listed in various tables differ considerably, partially due to the lack of distinction between the active metabolites and the inactive pyridoxic acid. Plant foods contain predominantly pyridoxine, which is relatively stable and suffers few losses during food preparation. Animal products contain predominantly the phosphate forms, all of which are very sensitive to heat and light. Milk stored in a clear glass bottle loses 50% of its B$_6$ under exposure to sunshine within a few hours, and the frying of meat causes an approximate 40% loss in B$_6$. On average, in Western nutrition, a 20% loss has to be assumed from preparation.

Vitamin B$_6$ requirements (B) depend on protein intake, hence an estimated need of 20 µg/g of protein. In the U.S., current recommendations are based on the **Estimated Average Requirements (EAR)** plus two standard deviations (SD) in order to cover the needs of 97.5% of the population. Since the actual SD for the B$_6$ EAR is unknown, it is estimated at 10%. The recommendations for adults are 1.3 mg/d until age 50, and above 50 1.5 and 1.7 mg/d for men and women, respectively. As marginal intakes have been shown to be common during the last trimester of pregnancy, the normal requirements are increased by an additional 0.6 mg/d in pregnant women. B$_6$ concentrations in mother's milk decline with insufficient vitamin B$_6$ intakes; therefore, an additional 0.7 mg/d is required during lactation. Intakes in 20–30% of adolescent females in the U.S. are marginal,

13–20% are deficient. In general, women of all age groups tend to not take the recommended amounts. Even though there are no studies providing proof to date, a serious undersupply during pregnancy and lactation may be assumed.

At early stages, **symptoms of vitamin B$_6$ deficiency** resemble those of niacin and riboflavin deficiency. Skin changes with stomatitis and dermatitis resembling pellagra dominate. Children who developed pyridoxine deficiency due to being fed autoclaved children's foods had seizures and altered EEGs (**C**). The latter is probably due to disturbed neurotransmitter metabolism in the brain since PLP has an important coenzyme function in amino acid decarboxylases. In advanced stages, peripheral neuropathy and demyelinization of nerve cells occur. Because of its involvement in heme synthesis, it also causes a hypochromic anemia that does not respond to iron supplementation.

Isolated B$_6$ deficiencies are extremely rare. Pyridoxine is used for treatment of various metabolic defects like homocysteinuria or sideroblastic anemia. Besides that, there are a multitude of pseudoscientific indications for some of which supplements even containing megadoses of pyridoxine are given (e. g., bodybuilding). Such uncontrolled use is not without problems: as opposed to other B vitamins, pyridoxine has a rather high level of chronic toxicity. After consumption of more than 150 mg/d for months, reversible peripheral neuropathy with problems walking, loss of reflexes, and disturbed sensation may be expected. The **UL** is 100 mg/d for adults.

A. Occurrence and Daily Requirement

The daily requirement of 1.5 mg B₆ is contained in:

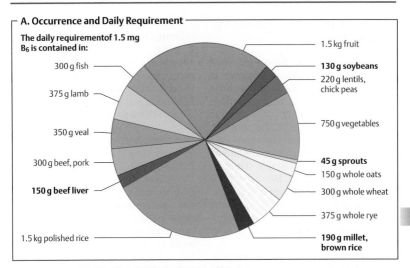

- 1.5 kg fruit
- **130 g soybeans**
- 220 g lentils, chick peas
- 750 g vegetables
- **45 g sprouts**
- 150 g whole oats
- 300 g whole wheat
- 375 g whole rye
- **190 g millet, brown rice**
- 1.5 kg polished rice
- 150 g beef liver
- 300 g beef, pork
- 350 g veal
- 375 g lamb
- 300 g fish

B. Recommended Intakes (DRI/AI*, 2000) and UL

Life Stage and Gender Group	Age	Pyridoxine		UL
		(mg/d)	(mg/kg)	(mg/d)
Infants	0 – 6 mo	0.1*	~ 0.014*	No supplements
	7 – 12 mo	0.3*	~ 0.033*	
Children	1 – 3 y	0.5		30
	4 – 8 y	0.6		40
Boys and girls	9 – 13 y	1.0		60
Adolescent males	14 – 18 y	1.3		80
Adolescent females	14 – 18 y	1.2		80
Adults	19 – 50 y	1.3		100
Men	>50 y	1.7		100
Women	>50 y	1.5		100
Pregnancy	14 – 18 y	1.9		80
	19 – 50 y	1.9		100
Lactation	14 – 18 y	2.0		80
	19 – 50 y	2.0		100

C. Deficiency Symptoms

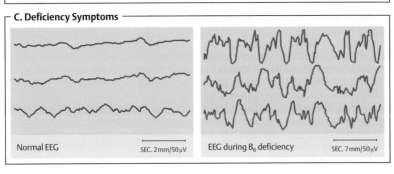

Normal EEG   SEC. 2 mm/50 µV

EEG during B₆ deficiency   SEC. 7 mm/50 µV

Cobalamin: Chemistry, Metabolism, and Functions

Cobalamin was not discovered until 1948; its structure became known in 1955. **Chemically**, cobalamin is a corrin ring system consisting of pyrrole rings that hold in their center a Co atom, to which variable ligands (R) are attached. Vitamin B_{12} is a general term used for a series of **corrinoids** (cobalt containing compounds) with a variable structure attached. Cyano- and hydroxycobalamin are used in supplements and pharmaceutical preparations; the naturally occurring active forms are 5′-adenosyl- and methylcobalamin.

In foods, vitamin B_{12} occurs protein-bound, as well as in free form. As food is ingested, the free B_{12} is bound to saliva glycoproteins, so-called **haptocorrins** or R-proteins (**A**). Protein-bound B_{12} is released by pepsin in the stomach, and some of it is again bound to haptocorrins in the proximal small intestine. The activity of pancreatic trypsin releases the B_{12} again, and it finally bonds to **intrinsic factor** (IF), which is produced in the parietal cells of the gastric mucosa. Once in the ileum, the cobalamin-IF-complex attaches to specific mucosal receptors that facilitate its active **absorption**. Passive diffusion is limited to high concentrations.

In the intestinal mucosa, B_{12} is bound to **transcobalamin II**, a plasma-binding protein that carries it through the bloodstream. Cellular uptake occurs through receptor-mediated endocytosis. The liver converts it to the active coenzyme forms adenosyl- and methylcobalamin. The liver also stores 60% of all the body's B_{12} (2–5 mg). Some of it is continually excreted via bile but is recirculated quite effectively through the enterohepatic circulation.

The **absorptive capacity** for vitamin B_{12} is limited by the IF/IF-receptor ratio (**B**). If there is too little IF, B_{12} is not absorbed. On the other hand, if IF is in excess, receptors are occupied—and the IF-cobalamin complex is unable to bind. Maximum active cobalamin absorption occurs with a single dose of ~10 µg.

As a **coenzyme**, vitamin B_{12} is involved in three metabolic reactions. In the mitochondria, adenosylcobalamin is the active form, in the cytosol it is methylcobalamin. When propionate is broken down in mitochondria, methylmalonyl-CoA is converted to succinyl-CoA, thus allowing the C3 body of the propionate to enter the citrate cycle. Also in the mitochondria, α-leucine is converted to β-leucine, exchanging an amino group for an H atom.

In the cytosol, enzyme-bound methylcobalamin is involved in the transfer of methyl groups for the synthesis of methionine from homocysteine. This reaction regenerates methyltetrahydrofolic acid, so that "active" tetrahydrofolic acid is formed. This is how B_{12} metabolism is related to folic acid metabolism (see p. 200).

A. Metabolism

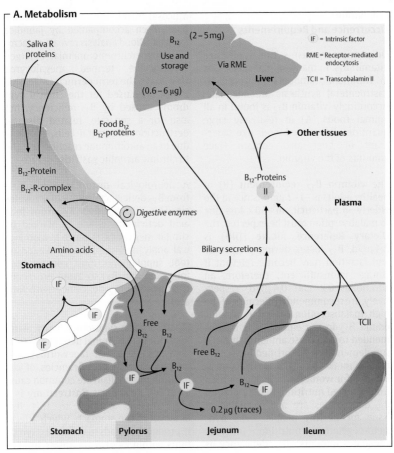

B. Absorption

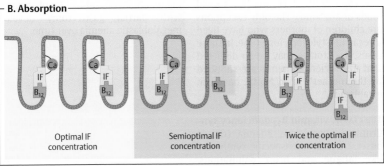

Cobalamin:
Occurrence and Requirements

Only microorganisms can synthesize vitamin B_{12}. In many animal species, as in ruminants, amounts produced by gastroenteral synthesis are adequate. Accordingly, vitamin B_{12} is found in all animal **foods** (**A**) in relatively large quantities. Fermented foods like sauerkraut or beer also contain trace amounts of the vitamin.

The **vitamin B_{12} requirement** (**B**) of healthy adults is ~1–2 µg/d. Since in the elderly, in particular, an ~50 % loss due to malabsorption must be expected, the **Dietary Reference Intake** (**DRI**) is 2.4 µg/d. B_{12} losses during pregnancy and lactation may become relevant if storage is insufficient; therefore, an additional 0.2 and 0.4 µg/d, respectively, are recommended. Because of the high malabsorption rates for protein-bound B_{12} in the elderly, it is recommended to give these amounts through supplementation or fortified foods. The median intake in the U.S. is estimated at 3.5 µg/d for women and 5 µg/d for men from a mixed nutrition. Hence, vitamin B_{12} deficiencies are not normally an issue for healthy people. Even ovo-lacto-vegetarian nutrition provides adequate amounts; B_{12} deficiency is rare even in strict vegans (no animal foods of any kind). The only exceptions are children of mothers who have lived a vegan lifestyle for a long time. In these cases, B_{12} storage may be so depleted that insufficient amounts are supplied by the mother's milk. No **UL** has been established.

The **classic vitamin B_{12} deficiency syndrome** is pernicious anemia (**C**). At onset, there are nonspecific symptoms like fatigue and heart palpitations. Mucosal membranes and skin become pale, often accompanied by jaundice (icterus). Blood analysis reveals a macrocytic, hyperchromic anemia: enlarged erythrocytes termed megalocytes. Nowadays, the term **pernicious anemia** is not only used for the clinical syndrome caused by B_{12} deficiency, but also for a separate, related disease: destruction of parietal cells, probably due to an autoimmune reaction, leading to chronic atrophic gastritis.

A neurological disturbance resulting from B_{12} deficiency is **funicular myelosis**. This **distinguishes B_{12} from folic acid deficiency**, which is marked by similar megaloblasts. Since hematological analysis is the primary diagnostic tool, supplements must contain both folic acid and B_{12} to avoid erroneous treatment of B_{12} deficiency with folic acid.

Malabsorption syndromes, particularly regarding the terminal ileum, intestinal parasites (e.g., fish tapeworms), and various congenital deficiencies of cobalamin metabolism are common causes of B_{12} deficiency. **Gastrectomy** is a more recent addition to this list. Removal of the stomach, which affects IF production, leads to deficiency symptoms within 2–10 years unless supplements are taken. Up to 18 % of patients with partial gastrectomy develop megaloblastic anemia over time.

A. Occurrence and Daily Requirement

The daily requirement of 3 µg vitamin B_{12} is contained in:

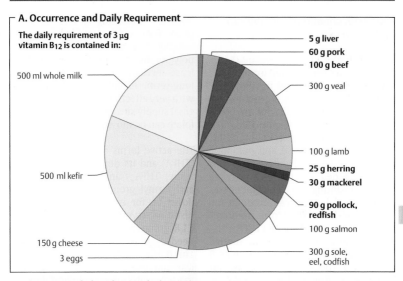

- 5 g liver
- 60 g pork
- **100 g beef**
- 300 g veal
- 100 g lamb
- **25 g herring**
- **30 g mackerel**
- **90 g pollock, redfish**
- 100 g salmon
- 300 g sole, eel, codfish
- 3 eggs
- 150 g cheese
- 500 ml kefir
- 500 ml whole milk

B. Recommended Intakes (DRI/AI*, 2000)

Life Stage and Gender Group	Age	Cobalamin (µg/d)	Cobalamin (µg/kg)
Infants	0 – 6 mo	0.4*	~ 0.05*
	7 – 12 mo	0.5*	~ 0.05*
Children	1 – 3 y	0.9	
	4 – 8 y	1.2	
Boys and girls	9 – 13 y	1.8	
	14 – 18 y	2.4	
Men and women	>19 y	2.4	
Pregnancy	14 – 50 y	2.6	
Lactation	14 – 50 y	2.8	

C. Deficiency Symptoms

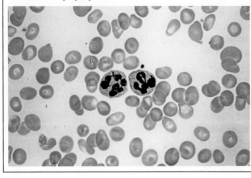

Megaloblastic anemia with hypersegmented granulocytes

Folic Acid: Chemistry, Metabolism, and Function

Folic acid, also known as folate (Latin. folium = leaf), was isolated from several tons of spinach leaves in 1941. The names folacin, vitamin Bc, vitamin B_9, and lactobacillus casei factor are obsolete and should no longer be used.

Chemically (A), it consists of pteridine, para-aminobenzoic acid, and glutamate (Pte-GLU). Additional glutamate groups may be added via the γ-carboxylate group, resulting in polyglutamates ($PteGLU_n$). Folic acid can occur in the reduced or the oxidized form, predominantly as tetrahydrofolate (THFA = H_4-PteGLU). In its hydrated form, methyl groups can be attached in positions 5 and/or 10 (both N atoms), as, for instance in 5-methyltetrahydrofolate, (H_3C-PteGLU). The same applies to methenyl-, formyl-, and formimine R-groups (abbreviation: R-PteGLU).

In order for $PteGLU_n$ to be **absorbed (B)**, γ-glutamyl carboxypeptidases, mucosa-bound and/or contained in intestinal secretions, have to degrade the polyglutamates to monoglutamates, which are then actively absorbed into the mucosa cells almost completely. In serum, 80% of folate occurs as methyltetrahydrofolate (H_3C-Pte-GLU). It is transported mostly loosely-bound to plasma proteins like albumin, transferrin, etc. A specific folate-binding protein, the concentration of which is controlled, transports oxidized folate to the liver, which turns it into tetrahydrofolate.

Enterohepatic circulation plays an important role in short-term regulation of folate homeostasis. Since folate concentrations are 10 times higher in bile than in serum, the folate circulating enterohepatically can be used to balance fluctuating levels between meals. Folic acid is stored in hepatic and peripheral tissue as nonmethylated polyglutamates. Their storage and release serves to maintain serum levels long-term. Excretion is mostly renal with very effective reabsorption in marginal supply situations. This way, loss of folate can be mostly prevented.

The active forms are **tetrahydrofolate** (THFA) and its derivatives. As a **coenzyme**, THFA transfers hydroxymethyl and formyl groups during the breakdown of, for example, homocysteine, histidine, tryptophan, and serine. The C1 R-groups transferred to the THFA are needed for purine and DNA synthesis. This is a fact exploited for pharmacological purposes: cytostatic drugs like methotrexate inhibit dihydrofolate reductase, which regenerates dihydrated folate to THFA. Thus, nucleic acid synthesis is interrupted, inhibiting cellular growth and reproduction. After homocysteine breakdown, THFA is also regenerated from methyl-PteGLU. Since vitamin B_{12} is involved in this reaction, B_{12} deficiency has direct consequences for the folate metabolism: since the active form (THFA) is missing, no further storage is possible, and serum levels of the inactive H_3C-Pte-GLU rise.

A. Chemistry

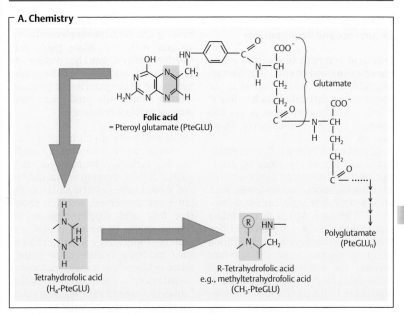

Folic acid
= Pteroyl glutamate (PteGLU)

Glutamate

Polyglutamate
(PteGLU$_n$)

Tetrahydrofolic acid
(H$_4$-PteGLU)

R-Tetrahydrofolic acid
e.g., methyltetrahydrofolic acid
(CH$_3$-PteGLU)

B. Metabolism

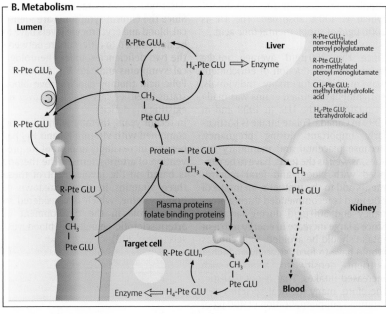

Lumen

R-Pte GLU$_n$

R-Pte GLU

R-Pte GLU

R-Pte GLU

CH$_3$
|
Pte GLU

Liver

R-Pte GLU$_n$

H$_4$-Pte GLU ⟹ Enzyme

CH$_3$
|
Pte GLU

Protein — Pte GLU
CH$_3$
|

Plasma proteins
folate binding proteins

Target cell

Enzyme ⟸ H$_4$-Pte GLU

R-Pte GLU$_n$

CH$_3$
|
Pte GLU

CH$_3$
|
Pte GLU

Kidney

Blood

R-Pte GLU$_n$:
non-methylated
pteroyl polyglutamate

R-Pte GLU:
non-methylated
pteroyl monoglutamate

CH$_3$-Pte GLU:
methyl tetrahydrofolic
acid

H$_4$-Pte GLU:
tetrahydrofolic acid

Folic Acid:
Occurrence and Requirements

Folic acid occurs in **foods** in all of the above-mentioned forms (**A**). Certain vegetables, like beans, spinach, or tomatoes are particularly rich in folate. For most people, liver, yeast, germs, and sprouts are more theoretical folate sources.

Folic acid requirements (**B**) were established as early as the 1960s by determining the minimum amounts required to maintain normal serum levels. With an added safety margin, current recommended intake is 400 µg **dietary folate equivalents** (DFE) per day from fortified foods, supplements, or both, in addition to consuming food folate. DFE take into account the lower bioavailability of folate from food (1 µg of food folate is equivalent to 0.5 µg of a folate supplement taken on an empty stomach). Only supplements contain the free folate, which is 100% absorbed. The **UL** is 1000 µg/d of supplemental folic acid.

Since the 250 µg/d average intake before the introduction of enrichment was marginal for many individuals, enrichment of refined grains was made mandatory in the U.S. in 1998 and in 1999 in Canada. Folate intake is particularly important during **pregnancy**. Because placental and mammary tissues, as well as the fetus, have to be supplied with blood, and fetal requirements add to the mother's, an intake of 600 µg/d is recommended during pregnancy and 500 µg/d during lactation. Since a large increase in energy nutrient intake should be avoided, food choices would have to focus strongly on higher nutrient density to achieve such increased intakes. That is not realistic; therefore, many medical societies recommend supplementation of 400 µg of folic acid per day for all women of childbearing age. Without supplementation, women with low folate pools may develop deficits quickly: particularly pregnancies with multiple babies, rapid succession of pregnancies, or pregnancies in adolescents predispose these women to folate deficiency.

Folate deficiency (**C**) during pregnancy is associated with a number of complications, including miscarriages, congenital defects, developmental defects, and neural tube defects. As far as the latter are concerned, research shows that folic acid supplementation, although unable to prevent neural tube defects completely, greatly reduces their incidence. Outside of pregnancy, folate deficiency, as it may develop due to malabsorption or insufficient intakes (nowadays mostly in developing countries) leads to **megaloblastic anemia**, as described above (vitamin B_{12}, p. 194). Since the clinical symptoms are identical, blood and erythrocyte levels have to be determined to differentiate between the two deficiencies, unless neurological symptoms indicate B_{12} deficiency. Folic acid therapy can improve blood status in either case and may cover up existing B_{12} deficits.

In recent years, therapy with folic acid combined with vitamin B_6 and B_{12} has become increasingly important for prevention of arteriosclerosis. The therapy is based on the involvement of these three vitamins in the breakdown of homocysteine, which is considered to play a role in the development of arteriosclerotic changes in blood vessels (see p. 200).

A. Occurrence and Daily Requirement

The daily requirement of 400 µg total folate is contained in:

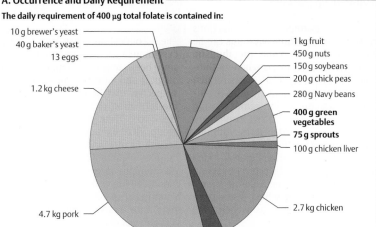

- 10 g brewer's yeast
- 40 g baker's yeast
- 13 eggs
- 1.2 kg cheese
- 4.7 kg pork
- 1 kg fruit
- 450 g nuts
- 150 g soybeans
- 200 g chick peas
- 280 g Navy beans
- **400 g green vegetables**
- **75 g sprouts**
- 100 g chicken liver
- 2.7 kg chicken
- 250 g liver

B. Recommended Intakes (DRI/AI*, 2000) and UL

Life Stage and Gender Group	Age	Dietary Folate Equivalent (µg/d)	Dietary Folate Equivalent (µg/kg)	UL (µg/d)
Infants	0 – 6 mo	65*	~ 9.4*	Could not be established
	7 – 12 mo	80*	~ 8.8*	
Children	1 – 3 y	150		300
	4 – 8 y	200		400
Boys and girls	9 – 13 y	300		600
	14 – 18 y	400		800
Men and women	>19 y	400		1000
Pregnancy	14 – 18 y	600		800
	19 – 50 y	600		1000
Lactation	14 – 18 y	500		800
	19 – 50 y	500		1000

C. Deficiency Symptoms

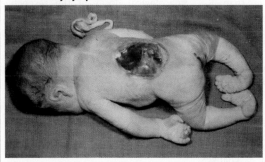

Neural tube defect
(Spina bifida)

B Vitamin Interactions

A current example for interactions between water-soluble vitamins can be found in **homocysteine metabolism.** Homocysteine (**A**) forms when methionine is demethylated (**B**). Methyl transferase, a B_{12}-dependent enzyme, regenerates methionine by remethylating homocysteine. The methyl groups are donated by 5-methyl-tetrahydrofolic acid (5-methyl-THF or H_3C-PteGLU—see p. 196). An additional pathway for homocysteine removal is its conversion to cysteine—using the enzyme cystathionine synthase, which uses pyridoxal phosphate (PLP) as a coenzyme (see p. 188).

Hence, the water-soluble B vitamins folic acid, B_{12}, and B_6 are all involved in this metabolism. A lack of these vitamins, theoretically even a lack of one of them, leads to elevated blood homocysteine levels. Blood homocysteine levels can, therefore, be used as a marker for folic acid, B_{12}, and B_6 status, respectively. Elevated blood levels can be corrected by supplementing these vitamins. As expected from the theoretical findings, supplementation with all three in combination is most effective for this purpose (**C**). Availability of folic acid seems to be more important for homocysteine metabolism than B_{12} and/or B_6 since folic acid yields the best results among single vitamin supplements.

Homocysteine is currently discussed as one of the causes of **atherosclerosis**. This was initially hypothesized based on the observation that patients with homocystinuria, a hereditary metabolic defect that leads to very high blood homocysteine levels, typically exhibit marked atherosclerotic changes. Patients usually die from the consequences (embolisms, etc.) before age 30.

The connection between homocysteinemia and atherosclerosis has since been confirmed in many epidemiological and case-control studies. It is suspected that homocysteine leads to the formation of reactive oxygen species (ROS) through its terminal thiol group. ROS enhance the secretion of growth factors, and thereby cell proliferation, in smooth vascular muscles. Additionally, larger numbers of white blood cells may migrate into the subendothelial space where they differentiate into macrophages. There, they could ingest oxidized LDL, which would turn them into fatty foam cells. The typical vascular degeneration follows: fibrous plaques form, consisting of foam cells, lymphocytes, lipids, and muscle cells, embedded in connective tissue.

The above is an example of another problem that could be improved by high fruit and vegetable nutrition that would supply high levels of folic acid. Vitamin B_6 seems to play a minor role in homocysteine metabolism, whereas sufficient vitamin B_{12} should generally be available due to the body's large storage capacity. For hereditary homocysteinemia, supplementation of pharmacological doses of the respective missing vitamin is indicated.

A. Chemistry

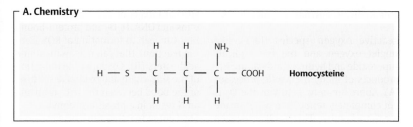

$$H - S - \underset{\underset{H}{\overset{\overset{H}{|}}{|}}{C} - \underset{\underset{H}{\overset{\overset{H}{|}}{|}}{C} - \underset{\underset{H}{\overset{\overset{NH_2}{|}}{|}}{C} - COOH \qquad \textbf{Homocysteine}$$

B. B Vitamin Interactions in Homocysteine Metabolism

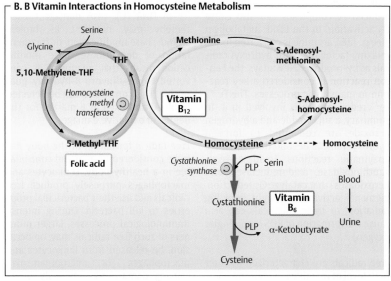

C. Supplementation Effects

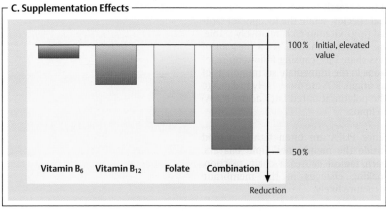

Free Radicals: Formation and Effects

Reactive oxygen species (ROS), like singlet oxygen and the free radicals superoxide and hydroxyl radical, are by-products of many metabolic processes (**A**). Approximately 3–10% of the O_2 is not completely reduced to water inside the mitochondria. This results in oxygen radicals. Auto-oxidation of quinones or reduced Fe-complexes can also cause O_2 activation. In the EDRF metabolism (see p. 128), arginine is converted to the relaxing factor NO, with hydroxyl radicals as by-products. Nowadays, the **Fenton reaction** is considered a key reaction in many toxic processes. The Fe^{3+}/Fe^{2+} redox system is involved in it. In summary, a superoxide and a hydrogen peroxide are converted to form a hydroxyl radical. Beyond that, there are enzymatic reactions (oxidases—e.g., xanthinoxidase, oxidoreductases, and peroxidases) that catalyze O_2 reduction. Pigments activated by light, ionizing radiation, or toxic chemicals can also cause the formation of ROS (e.g., singlet oxygen).

Free radicals are characterized by their **high level of reactivity**, which, however, differs greatly between the various radical species: while the tocopherol radical (e.g., vitamin E) is relatively stable, the hydroxyl radical has a lifespan of less than 1 µs, causing follow-up reactions in the immediate surroundings of its origin. ROS are most likely to damage the polyunsaturated fatty acids (PUFA) in lipids.

Since PUFA are often tightly packed inside the membranes' lipid bilayers, each radical causes a chain reaction, making changes in the **membrane** structure likely.

Further targets of free radicals are proteins and DNA. H_2O_2 and protein-bound Fe^{2+} can lead to formation of ROS (Fenton reaction), that can react with amino acid esters (**B**). Oxidative deamination of the side-chain and oxidative splitting of the bond between the α-C-atom and an N result in a protein carbonyl.

The Fenton reaction can cause hydroxyl radicals to form in the immediate vicinity of **DNA** (**C**). DNA damage caused thereby may manifest as broken strands, base modification, or fragmentation of deoxyribose. Base modification means that guanosine is converted to 7,8-dihydro-8-hydroxy guanosine. This compound can be detected in blood and used as a marker for the degree of oxidative damage.

Free radical formation in the body has to be considered normal and controllable in a healthy body. Leukocytes and macrophages purposely produce free radicals and use their bactericidal properties to kill bacteria. During intense immunological processes, larger numbers of such free radicals may, on occasion, be released from leukocytes and macrophages (or microorganisms), causing damage to previously intact structures.

A. Free Radical Formation

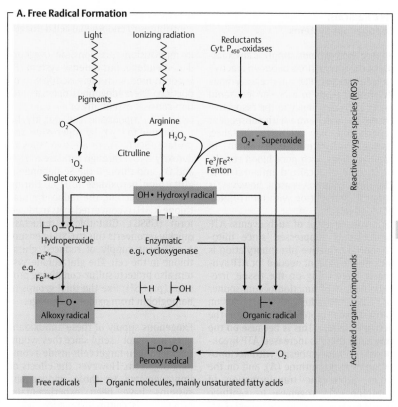

B. Damage to Proteins

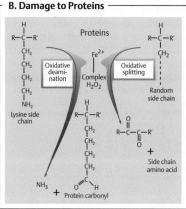

C. DNA Damage

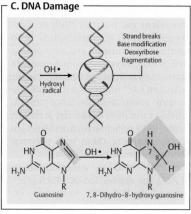

Free Radicals:
Endogenous Systems

Suppression of blood supply is an example of the interactions between reactive oxygen species (ROS) and endogenous defense. It leads to more or less rapid onset of O_2 deficiency in the respective tissue. Such **ischemia** with subsequent **reperfusion** may occur, for instance, during short-term muscle strain, in capillary beds with poor blood supply, or in case of localized inflammation. The most common reason, however, is surgical intervention with interruption of blood flow.

As a consequence of such events, ATP synthesis is suppressed since mitochondrial oxidative phosphorylation is lacking the oxidant needed for ATP synthesis. Depending on the tissue, irreversible loss of function occurs sooner or later. Paradoxically, reperfusion causes even more damage than the actual ischemia. This is because on the one hand there is increased ATP breakdown (no neosynthesis) with accumulation of hypoxanthine (**A**), and on the other, proteolytic transformation of xanthine dehydrogenase to xanthine oxidase (XO), due to increased Ca^{2+} influx into the cell (malfunction of ATP-dependent ion pumps). With renewed oxygen supply, XO metabolizes hypoxanthine to xanthine and uric acid, as well as ROS. Subsequent lipid peroxidation causes membrane damage, causing increased Ca^{2+} influx into the cells. This in turn stimulates phospholipase A_2, causing formation of platelet activation factor (PAF), which in turn activates leukocytes, turning them into polymorphonuclear leukocytes (PMN).

The PMN bind to adhesion factors (ICAM), the expression of which is also induced by ROS. ROS formation, due to activated PMN and proteases, further contributes to endothelial cell damage.

In reperfusion situations, an overburdened **endogenous defense system** (**B**) is confronted with increased ROS production. The endogenous defense system consists essentially of enzyme systems (**C**). Superoxide can quickly be dismutated to H_2O_2 by **superoxide dismutase** (SOD). There are two ways to detoxify H_2O_2: through **catalase** to H_2O and O_2, and through the Se-dependent **glutathion peroxidase** to H_2O. During the latter reaction, the reduced glutathione (GSH) is converted to its oxidized form (GSSG). Glutathione reductase quickly reconverts this to GSH to ensure a sufficient supply of reduced glutathione in the cell. The glutathione system also protects sulfur-containing proteins (prot-SH) like the thiol groups in hemoglobin from oxidative damage.

Exogenous supply of these antioxidant enzymes is not useful since they would not reach their target cells inside a complex organism. However, the effects of improvements to those endogenous systems have been experimentally proven: it is common practice, when conserving certain organs for transplantation, to add an oxidant mixture (containing SOD and allopurinol, among others, to inhibit xanthine oxidase). This greatly improves the organ's chance of survival after reperfusion (i.e., after transplantation).

A. Ischemia and Reperfusion

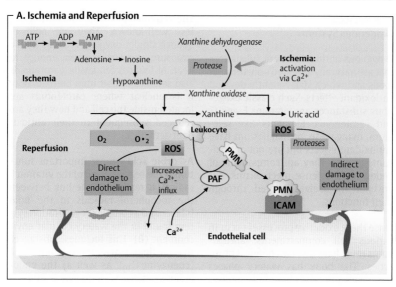

B. Balance Between Production and Defense

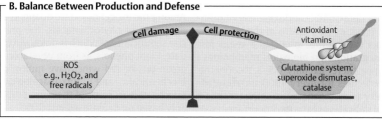

C. Endogenous Defense Mechanism

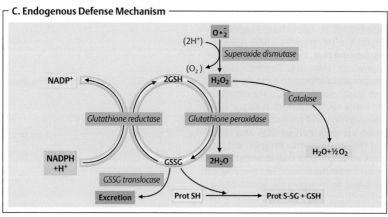

Free Radicals:
Exogenous Systems

Exogenous antioxidants are substances that are naturally supplied only through foods and which subsequently develop antioxidant effects. Such **classic exogenous substances** are vitamins E and C, and carotenoids. Elements like selenium, manganese, or magnesium have antioxidant effects but are not antioxidants proper. They are components of endogenous defense mechanisms, but are not themselves altered through their functions.

Since these oxidative processes occur in various cell compartments, antioxidants must have diverse chemical properties. The body has watery phases (e.g., cytosol) and lipophilic phases (e.g., all membranes). The most important lipid-soluble antioxidant is vitamin E. The long side-chains of the **tocopherols** (see p. 156) predestine them for integration into biological membranes. Since there are only 0.5–3 tocopherol molecules for every 1000 unsaturated fatty acids, regeneration of the tocopherol radical is of extreme importance (see below).

Tocopherols limit lipid peroxidation in membranes by quenching singlet oxygen and/or interrupting chain reactions (**A**). Beyond that, they are necessary for membrane integrity. Recent research also points to effects on gene expression and intracellular signal transduction. For instance, transcription factor NFkB (involved in viral reproduction, among others) is activated by ROS and inhibited by tocopherol. Protein kinase C plays an important role in intracellular signal transduction. The enzyme is inhibited by tocopherols, which reduce cell proliferation. Vitamin E's anticancer effect may be due to this activity.

The activities of **carotenoids** are much less well-known. They are able to quench singlet oxygen produced by UV exposure, converting their energy to heat. At low oxygen levels, carotenoids also seem to inhibit lipid peroxidation. It is unclear where carotenoids are located inside the cell and how they are reduced subsequent to their antioxidant activities.

Ascorbic acid's most important function is the regeneration of the vitamin E radical. It represents the link between the tocopherol radicals in the lipid bilayer and a complex regeneration system found in the watery cellular environment (**B**). This includes substances like α-lipoic acid and ubiquinone (coenzyme Q_{10}), as well as the endogenous defense systems (see p. 204).

Among the exogenous antioxidants is a multitude of phytochemicals, the precise significance of which is unknown to date. Plant phenols, as from vegetables, green tea, or red wine, have multiple, biochemical and pharmacological effects; at least some of them are probably based on defense against ROS.

A. Lipid Membrane Quenching Mechanisms

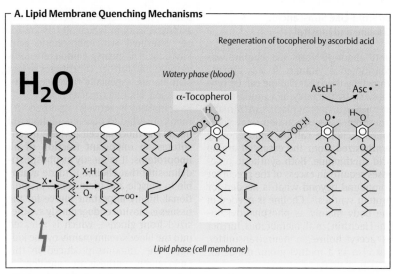

Regeneration of tocopherol by ascorbid acid

Watery phase (blood)

α-Tocopherol

AscH⁻   Asc•⁻

H_2O

Lipid phase (cell membrane)

B. Vitamin E Regeneration

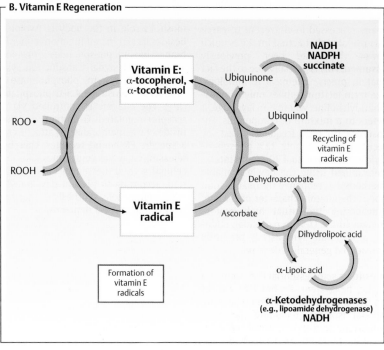

Vitamin-Like Substances:
Choline and Inositol

Until about 40 years ago, **choline** was considered a vitamin. It was already known by then that choline can be synthesized by the body in a similar manner as niacin: just as niacin can be made from the essential amino acid tryptophan, choline can be endogenously synthesized from the essential amino acid methionine. Both synthetic processes require an excess of the precursor compound beyond what is needed for protein synthesis. Choline is needed in the body mainly as phosphatidylcholine (**lecithin**) in all membranes, further as **acetylcholine**, a neurotransmitter, but also as a methyl group donor for intermediate metabolism.

Although choline is abundant in **foods** and lecithin is used as an additive in many processed foods, recent research has revealed that **actual intake** is much lower than had been previously assumed. This is partially due to the fact that in precise chemical terminology, the term lecithin applies only to phosphatidylcholine, whereas in lay usage, it refers to a mixture of compounds. For instance, the most frequently used soy lecithin contains only 22% phosphatidylcholine. The actual 300 mg/d intake, determined using the newly available methods, has reopened the old question about the vitamin character of choline; considering the usual high protein intakes in the U.S., in particular, endogenous choline synthesis is presently considered generally adequate.

Inositol, a semi-essential B vitamin, is a cyclic, hexavalent alcohol that carries an OH-group at each carbon. There are several isomers, including the most important: free-form inositol and myo-inositol. In foods, particularly in the outer layers of cereals, it occurs mostly as phytic acid, in which all OH-groups are esterified with phosphoric acid. Phytic acid is nearly completely indigestible, and further, contributes to loss of minerals, especially trace elements, by its ion-binding capacity.

Free inositol is actively absorbed (**A**), then converted to phosphatidylinositol inside the mucosal cells, where it constitutes an important **fraction of all lipoproteins**. It is mostly as phosphatidylinositol that choline is made available to muscle and brain cells. An additional, highly important source for the tissues is inositol endogenously synthesized from glucose, which is released into the bloodstream mainly by the kidneys. The amounts produced in this endogenous synthesis are considerably higher than any potential intakes from foods.

Inositol's role in the body is twofold: besides its significant function in membranes, inositol phosphatides represent an important signal transduction system. In this system, phospholipase C produces inositol-1,4,5-triphosphate (IP_3). The enzyme is controlled via a receptor-regulated G-protein on the inside of the membrane. IP_3 attaches to a specific ER-bound receptor, thereby releasing Ca, which contributes to intracellular second messenger Ca. In addition, according to present-day knowledge, endogenous synthesis of inositol is sufficient to meet demands.

A. Inositol and Inositol Phosphate

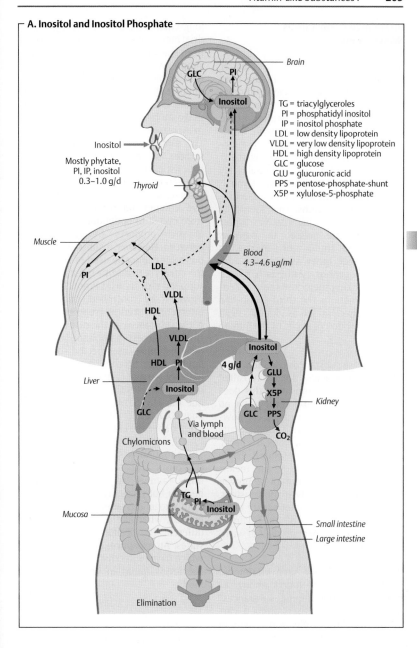

Brain

GLC → PI
Inositol

TG = triacylglyceroles
PI = phosphatidyl inositol
IP = inositol phosphate
LDL = low density lipoprotein
VLDL = very low density lipoprotein
HDL = high density lipoprotein
GLC = glucose
GLU = glucuronic acid
PPS = pentose-phosphate-shunt
X5P = xylulose-5-phosphate

Inositol →
Mostly phytate,
PI, IP, inositol
0.3–1.0 g/d

Thyroid

Muscle

PI

LDL
?
VLDL
HDL

Blood
4.3–4.6 µg/ml

VLDL
HDL   PI   Inositol   4 g/d   GLU

Liver   X5P

GLC   GLC   PPS   *Kidney*

CO_2

Chylomicrons

Via lymph
and blood

TG PI
Mucosa   Inositol

Small intestine
Large intestine

Elimination

Vitamin-Like Substances: Nonvitamins

In the early stages of vitamin research, before an exact meaning of the term "vitamins" was defined, newly discovered substances were frequently assigned vitamin properties without their actual effects being known. This is why, even today, a number of "pseudovitamins" still exist (**B**). Among them, for instance, are the essential fatty acids, which used to be called vitamin F. While they continue to be essential, they are not vitamins. This should be clear from the quantitative aspect alone—they are needed in gram as opposed to milli- or microgram amounts. For other substances, adequate endogenous synthesis has been shown, making them lose their "essential" designation. The third group had been falsely classified as vitamins even though they do not occur in the human body.

Even if those substances (excluding the essential fatty acids) are today called nonvitamins or vitaminoids, this does not necessarily mean that they have no metabolic effects. Since they are nowadays sold mostly as food supplements with claimed pharmacological effects, they ought to be measured by a pharmacological yardstick. This means in short: effects that cannot be proven in a double-blind study are nonexistent. Since nonvitamins do not satisfy these strict criteria, most of the claimed effects must be a mere product of wishful thinking.

Prime examples for such vitaminoid preparations can be found among so-called "non-drug doping substances" propagated in the fitness arena. **L-carnitine (B)** plays a role in transport of long-chain fatty acids at the mitochondrial membrane. The sales pitch derived from this fact sounds as logical as it is simple: with increased energy metabolism (exercise), fatty acids have to undergo β-oxidation; therefore, optimizing fatty acid transport mechanisms make more energy available, resulting in increased performance.

The sales pitch for many other substances sold today is based on similarly simplistic arguments. Since they are not registered as pharmaceuticals, exact sales figures are unknown: in competitive athletics and in the fitness arena—from cyclist to bodybuilder—non-users of such products are few and far between. However, a substance's metabolic role cannot be used to extrapolate the effects of that same substance when supplied exogenously. Proof can only be provided by controlled, double-blind intervention studies (supplementation of the substance): in the case of L-carnitine, the success in unblinded studies is overwhelming—as expected—but nil in double-blind studies. Recent studies have shown that carnitine supplements do increase carnitine plasma levels but not muscle carnitine levels. Since it does not reach its target tissue, it simply cannot have the claimed effect.

The situation is similar for coenzyme Q_{10}, orotic acid ("vitamin B_{13}"), creatinine, taurine, and many others. A healthy body usually does not benefit from exogenous supply of such compounds, whereas the situation may be different in specific, defined disease states. An exception are bioflavonoids, which have protective effects already at the levels found in bioflavonoid-rich foods.

A. Nonvitamins

Nonvitamins
Essential, but incorrect designation, e.g., fatty acids
Adequate endogenous synthesis e.g., coenzyme Q
Not naturally present in the human body e.g., bioflavonoids
"Pharmacological" effects of high dosages
Yes
?
?
Required from foods
Yes, essential
No
?

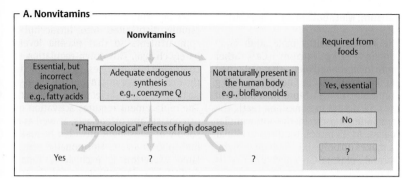

B. Structures of Selected Nonvitamins

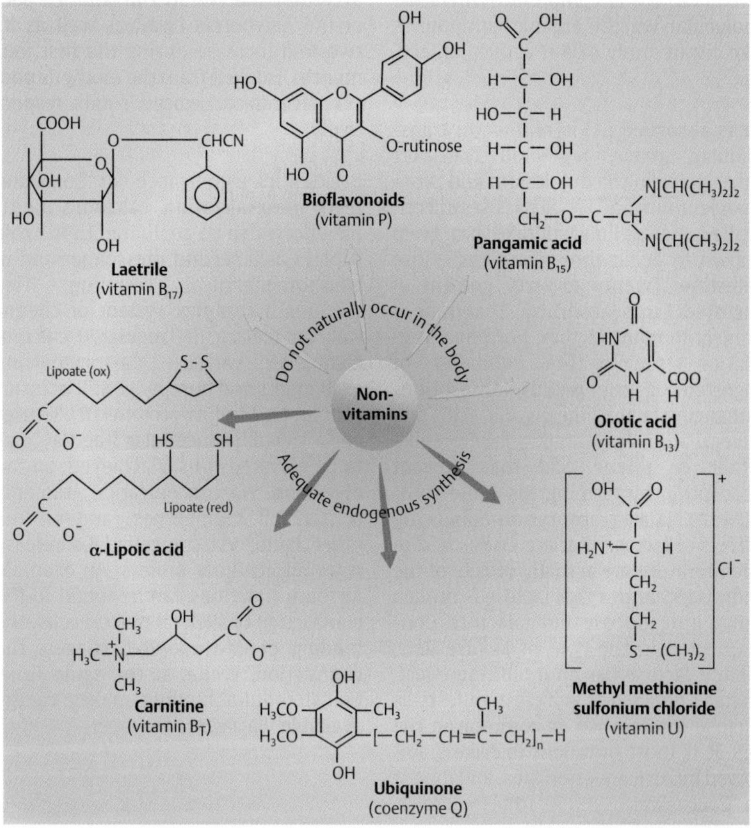

Laetrile
(vitamin B17)
Bioflavonoids
(vitamin P)
O-rutinose
Pangamic acid
(vitamin B15)
Do not naturally occur in the body
Non-vitamins
Adequate endogenous synthesis
Lipoate (ox)
Lipoate (red)
α-Lipoic acid
Orotic acid
(vitamin B13)
Methyl methionine sulfonium chloride
(vitamin U)
Carnitine
(vitamin BT)
Ubiquinone
(coenzyme Q)

Calcium: Metabolism and Functions

The average healthy male adult body contains ≥1 kg calcium (Ca)—rather more in big-boned men—that of women ~800 g, and of a newborn ~30 g (1 mmol = 40 mg). More than 99.5 % of the Ca is found in bones and teeth, the remainder mostly in the intracellular spaces. At 35 mmol, total extracellular Ca makes up only ~0.1 % of body weight. Normal plasma-Ca concentration is 2.5 mmol/L, 47 % of that protein-bound, mainly to albumin. Of the remaining "free" Ca, 6 % is complexed with low-molecular-weight organic compounds like citrate; only 47 % is active, ionized, Ca^{2+}.

Ca is **absorbed** (**A**) in two ways: transcellular, active, regulated transport takes place in the duodenum and proximal jejunum and while passive, uncontrolled, paracellular uptake has been shown to occur throughout the entire intestine. Twenty to sixty percent of ingested Ca is absorbed. That rate is subject to many factors: hormonal regulation (see p. 214), solubility of ingested Ca compounds, absorption-enhancing factors like organic acids and several amino acids, and inhibitors like oxalic or phytic acid that prevent absorption by forming insoluble complexes. The absorption-enhancing effects of lactose that are often cited in the literature are actually effects of the monosaccharides that lactose is broken down into, glucose and galactose. Consequently, in the case of lactase deficiency, lactose has an inhibiting effect. Lactase deficiency, which manifests as **lactose intolerance**, is common in the U.S. It is most prevalent in Asians, followed by African Americans, and lowest in Caucasians (~85/50/10 % incidence, respectively, 25 % overall).

After absorption into the blood, Ca is rapidly distributed into intracellular compartments so that plasma levels barely change. This down-regulation is controlled by hormones. The skeleton is the **main storage organ** for Ca. Each day, up to 1000 mg of skeletal Ca is replaced. The replacement requires activation of osteoblasts and osteoclasts, as well as a supply of phosphate provided by alkaline phosphatase. Hormonally regulated **excretion** is exclusively renal. Additionally, large amounts of Ca are lost through pancreatic and biliary excretion and sweat. The large Ca pool of the newborn's body, as well as its two-fold increase during the first four months, is taken from the mother's pool via placenta and mother's milk, respectively.

Besides its significance for bone and teeth **mineralization**, calcium's multiple effects can be attributed to the **role** it plays as a **second messenger** and in **electromechanical coupling**. This requires a complex system of chemically or electrically regulated calcium channels, various Ca-transporting exchangers and pumps, as well as intracellular Ca-binding proteins (**B**). To trigger a signal, intracellular free Ca^{2+} has to be elevated; this is achieved, on the one hand, via concentration gradients across cell membranes; and on the other hand, via controlled Ca release from intracellular buffers. An example for both functions can be found in the contraction of skeletal muscle cells: the binding of Ca-troponin C triggers the contraction, while, at the same time, Ca-calmodulin binding makes energy available via a cascade.

A. Calcium Metabolism

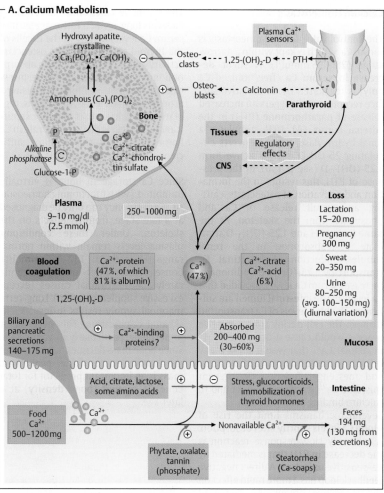

B. Calmodulin, a Ca-Binding Protein

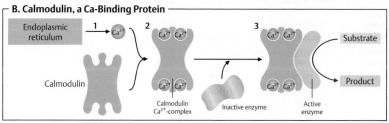

Calcium Homeostasis

The control value for Ca homeostasis is serum Ca, which is kept within a narrow range (2.2–2.6 mmol/l). A slight **decrease in serum Ca** (free, ionized Ca only) is registered by Ca-sensitive surface receptors and triggers an increased release of **parathormone** (PTH) in the adrenal cortex (**A**). PTH stimulates a renal hydroxylase, which converts circulating 25-OH-D into its active form **1,25-(OH)$_2$-D** (see p. 150). In the presence of PTH, this results in the formation and activation of osteoclasts, causing an overall release of Ca and phosphate from the **skeleton**. At the same time, PTH and 1,25-(OH)$_2$-D stimulate Ca-reabsorption in the **renal tubules**. Induction of **intestinal Ca transport** by 1,25-(OH)$_2$-D additionally increases serum Ca levels, provided that Ca levels in the intestinal lumen are sufficient. The high levels of Ca transported through the cell during this absorptive process would cause a drastic increase in cellular Ca^{2+} that would affect many cellular processes due to calcium's second messenger function. To prevent this, free Ca^{2+} is immediately bound to calcium binding protein (CaBP).

Several mechanisms limit the **rise of blood Ca levels** shortly after absorption. A relatively slow-response reaction is the **decrease in PTH** that is mediated by Ca-sensitive receptors. A direct negative feedback loop has a more rapid effect on the respective organs. An increased supply of Ca and phosphate **inhibits osteoclast activity**. The rise of free Ca in the blood has several **renal** effects: inhibition of 1-hydroxylase, reduction of glomerular filtration rates, diuretic effects in the proximal tubules, and inhibition of antidiuretic hormone (ADH). This probably involves a Ca-sensitive receptor on the renal cell surface.

The hormone **calcitonin** affects blood Ca levels long-term. It forms at elevated serum Ca levels mainly in the C-cells of the thyroid gland. It inhibits osteoclast activity and thereby induces Ca absorption into bone. At the same time, intestinal Ca transport is inhibited, causing a drop in serum Ca levels. In humans, regulation via calcitonin is of minor significance. PTH levels play a major role in Ca homeostasis, and this requires sufficient availability of vitamin D.

Since Ca storage in bone is virtually unlimited, (with functioning homeostasis) Ca deficiency can only be diagnosed at a late stage, from its effects on the skeleton. Under these conditions, plasma levels remain within normal range (ionized Ca: 1.12–1.23 mmol/l). Consequently, hyper- or hypocalcemia rarely has nutritional causes (except excessive supplementation). Long-term marginal supply results in insufficient skeletal calcification. This is of major importance, particularly in youngsters. Since bone mass declines naturally as of the fourth decade of life, **peak bone mass** is an important predictor for total bone Ca content (**bone density**) at a later age.

A. Calcium Homeostasis

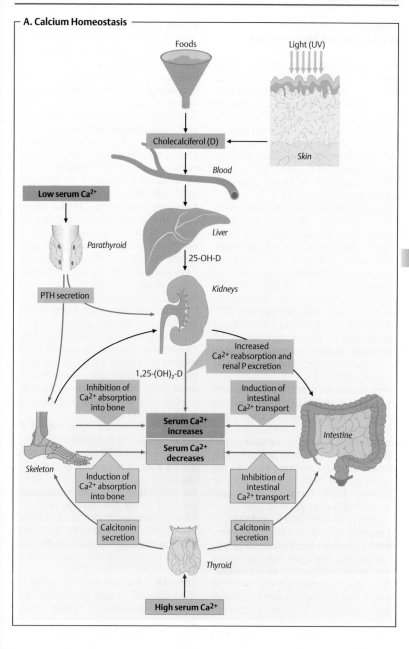

Foods

Light (UV)

Cholecalciferol (D)

Skin

Blood

Low serum Ca²⁺

Parathyroid

Liver

25-OH-D

PTH secretion

Kidneys

Increased Ca²⁺ reabsorption and renal P excretion

1,25-(OH)₂-D

Inhibition of Ca²⁺ absorption into bone

Induction of intestinal Ca²⁺ transport

Serum Ca²⁺ increases

Serum Ca²⁺ decreases

Intestine

Skeleton

Induction of Ca²⁺ absorption into bone

Inhibition of intestinal Ca²⁺ transport

Calcitonin secretion

Calcitonin secretion

Thyroid

High serum Ca²⁺

Calcium:
Occurrence and Requirements

Ca is found mostly in milk and dairy products, several vegetables, herbs, and nuts (**A**). Muscle meats, fish, and fruit are low in Ca. According to the USDA, in 1994, 73 % of food Ca intake in the U.S. stemmed from dairy, 9 % from vegetables and 5 % from grain products. Even though grains contain little calcium, they constitute a major source of Ca in ethnic diets rich in them (Mexican-American, Puerto Rican).

Milk contains ~120 mg Ca/l. Milk products have higher contents, e. g., hard cheeses like Swiss cheese (~900 mg/100 g)—the most Ca-rich food is old, dehydrated Parmesan with ~1200 mg/100 g. Processed cheeses like American cheese contain 500–550 mg/100 g. Low-Ca exceptions are some dairy products like cottage cheese (32–68 mg/100 g) and ricotta (115–150 mg/100 g). Except in cottage cheese, fat content tends to be inversely correlated to cheese Ca content: the higher the fat content, the less Ca.

Some vegetables contain large amounts of Ca. Green kitchen herbs like basil (up to 1000 mg/100 g), parsley, chives, and chervil contain even more Ca, but they do not play a large quantitative role. Pine nuts, almonds, and sesame seeds are also good Ca sources (225–785 mg Ca/100 g)—but high in fat—as well as sardines, most forms of tofu, and Ca-fortified orange juice.

Because of Ca homeostasis and the lack of measurable parameters, **Ca requirements** (**B**) cannot be determined by balance studies. Therefore, current recommendations are based on **AI**, not on **EAR**. Even though humans are able to adjust to very low calcium intakes (<200 mg) for short periods, it has to be assumed that the **minimum intake** for an adult should not fall below 500 mg/d long-term. A safety margin is necessary to account for individual variability. The present **dietary recommendations** take into account that more Ca (1300 mg/d) is needed for maximum skeletal calcification during the growth phase; 1000 mg/d are recommended as a **maintenance dose** until age 50, whereupon a 200 mg increase appears necessary to counteract bone loss. Many scientists do not consider these recommended amounts to be "optimal": the NIH, for instance, recommends up to 1500 mg Ca/d for adolescents and women after menopause. It is assumed that an **optimal Ca supply** during all phases of life, particularly before age 35, contributes to a positive Ca balance and thereby has a preventive effect for osteoporosis.

Actual intakes deviate greatly from these recommendations. Mean intakes in males and females above nine years of age were 865 and 625 mg/d (21.6 and 15.6 mmol), respectively, in 1994. Men's intakes tend to be closer to adequate, with adolescents and elderly women most likely to be deficient. Approximately 25% of women consume no more than 300 mg/d.

The most important **symptom of Ca deficiency** today is osteoporosis (**C**). It results in vertebral fractures in women, mostly after menopause, and at a higher age in hip fractures, also in men. Out of the 100 000 women with hip fractures per year in the U.S., 50 000 never get back on their feet. Anorectics and highly competitive female athletes frequently develop osteoporosis much earlier, due mostly to cessation of estrogen production.

The **UL** for adults is 2500 mg (62.5 mmol/d). Excessive intakes may lead to hypercalcemia, kidney stones, and renal insufficiency.

A. Occurrence and Daily Requirement

The daily requirement of 1000 mg Ca is contained in:

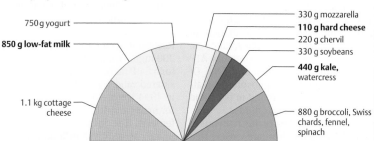

- 750 g yogurt
- **850 g low-fat milk**
- 1.1 kg cottage cheese
- 330 g mozzarella
- **110 g hard cheese**
- 220 g chervil
- 330 g soybeans
- **440 g kale,** watercress
- 880 g broccoli, Swiss chards, fennel, spinach

B. Adequate Intakes (AI, 1999) and UL

Life Stage and Gender Group	Age	Calcium		UL
		(mg/d)	(mmol/d)	(mg/d)
Infants	0 – 6 mo	210	5.3	Not possible
	7 – 12 mo	270	6.8	to establish
Children	1 – 3 y	500	12.5	2500
	4 – 8 y	800	20	2500
Boys and girls	9 – 18 y	1300	32.5	2500
Adults	19 – 50 y	1000	25	2500
	>50 y	1200	30	2500
Pregnancy and lactation	14 – 18 y	1300	32.5	2500
	19 – 50 y	1000	25	2500

C. Deficiency Symptoms

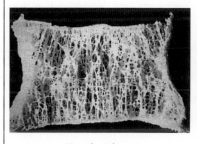

Normal vertebra

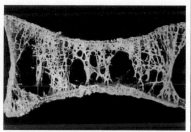

Osteoporosis

Phosphorus

Phosphorus (P, 1 mmol ≈31 mg) occurs in the body exclusively as phosphate and is involved in the formation of hydroxyl apatite (Ca phosphate) in bone, as well as organic esters like ATP and phospholipids, DNA, and RNA. Of the ~700 g total body phosphorus (calculated as P), 85 % is found in bone and only 1 % in extracellular fluids.

Even though **regulatory mechanisms** of phosphate metabolism are closely tied in with Ca homeostasis, plasma phosphate levels fluctuate over a wider range (0.7–1.5 mmol/l). Since increased plasma phosphate levels (**A**) reduce the levels of free, ionized Ca due to the solubility product, they cause increased PTH secretion, which in turn leads to increased renal phosphate excretion; the expected resulting formation of 1,25-$(OH)_2$-D, however, is inhibited by the high phosphate levels. Lowered 1,25-$(OH)_2$-D concentrations reduce intestinal phosphate absorption and decrease phosphate release from bones. These interactions ensure that phosphate levels can be down-regulated without a severe impact on Ca metabolism. At persistently elevated levels, the increase in PTH and decrease in a 1,25-$(OH)_2$-D have consequences: bone loss, which can, in extreme cases, even lead to spontaneous fractures. This syndrome, termed "secondary hyperparathyroidism" occurs mostly in cases of renal insufficiency, when renal phosphate excretion is impaired.

P occurs in all **foods** (**B**) as phosphate. Meat and fish contain ~200 mg/100 g (figures given as P), milk products up to 1100 mg/100 g. Processed cheese is very high-phosphate, since phosphates are used for processing. Cereal flours contain 100–400 mg/100 g, depending on the degree of refinement; however, the P contained in the outer layers is bound to phytate and is, therefore, poorly absorbed.

Recommended P intakes for adults are 700 mg/d (**C**). Older recommendations for a Ca:P ratio of 1:1 are no longer considered valid. Mean P intakes in the U.S. in 1994 were ~1500 mg (48.2 mmol)/d for males and 1025 mg (33 mmol)/d for females. The increasing use of phosphates as additives in food processing over the past two decades and increased consumption of processed foods contributes to increasingly high intakes. P intakes usually exceed Ca intakes (Ca:P ratio 1:1.7 = 0.59). P is, therefore, not considered a critical mineral. The **UL** is 4 g/d. Exclusive infant nutrition from mother's milk constitutes a special case: for exclusively breast-fed infants the limiting factor for bone mineralization is P, not Ca. The Ca:P ratio in mother's milk is ~2:1, preventing renal P overload in the infants' immature kidneys.

Alimentary **phosphate deficiencies** are unknown. Deficiency symptoms have been reported only as a result of parenteral nutrition and from daily use of antacids containing aluminum. Early symptoms are generalized physical weakness; long-term effects on the skeleton are likely.

A. Regulation of Plasma Phosphate Levels

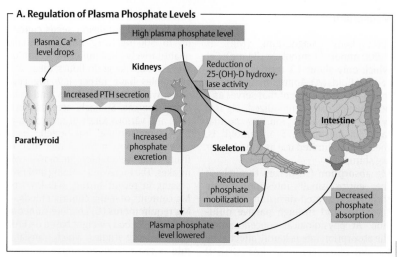

B. Occurrence

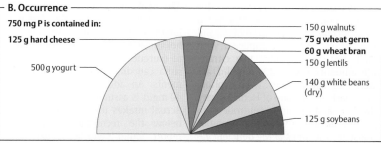

750 mg P is contained in:

125 g hard cheese

500 g yogurt

- 150 g walnuts
- **75 g wheat germ**
- **60 g wheat bran**
- 150 g lentils
- 140 g white beans (dry)
- 125 g soybeans

C. Recommended Intakes (DRI/AI*, 1999) and UL

Life Stage and Gender Group	Age	Phosphorus (mg/d)	Phosphorus (mmol/d)	UL (mg/d)
Infants	0 – 6 mo	100*	3.2	No supplements
	7 – 12 mo	275*	8.9	
Children	1 – 3 y	460	14.8	3000
	4 – 8 y	500	16.1	3000
Adolescents	9 – 18 y	1250	40.3	4000
Adults	19 – 70 y	700	22.6	4000
	> 70 y	700	22.6	3000
Pregnancy	14 – 18 y	1250	40.3	3500
	19 – 50 y	700	22.6	3500
Lactation	14 – 18 y	1250	40.3	4000
	19 – 50 y	700	22.6	4000

Magnesium

Total body magnesium (Mg) is ~1000 mmol (1 mmol = 24 mg), of which only about 1 % resides in extracellular fluids (**A**). Approximately 65 % is found in bone—some of that serves as a pool, which can be mobilized. Mg is a typical intracellular ion. Its normal range in plasma (0.75–1.1 mmol/l) is, therefore, of limited use as a marker for Mg status.

Mg **absorption** (**A**) occurs throughout the entire small intestine mostly through facilitated diffusion, which is saturable, and through passive diffusion. At physiological concentrations, the absorption rate is hardly affected by Ca and phosphate, and $1,25-(OH)_2$-D does not seem to be very relevant for Mg absorption. Since >60 % of the Mg in blood prevails as free, ionized Mg^{2+}, and an additional 10% is complexed with small organic molecules like citrate, large amounts of Mg (~200 mmol/d) are filtered by the kidneys. Reabsorption, particularly in the loop of Henle, is very effective and tightly controlled to ensure that urinary excretion becomes almost zero at times of Mg deficiency.

Through its **function** as a **cofactor** for ~300 enzymes, Mg is involved in nearly all aspects of anabolic and catabolic metabolism. In many reactions, Mg^{2+} occurs as an ATP-Mg^{2+} complex that forms during reactions between enzymes and substrates and enables transphosphorylation. Many other effects of Mg are based on its resemblance to Ca. Therefore, Mg is considered **calcium's** physiological **antagonist**. Mg modulates the influx of extracellular Ca through specific Ca channels, as well as calcium's intracellular effects. Intracellular Mg^{2+} also affects K^+ channels, particularly in the heart muscle.

Few **foods** are Mg-rich (**B**). Wheat germ and bran and sunflower seeds contain up to 500 mg/100 g but are usually quantitatively insignificant. Common staple foods like grain flours, meat, and vegetables have rather low Mg contents; whole-grain products tend to be better sources. Spinach, acorn squash, tofu, and various kinds of nuts contain 85–130 mg/serving. All green, leafy vegetables contain Mg. A diet high in fruits and vegetables increases Mg intakes. The increased refining and processing in recent history has lowered Mg contents of many common foods.

Mg requirements (**C**) are determined at 3–4.5 mg/kg body weight based on **EAR**, using balance studies, which translates into a recommended intake of 400–420 mg/d and 310–320 mg/d for men and women, respectively. Additional losses through profuse sweating, alcohol abuse (renal wasting), or regular use of diuretics that lead to hypermagnesuria can drastically increase requirements. An additional requirement of 40 mg/d is assumed during pregnancy. **Actual intakes** tend to remain slightly below the recommendations; some reports found lower levels, particularly among minorities. In general, Mg is not considered a problem mineral; rather, a marginal supply situation is assumed to exist in all age groups.

Symptoms of classic magnesium deficiency—neuromuscular disturbances, including tetany—are not to be expected with Western nutrition. Preventive and therapeutic effects of optimal intakes or even elevated Mg pools, for cardio-therapeutic purposes, prevention of certain muscle cramps, or inhibition of uterine contractions have much greater relevance. Toxicity occurs only from nonfood sources. The **UL** for adults is 350 mg of supplemental Mg.

A. Uptake and Distribution

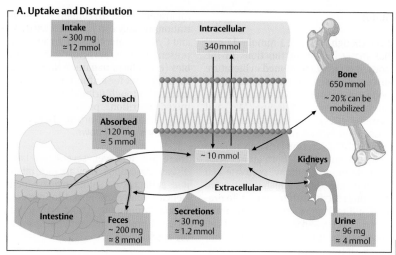

B. Occurrence and Daily Requirement

The daily requirement of 350 mg magnesium is contained in:

- 200 g nuts
- 1 kg fish
- 1.2 kg meat
- 250 g rolled oats
- **150 g cereal germs**
- **60 g wheat bran**
- 75 g sunflower seeds
- 200 g beans (dry)
- 1.2 kg vegetables
- 500 g spinach

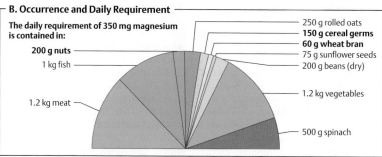

C. Recommended Intakes (DRI/AI*, 1999) and UL

Life Stage and Gender Group	Age	Magnesium		UL
		(mg/d)	(mmol/d)	(mg/d)
Infants	0 – 6 mo	30*	1.1	ND
	7 – 12 mo	75*	3.1	ND
Children	1 – 3 y	80	3.3	65
	4 – 8 y	130	5.4	110
Boys and girls	9 – 13 y	240	10.0	350
Adolescent males	14 – 18 y	410	17.1	350
Adolescent females	14 – 18 y	360	15.0	350
Men	19 – 30 y	400	16.7	350
	> 31 y	420	17.5	350
Women	19 – 30 y	310	13.3	350
	> 31 y	320	13.3	350
Pregnancy	14 – 18 y	400	16.7	350
	19 – 30 y	350	15.0	350
	31 – 50 y	360	15.0	350
Lactation	14 – 18 y	360	15.0	350
	19 – 30 y	310	13.3	350
	31 – 50 y	320	13.3	350

Sulfur

Even though sulfur (S, 1 mmol = 32 mg) has many important functions in the body, it is rarely mentioned in literature discussing essential nutrients. Since the body's main sources of S are the sulfurous amino acids methionine (Met) and cysteine (Cys), the mechanism of S absorption is that of the amino acids (see p. 124). **Excretion** is mainly renal as inorganic sulfate (**A**). Both amino acids degrade to form sulfonyl pyruvate and sulfur dioxide (SO_2), which is converted to highly reactive sulfite (SO_3^{2-}). To prevent sulfite from reacting with thiamin, proteins, NAD, and other important cell components, it has to be quickly eliminated. Intracellular sulfite concentrations are kept at very low levels by sulfite oxidase: the product, sulfate (SO_4^{2-}), is nontoxic and is filtered out by the kidneys. Small amounts of sulfite may be taken up with foods, since a number of products are "sulfured" (treated with SO_2) to prevent oxidative and microbial decomposition.

An alternative pathway of cysteine degradation leads to taurine, which is subsequently conjugated with bile acids. Degradation of sulfurous glycosaminoglycans (GAGs) also yields sulfate directly, with specialized sulfatases splitting the sulfate off the ring. Before certain compounds, like steroids, can be excreted, they have to be esterified with sulfuric acid. Therefore, ~10 % of the S in urine occurs in ester sulfate form (e.g., estrone sulfate).

Besides providing S for the endogenous synthesis of a multitude of sulfurous substances (e.g., heparin, cerebrosides), the sulfurous amino acids Met and Cys are important for the structure of proteins (e.g., disulfide bridges).

All protein **foods** (**B**) contain S. Concentrations usually correlate well with Met and Cys contents. Nonprotein S may be present in foods, particularly in vegetables (e.g., allicin in garlic). No **requirements** are set for sulfur. 1.0–1.3 g S/d is excreted through urine during normal, mixed nutrition, probably reflecting daily amounts absorbed. **Deficiency symptoms** are unknown.

There are, however, several S-related disease conditions. They are rare, inherited sulfatase or sulfite oxidase deficiencies, which are linked to impaired mental function. Using a low-S, reduced-protein diet would be a sensible approach here.

Toxic reactions to sulfurous substances are common. For instance, hydrogen sulfide (H_2S), but also excessive use of S as a laxative, can cause sulfhemoglobinemia, irreversibly damaging hemoglobin and making it unable to transport O_2. Another common reaction is pseudoallergic: 1–5 % of asthmatics react to sulfite. In these cases, only rigorous avoidance of all foods produced with sulfur additives provides relief. Since nowadays, many semifinished foods are preserved with sulfur compounds, in extreme cases, patients may have to avoid all industrially prepared foods.

A. Metabolism

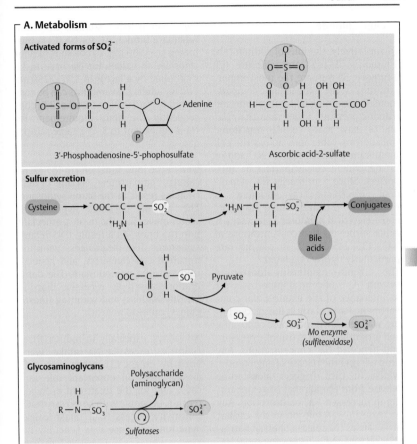

B. Occurrence

The amount of sulfur equivalent to daily
urinary sulfur excretion (1000 mg) is contained in:

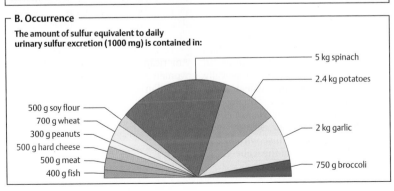

Sodium Chloride

Quantitatively, the ions of sodium (Na, 1 mmol = 23 mg) and chlorine (Cl, 1 mmol = 35 mg) are the most important ions of the extracellular compartment, determining its total volume and osmotic pressure. Other than that, Na^+ and Cl^- have many cellular **functions**: transporting other ions across the cell membrane usually requires Na^+ and/or Cl^--dependent cotransporters or antiporters. Since a primarily Na^+-dependent electrochemical gradient is needed for transmembrane transport and electrical membrane processes, it is not surprising that concentrations of Na^+ (135–145 mmol/l in plasma) are particularly tightly regulated.

The **renin-angiotensin-aldosterone system (A)** is of central importance for maintenance of the extracellular compartment. Particularly in the venous lining, wall tension is measured constantly and is tightly linked to osmotic pressure and hence to Na^+ concentrations. Any drop triggers the release of angiotensin, which in turn triggers aldosterone release from the adrenal cortex resulting in increased Na^+ reabsorption. Any increase in wall tension in the cardiac atria causes the release of atrial natriuretic factor (ANF)—increasing renal Na^+ excretion.

Staple foods (B) contain relatively little Na^+ and Cl^- (meat and vegetables ~100 mg Na/100 g, only traces in grains). Food processing drastically increases Na content: wheat flour <5 mg Na/100 g, bread >500 mg Na/100 g. "Good" sources of Na are abundant today: cheese or salami with >2.0 g/100 g, salted codfish with >7.0 g/100 g are just the tip of the iceberg.

Based on balance studies, the adult **Adequate Intake (AI)** for Na **(C)** is estimated at ~1500 mg. To obtain values for chloride, all values for Na have to be multiplied by a factor of 1.5 (~2250 mg Cl/d for adults). Na amounts can be converted to NaCl using a factor of 2.5; consequently the daily requirement for Na is equivalent to 3.75 g table salt per day.

Due to the ions' functions in the extracellular compartment, **Na and Cl deficiencies** result in the same symptoms. The plasma becomes hypoosmolar. Water moves into the tissues, especially into the brain. As a result, CNS-related symptoms like headaches, vomiting, impaired consciousness, and generalized seizures predominate. The dehydration caused by excessive diarrhea (mostly Na loss) and vomiting (mostly Cl loss) can lead to death.

Nowadays, especially in industrialized countries, **excessive Na intake** (worsened by excess Cl) rather than deficiency, plays an important role as a cause and for the treatment of hypertension. In people with hereditary NaCl-sensitivity, excess NaCl intake causes hypertension. Since it is generally not known who is "salt-sensitive," an overall reduction of NaCl intake (<6 g NaCl/d) is desirable as a preventive measure. The **UL** for Na is 2.3 g and for Cl 3.5 g (= 5.8 g table salt). In 2003, >95 % of American men and 70 % of American women 31–50 years old (90 and 50 % in Canadians) consumed NaCl in excess of the UL.

A. Regulation of Na Metabolism

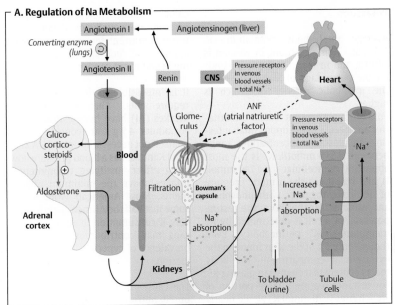

B. Occurrence and Daily Sodium Requirement

The estimated daily requirement of 550 mg sodium is contained in:

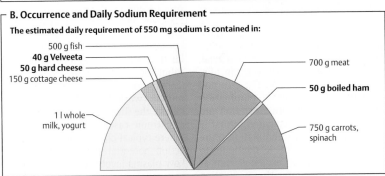

- 500 g fish
- **40 g Velveeta**
- **50 g hard cheese**
- 150 g cottage cheese
- 1 l whole milk, yogurt
- 700 g meat
- **50 g boiled ham**
- 750 g carrots, spinach

C. Adequate Intakes for Sodium and Chloride (AI, 2004) and UL

Life Stage and Gender Group	Age	AI			UL		
		Na (g/d)	CL (g/d)	NaCl (mmol/d)	Na (g/d)	CL (g/d)	NaCl (mmol/d)
Infants	0 – 6 mo	0.12	0.18	5			
	7 – 12 mo	0.37	0.57	16			
Children	1 – 3 y	1.0	1.5	42	1.5	2.3	65
	4 – 8 y	1.2	1.9	53	1.9	2.9	83
Adolescents	9 – 13 y	1.5	2.3	65	2.2	3.4	95
	14 – 18 y	1.5	2.3	65	2.3	3.6	100
Adults	19 – 50 y	1.5	2.3	65	2.3	3.6	100
	50 – 70 y	1.3	2.0	55	2.3	3.6	100
	≥ 70 y	1.2	1.8	50	2.3	3.6	100

Potassium

Average total body potassium (K, 1 mmol ~39 mg) content in women is ~100 g, and in men ~150 g. It depends on the percentage of lean body mass, the metabolic activity of which is higher.

Potassium **absorption** is near quantitative and occurs in the upper small intestine. In plasma, concentrations range between 3.5–5 mmol/l. K^+ is the most abundant intracellular ion (140 mmol/l), and maintains the osmotic pressure of our cells, together with phosphate and proteins. Furthermore, the resting potential of a cell is determined by its membrane's K^+ permeability. Even though only 2% of the K^+ is found in the extracellular compartment, the body reacts acutely to a change in plasma K^+. For instance, eating a large portion of French fries (~70 mmol K) would nearly double the plasma K^+ level—a deadly rise. Since only ~50% of this K^+ shows up in the urine postprandially, rapid transport of incoming K^+ into the intracellular compartment is crucial. After a meal, this is achieved primarily by insulin, which activates Na^+-K^+-ATPase to pull K^+ into the cells. Renal **elimination** occurs primarily by active secretion into the distal tubules—regulated primarily by aldosterone. This elimination route has the advantage that K^+ continues to be at least partially excreted even at reduced filtration rates, thus preventing life-threatening blood K^+ levels for a while even under such reduced filtration conditions.

K is found in all **foods** (A). Good sources are several vegetables like spinach, Swiss chard, or winter squash, as well as certain fruits. The most well-known is the banana: while it is true that it contains 250 mg K/100 g, it also has a high caloric content. Therefore, other types of fruit are equally good sources in terms of nutrient density. The following applies to all foods: washing and cooking in water can cause great K losses.

It is impossible to determine exact K requirements. Therefore, **Adequate Intakes** (**AI**) have been estimated (**B**). For adults, 4.7 g K are considered adequate, if not necessarily optimal. A high-level K intake has a blood pressure-lowering effect—justifying recommended intakes above the minimum requirements. Most American women consume just half the AI, men slightly more. Low K consumption in African Americans may contribute to the greater prevalence of hypertension in this population.

The causes of **K deficiency** are rarely purely nutritional. Massive K losses can result from diarrhea, or from abuse of laxatives and diuretics. Excessive licorice consumption can also induce hypokalemia: licorice has effects similar to those of aldosterone, enhancing tubular K secretion in the kidneys. Clinical symptoms manifest in skeletal muscle (weakness, paresis in extreme cases), the digestive tract (obstipation, in extreme cases ileus), and the heart, where typical changes of heart muscle action potential can be observed (**C**). Low plasma levels even if >6.5 mmol/l may cause acute emergencies (arrhythmias, even possible fibrillation). Acidosis (as in diabetic coma), digitalis poisoning, and kidney failure can lead to life-threatening **hyperkalemia**. There is currently no **UL** set for potassium.

A. Occurrence and Daily Requirement

The daily requirement of 2000 mg potassium is contained in:

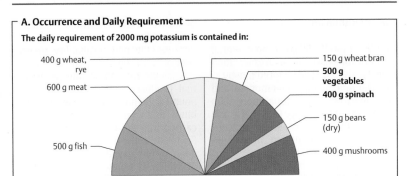

- 400 g wheat, rye
- 600 g meat
- 500 g fish
- 150 g wheat bran
- **500 g vegetables**
- **400 g spinach**
- 150 g beans (dry)
- 400 g mushrooms

B. Adequate Intakes (AI, 2004)

Life Stage and Gender Group	Age	Potassium	
		(mg/d)	(mmol/d)
Infants	0 – 6 mo	0.4	10
	7 – 12 mo	0.7	18
Children	1 – 3 y	3.0	77
	4 – 8 y	3.8	97
Adolescents	9 – 13 y	4.5	115
	14 – 18 y	4.7	120
Adults	≥ 19 y	4.7	120
Lactation	14 – 50 y	5.1	120

C. Deficiency Symptoms

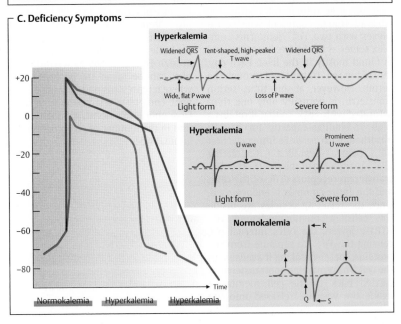

Hyperkalemia

Widened QRS   Tent-shaped, high-peaked T wave   Widened QRS

Wide, flat P wave   Loss of P wave

Light form   Severe form

Hyperkalemia

U wave   Prominent U wave

Light form   Severe form

Normokalemia

P   R   T   Q   S

+20   0   −20   −40   −60   −80   Time

Normokalemia   Hyperkalemia   Hyperkalemia

Iron: Metabolism

Iron (Fe, 1 µmol ≈56 µg) is an essential nutrient for nearly all organisms. Total body Fe is 2.5–4 g; Fe is stored mostly in the liver, spleen, intestinal mucosa, and bone marrow. At any time, more than two-thirds of total body Fe is in use as a cofactor of hemoglobin. Serum concentrations are 11–25 µmol/l in women and 12–30 µmol/l in men.

Fe **metabolism (A)** represents a complex interplay between intra- and extracellular proteins through which the needed amounts can be provided long-term, even in situations of minimal supply and poor availability, regardless of limited storage and large daily turnover rates. The average nutritional Fe supply is ~10–15 kg Fe/d, with a small amount added from biliary secretions. Only ~0.5–2 mg/d are absorbed and circulate in serum as **Fe-transferrin**. Fe-transferrin is a serum glycoprotein, which complexes with two Fe_3^{2+} ions. This complex serves as the body's Fe storage and is found mostly in the liver. Each day, 20–24 mg Fe is transported through the serum. However, at any time, serum transferrin is normally only one third saturated with Fe_3^{2+}, so that it retains a high Fe-binding capacity for any Fe absorbed in excess or Fe from cells that are being degraded. Circulating $(Fe_3^{2+})_2$-transferrin binds to the **Fe-transferrin receptors** (TfR) of the cells, and the entire complex is endocytosed. Once the resulting vesicles are inside the cells, a membrane-bound H^+-ATPase lowers the cell's internal pH, causing the Fe_3^{2+} to separate from the proteins, thereby making it available to the cell. The remaining apotransferrin is carried back to the cell membrane inside the vesicles, released into the bloodstream and now available again to transport Fe.

Because of its poor availability, **absorption** of Fe in the proximal small intestine is extremely important (**B**). In animal products, most of the Fe occurs bound to hemoglobin (heme Fe), which binds to an unknown receptor and is carried into the mucosa cells as heme Fe. Inside cells, the complex is broken down by hemoxygenase, the expression of which is upregulated when Fe is scarce. Nonheme Fe is reduced to Fe^{2+} by reductants like ascorbic acid, in the intestinal lumen (requires stomach HCl) and is absorbed through a special receptor. Heme and nonheme Fe is oxidized to Fe^{3+}, carried through the basolateral membrane and bound to apoferritin. To prevent oxidation of cell lipids, for example, free Fe must be bound to **ferritin** in all cells with high Fe content.

Because of variations in nutritional supply, enterocytes are exposed to large variations in free Fe. Those variations are buffered by rapid ferritin induction at high Fe levels. The Fe-ferritin complex can be taken up by lysosomes, where it represents part of the body's Fe pool. Long-term adaptation to varying Fe supply levels occurs through variation in the number of receptors on the luminal side.

A. Metabolism

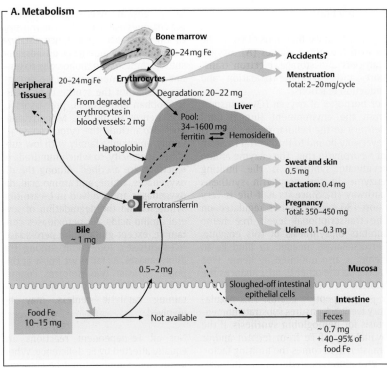

Bone marrow 20–24 mg Fe

Accidents?

Menstruation Total: 2–20 mg/cycle

Erythrocytes

20–24 mg Fe

Peripheral tissues

Degradation: 20–22 mg

From degraded erythrocytes in blood vessels: 2 mg

Liver

Pool: 34–1600 mg ferritin ⇌ Hemosiderin

Haptoglobin

Sweat and skin 0.5 mg

Lactation: 0.4 mg

Pregnancy Total: 350–450 mg

Urine: 0.1–0.3 mg

Ferrotransferrin

Bile ~ 1 mg

0.5–2 mg

Mucosa

Sloughed-off intestinal epithelial cells

Intestine

Food Fe 10–15 mg

Not available

Feces ~ 0.7 mg + 40–95% of food Fe

B. Absorption

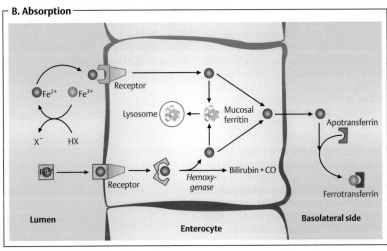

Fe^{2+} Fe^{3+}

X^- HX

Receptor

Lysosome

Mucosal ferritin

Apotransferrin

Fe^{3+}

Receptor

Hemoxy-genase

Bilirubin + CO

Ferrotransferrin

Lumen

Enterocyte

Basolateral side

Iron: Functions

The biochemical functions of Fe can be divided into three classes (**A**): oxygen transport and storage, electron transport, and enzymatic oxidation and reduction reactions.

For purposes of oxygen (O_2) transport from the environment (lungs) until delivery to the cellular oxidases, O_2 is reversibly bound to the central Fe atom of a porphyrin ring. The enzyme amino levulinate synthase is the limiting enzyme in the porphyrin synthesis pathway (**B**). Since its half-life is very short (80 minutes), it is regulated on the transcriptional level: free heme inhibits biosynthesis of this enzyme. Ferrochelatase, needed to bind Fe to heme, is also inhibited by heme. Free heme, on the other hand, enhances the protein synthesis of hemoglobin (2 α-, 2 β-) polypeptide chains. This regulatory feedback ensures substrate homeostasis for **hemoglobin synthesis**. If the availability of Fe from ferritin and/or transferrin becomes the limiting factor, erythropoiesis is reduced causing anemia.

Myoglobin found in the cytoplasm of muscle cells also contains heme but only one polypeptide chain. It facilitates O_2 transfer from the capillary erythrocytes to cytoplasm and mitochondria. During conditions of Fe deficiency, myoglobin is drastically reduced, becoming a limiting factor for muscle contractions, which are highly O_2-dependent.

The **electron transport chain** of the inner mitochondrial membrane transfers electrons to O_2. It consists of three firmly attached enzyme complexes, as well as two mobile transfer molecules, ubiquinone and cytochrome C. Altogether, 40 different proteins are involved in this process.

Many substrate-oxidizing and -reducing enzymes use Fe for electron transfer. **Oxidoreductases**, for instance, catalyze the oxidation of aldehydes or inorganic sulfites. Amino acid monooxygenases— one of many **monooxygenase** groups, are needed for the synthesis of 5-OH-tryptophan and L-dopa, precursors of CNS neurotransmitters. Monooxygenases also include the cytochrome P_{450} family, an enzyme family with low substrate specificity, to which hundreds of reactions are ascribed. Among the dioxygenases, amine, and amino acid, **dioxygenases** are involved in L-carnitine synthesis and the degradation of several amino acids. All peroxidases contain Fe, except glutathione peroxidase. NO-synthases, too, count among the dioxygenases. As far as we know at this point, at least two isoforms contain heme-Fe; additional nonheme Fe-containing catalytic centers may be involved.

Not all Fe-dependent reactions are equally affected by Fe deficiency. When insufficient supply cannot be compensated by increased absorption or improved recycling, pools are emptied first. Reduced erythropoiesis follows. Only thereafter is the activity of Fe-dependent enzymes affected.

A. Function

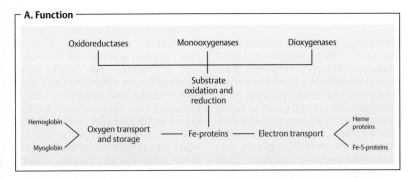

```
Oxidoreductases        Monooxygenases        Dioxygenases
        └──────────────────┼──────────────────┘
                  Substrate
                  oxidation and
                  reduction
                       │
Hemoglobin ┐                                    ┌ Heme
           ├─ Oxygen transport ── Fe-proteins ── Electron transport ─┤  proteins
Myoglobin ─┘    and storage                     └ Fe-S-proteins
```

B. Heme Iron Metabolism

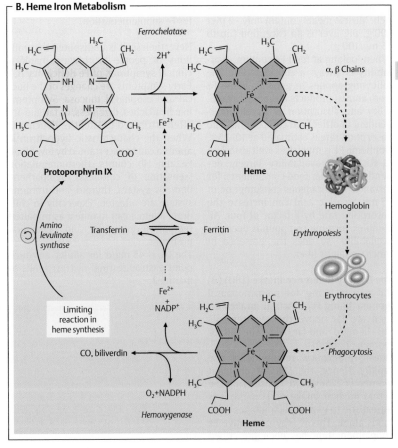

Ferrochelatase

Protoporphyrin IX → 2H⁺ / Fe²⁺ → **Heme**

α, β Chains

Amino levulinate synthase

Transferrin ⇌ Ferritin

Limiting reaction in heme synthesis

Fe²⁺ + NADP⁺

CO, biliverdin ← O₂ + NADPH

Hemoxygenase

Heme

Hemoglobin

Erythropoiesis

Erythrocytes

Phagocytosis

Iron: Occurrence and Requirements

Even though Fe is found in most **foods** (**A**), most of them contain only small amounts. Contents in fruit or milk products are negligible, whereas certain vegetables and cereal products (e.g., rolled oats, 4.6 mg/100 g) can be rather good sources. With cereals, the content decreases with increasing refinement: Fe content in white flour is only one-third of the whole-grain content. Even though Fe is contained in myoglobin, meat products are not necessarily Fe-rich. Muscle meats contain only ~2 mg/100 g; pig liver is an exception (up to 15 mg/100 g).

When looking at food Fe content, **availability** is always a consideration. The following applies in general: heme Fe from animal products has better availability and absorption is largely independent of other food components. The absorption rate is estimated at 10–25%. Nonheme Fe is much less well absorbed (3–8%), with availability largely dependent on other food components: for instance, simultaneous consumption of 75 mg ascorbic acid can increase the absorption rate by a factor of four. All complex-forming compounds decrease availability; so does the presence of much Ca salt or fiber.

The **Dietary Reference Intake (DRI) (B)** for men is 10 mg, for premenopausal women 18 mg Fe/d. **Actual intakes** for men are far above the requirements (16–18 mg/d) and far below the DRI for women (12 mg/d).

During pregnancy, requirements rise rapidly. Hence, the DRI for pregnant women is 27 mg Fe/d. Considering the actual median intake of 11 mg/d, it is unrealistic to expect such intakes from foods alone. This is why preventive Fe supplementation has been prescribed for pregnant women for decades. Many findings contraindicate this practice: for example, the incidence of pregnancy-related hypertension correlates with hemoglobin (Hb) levels. Some more recent evidence indicates that high Fe intakes may induce free radical formation in various tissues. The cancer-preventive effects of fiber may be based on fiber's Fe-binding capacity, which lowers the levels of free Fe atoms in the colon. The fact that the absorption rate increases manifold during low Fe intake casts doubt on the rationale for Fe supplementation.

Nevertheless, it is undisputed that millions of people worldwide manifest clinical **symptoms of Fe deficiency (C)**. Early symptoms are changes of the buccal and esophagal mucosa. Symptoms like headaches, dizziness, or fatigue are often attributed to latent Fe deficiency. When the characteristic **hypochromic anemia** can be ascertained by low blood Fe and Hb counts, thermoregulation (sensation of coldness), sympathetic nervous system, thyroid, and immune system are affected. Especially in children, anemia can manifest as impaired mental development and behavioral problems.

The **UL** is 45 mg/d for adults, at which point gastrointestinal distress tends to manifest.

A. Occurrence and Daily Requirement

The daily requirement of 50 mg iron is contained in:

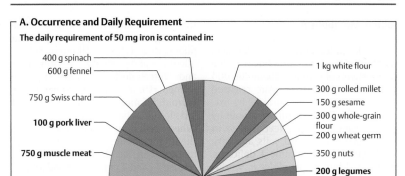

- 400 g spinach
- 600 g fennel
- 750 g Swiss chard
- **100 g pork liver**
- **750 g muscle meat**
- 1 kg white flour
- 300 g rolled millet
- 150 g sesame
- 300 g whole-grain flour
- 200 g wheat germ
- 350 g nuts
- **200 g legumes**

B. Recommended Intakes (DRI/AI*, 2002) and UL

Life Stage and Gender Group	Age	Iron (mg/d)	UL (mg/d)
Infants	0– 6 mo	0.27*	40
	7– 12 mo	11	40
Children	1– 3 y	7	40
	4– 8 y	10	40
Boys and girls	9– 13 y	8	40
Boys	14– 18 y	11	45
Girls	14– 18 y	15	45
Premenopausal women		18	45
Men and post-menopausal women	≥ 19 y	8	45
Pregnancy	14– 50 y	27	45
Lactation	14– 18 y	10	45
	19– 50 y	9	45

C. Deficiency Symptoms

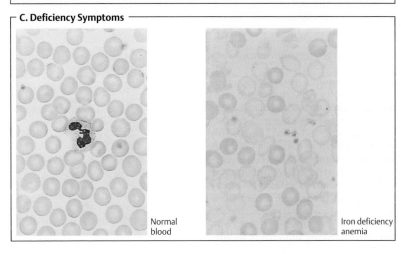

Normal blood

Iron deficiency anemia

Iodine: Metabolism

Iodine (I, 1 μmol = 127 μg) occurs in soil, plants, and sea water as iodide (I^-). Due to the effects of sunlight, about 400 000 metric tons of volatile I_2 are released from the large marine surfaces by oxidation daily. This I is returned to soils by rain—closing the cycle. Nevertheless, in many parts of the world, soils, and with them crops have become I deficient, putting ~1 billion people/year worldwide at risk of I deficiency diseases. I deficiency is the most common cause of avoidable mental defects.

These epidemiological findings are surprising, especially considering the effective I recycling in human **metabolism** (**A**). Nearly 100% of the daily intake of ~200 μg I (predominantly as I^-, intakes fluctuate greatly) is absorbed. Only a minimal percentage of all total body I (10–20 mg) is found in the extracellular compartment (250 μg); ~50% is in the thyroid, the remainder in the intracellular compartment. Some (less significant) storage occurs in salivary glands, gastric mucosa, and the lactating breast. I is actively and rapidly absorbed into the thyroid—a process inhibited by thiocyanate (e.g., in cigarette smoke). Excess I is excreted, mainly renally.

Inside the **thyroid**, several complex synthesis pathways occur in separate compartments. The thyroid follicles (**B**) consist of a single layer of thyrocytes that surrounds a colloid-filled lumen. This colloid functions as the site of synthesis and storage for thyroid hormones. Thyroglobulin is synthesized in thyrocytes and released into the colloid by exocytosis. Also in the colloid, a peroxidase oxidizes I^- to $I°$, which is shuttled out by the exocytotic vesicles, together with the protein. During subsequent **iodina-tion**, I is integrated into tyrosyl residues of thyroglobulin, resulting in mono-and diiodinated tyrosyl. Through subsequent coupling, **triiodo-L-thyronine** T_3 and **tetraiodo-L-thyronine** T_4 are formed (**C**). Without incoming I, the thyroid hormone pool in the colloid lasts for up to two months.

When needed, thyrocytes pick up all of the thyroglobulin via endocytosis, proteolyze it inside their lysosomes, and release T_3 and T_4 into the bloodstream. The excess I from remaining mono- and diiodinated tyrosine is recycled inside the cells. To prevent renal filtration, in plasma T_3 and T_4 (also referred to as thyroxine) are bound to proteins, mainly thyroxine-binding globulin (TBG), which is synthesized in the liver. Beyond that, the thyroid synthesizes mostly the relatively inactive T_4; its concentration is 20 times higher in plasma compared to T_3. Inside the target cells, T_4 is converted to the active form, T_3, releasing one molecule of I_2. This iodine again leaves the cell as I^- and is recycled. Due to the controlled conversion of T_4 to T_3, its effective binding to plasma proteins, and its long half-life (seven days), T_4 can be considered an important thyroid hormone pool.

A. Metabolism

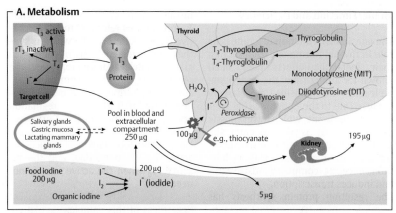

B. Thyroid Follicle

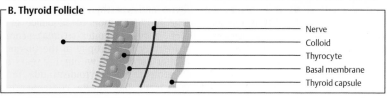

- Nerve
- Colloid
- Thyrocyte
- Basal membrane
- Thyroid capsule

C. Thyroid Hormone Structures

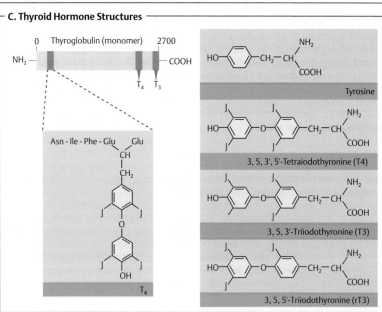

Thyroglobulin (monomer)

Asn - Ile - Phe - Glu - Glu

T_4

Tyrosine

3, 5, 3', 5'-Tetraiodothyronine (T4)

3, 5, 3'-Triiodothyronine (T3)

3, 5, 5'-Triiodothyronine (rT3)

Iodine: Function and Deficiency

The only known **function** of iodine is its role in thyroid hormones. Even though their metabolic effects have been known for a long time, the underlying molecular mechanisms are largely unclear. Due to the lipophilic character of T_3, the hormone, which forms mostly inside cells (**A**), is able to enter the nucleus, where it binds to a specific T_3 receptor. In many cells, this T_3-hormone-receptor complex binds to DNA and induces transcription.

The resulting protein synthesis has multiple **consequences**. Basal metabolism, and with it O_2 use, is increased in most tissues. ATP hydrolysis and sympathetic nervous system activation increase body temperature. The entire carbohydrate metabolism is stimulated; additionally, lipolysis may be enhanced. Normal maturation and development of the nervous system, and also of bones and other tissues, are thyroid hormone-dependent—in some cases through synergistic effects on growth hormone. Some of the interactions with catecholamines (e.g., adrenaline) occur via altered numbers of α-and β-receptors in various tissues. In the heart, for instance, this results in a positive chronotropic effect.

Because of their manifold effects on the entire metabolism, the activity of thyroid hormones must be strictly **regulated** (**B**). Basically, this regulation takes place on three levels: THR (thyrotropin-releasing hormone), formed in the hypothalamus, induces the release of TSH (thyroid stimulating hormone) by the pineal gland. TSH in turn stimulates all thyroidal synthesis and secretion processes for T_3/T_4. This **neuroendocrine axis** in turn is influenced by a multitude of factors: cold and stress, for instance, increase TRH secretion, while T_4 inhibits TSH release through a negative feedback loop via T_3, which is synthesized inside the cells of the pineal gland. **Iodide availability** represents the second level: lower concentrations of I^- stimulate hormone synthesis independently of TSH. Lastly, regulation occurs in each individual cell: the two different deiodases, individually regulated by various factors, produce the active T_3, when needed, and the inactive rT_3 when the active form is not needed.

Regardless of this complex regulation, hypo- and hyperthyroidism are not rare. The most common consequence of I deficiency (**C**) is goiter (struma), a compensatory hypertrophy of the thyroid. Goiter normalizes within 1–2 years of treatment. Hypothyroidism due to I deficiency has severe consequences, especially in neonates. Early symptoms are, among others, unwillingness to drink and obstipation. Later, retarded growth and CNS impairment become apparent. The full-blown syndrome is called **cretinism**. According to the WHO, at least 30 million people worldwide have varying degrees of preventable brain damage due to the effects of I deficiency during fetal brain development; beyond that, ~1.5 million people are at risk of I deficiency. Cretinism was common in certain areas of the U.S. until table salt was fortified with I^- (76 μg/g salt). In many countries, including the U.S., screening of neonates for TSH is mandatory. One in 5000 children in the U.S. is born with congenital hypothyroidism. In most cases, the development of cretinism can be largely prevented by timely thyroid hormone replacement therapy.

A. Function

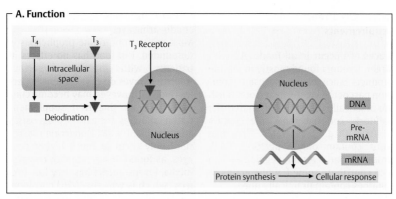

B. Thyroid Hormone Regulation

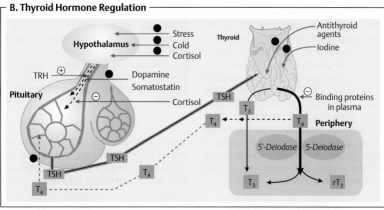

C. Iodine Deficiency

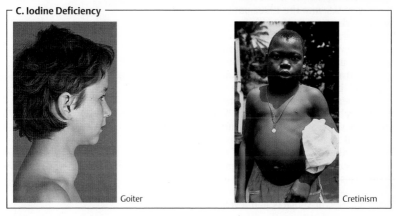

Goiter

Cretinism

Iodine: Occurrence and Requirements

Traces of I occur in all foods (**A**), with larger amounts found mostly in marine products. Since seaweeds are not a common part of the Western diet, ocean fish are practically the only good source of I: haddock, cod fish, and sole contain >140 µg/100 g. Freshwater fish like trout contain only 2 µg/100 g. Milk products and certain vegetables can also contribute some I, while grains or potatoes contain practically none.

The **DRI** for iodine for adults is 150 µg/d, with large increases needed during pregnancy (**B**). Fifty micrograms is considered sufficient to prevent the development of goiter. In the U.S., the estimated consumption (excluding iodized table salt) is 190–300 µg/d. These relatively high intakes are due to the common use of I in food processing (dairy, baked goods, food coloring). The recent wider use of bromides has reduced these intakes somewhat, and pregnant women especially need to ensure adequate iodide intakes.

Goiter was epidemic in the mid- and northwest U.S. into the 1920s until one of the earliest successful U.S. fortification programs, iodine fortification of table salt, was begun in 1924. Common vitamin/mineral supplements contain 150 µg I/d as a daily dose. Iodine supply may still be critical in some people, among them those who consume noniodized table salt from health food stores. A six-year government survey concluded in 1994 found a decrease in urinary iodine by more than half over the previous 20 years (to 145 µg/L). While this is still safely above deficiency levels, it requires monitoring. After all, 12 % of subjects had levels of <50 µg/L, including 16.5 % of women of childbearing age.

Most criticism of iodine prophylaxis is unfounded. I in food has no effects in patients with manifest hyperthyroidism (Graves disease). Latent hyperthyroidism, however, may become clinically relevant due to I supplementation, allowing for earlier diagnosis. I allergies like I acne (*Iododerma tuberosum*) only occur at much higher dosages, as found in I-containing contrast media, for instance. I has very low toxicity, which is why the WHO considers intakes of ≤1 mg (= 50 g iodized table salt) as harmless. Suggesting higher table salt intake—while improving I intake—would be counterproductive in that it would increase already high salt intakes, thereby contributing to hypertension.

The **UL** for iodine is set at 1.1 mg/d for adults.

Worldwide, about 1 billion people are affected by iodine deficiency, which could be prevented by proper fortification of salt, vegetable oils, water, or by supplements.

A. Occurrence and Daily Requirement

The daily requirement of 200 μg iodine is contained in:

- **48 g haddock**
- **76 g pollock**
- **104 g sole**
- 154 g blue mussels
- **166 g cod**
- 270 g redfish
- 340 g oysters
- 380 g herring, halibut
- 400 g tuna
- 2.1 kg rye bread
- 1 kg spinach

B. Recommended Intakes (DRI/AI*, 2002) and UL

Life Stage and Gender Group	Age	DRI/AI* (μg/d)	UL (μg/d)
Infants	0 – 6 mo	110*	ND
	7 – 12 mo	130*	ND
Children	1 – 3 y	90	200
	4 – 8 y	90	300
Adolescents	9 – 13 y	120	600
	14 – 18 y	150	900
Men and women	>19 y	150	1100
Pregnancy	14 – 18 y	220	900
	19 – 50 y	220	1100
Lactation	14 – 18 y	290	900
	19 – 50 y	290	1100

C. Iodine Deficient Regions

Approximately one billion people are affected by iodine deficiency

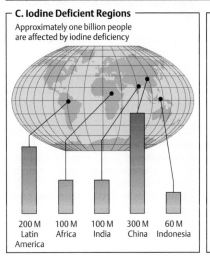

| 200 M Latin America | 100 M Africa | 100 M India | 300 M China | 60 M Indonesia |

D. Iodine Deficiency Prevention

Iodine deficiency prevention, using all sources of salt:

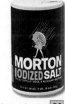

Salt used in households and restaurants	20
Industrially produced baked goods	50
Cheese and cured meats	30
All finished products and preserves	40
	140
Plus natural food iodine content	60
Total	200

(μg)

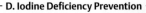

Fluorine

Fluorine (F, 1 mmol ≈19 mg) is a highly reactive chemical element.

F **absorption** (**A**) strongly depends on the compounds in which it is supplied; 25 % of F in watery solutions is absorbed in the stomach, the remainder almost completely in the small intestine. F levels in saliva are similar to F concentrations in blood; some of it participates in enteral circulation. The kidneys are the main excretory organ; losses through fecal matter and sweat amount to less than 10 %.

Due to low F availability from soils and rock, F contents in **foods** tend to be very low. Shrimp and other crustaceans, as well as meat and dairy products, are most likely to contribute to fluoride intake. Black tea contains ~1 mg of easily available F/l. Recommended F intakes (4 and 3 mg/d in men and women, respectively) include all sources, foods, supplements, and drinking water. Without fluoridation of drinking water and toothpaste, **actual intakes** would be 0.1–0.5 mg/d, far below recommended values. No deficiency symptoms have been observed at those levels. Since actual intakes are difficult to determine, the **Adequate Intakes** (**B**) are based on those intake levels that provide maximum protection against caries without causing unwanted a side effects (including moderate fluorosis). In 1986, 15 % of U.S. children under five and 8 % of those between five and 17 used fluoride supplements (available on prescription only).

Oral **fluoride supplementation** is particularly important during pregnancy, lactation, and during the first years of life.

Due to the **therapeutic range** of fluoride, multiple level prophylaxis is not advisable. Since infants should not be given table salt, the only alternative for them, if tap water is not fluoridated or not used, would be fluoride tablets (0.25 mg/d). After the third year of life, one can switch to the exclusive use of fluoridated table salt. F content in drinking water should also be taken into account. In many parts of the U.S., drinking water is routinely fluoridated (**C**) and contains between 0.4 mg/l (unfluoridated) and 0.7–1.1 mg/l F (fluoridated). If the drinking water contains >0.3 mg/l, supplementation should be reduced by one-half; if it contains >0.75 mg/l, no supplements should be taken. Replacement of water intake by soft drink consumption has increasingly reduced children's F intakes lately. On the other hand, frequent swallowing of fluoridated toothpaste by small children is a hard-to-asses risk factor for excessive intakes.

The most important **side effect** of excessive F intake is dental fluorosis, which may occur in children at dosages as low as twice the AI. According to Canadian government reports, 20–75 % of North Americans in fluoridated communities and 12–45 % in nonfluoridated communities have dental fluorosis, albeit mostly very mild forms. The most high-risk age group is children between seven months and four years of age. Skeletal fluorosis, which has been observed after many years of fluoride intakes of 10–25 mg/d is of a more theoretical nature. It should be noted that chronically toxic dosages can be obtained easily through combination of various prophylactic measures with drinking water fluoridation.

A. Metabolism

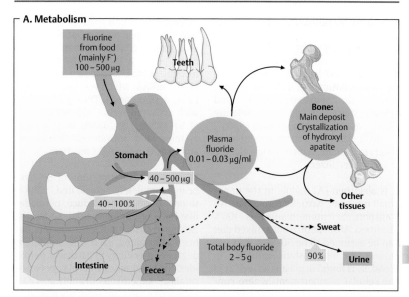

B. Adequate Intakes (AI, 1999) and UL

Life Stage and Gender Group	Age	Fluoride (mg/d)	UL (mg/d)
Infants	0 – 6 mo	0.01	0.7
	7 – 12 mo	0.5	0.9
Children	1 – 3 y	0.7	1.3
	4 – 8 y	2	2.2
Adolescents	9 – 13 y	2	10
	14 – 18 y	3	10
Males	>18 y	4	10
Females	>18 y	3	10
Pregnancy and lactation	14 – 50 y	3	10

C. Percentage of U.S. Population Receiving Fluoridated Water (2001)

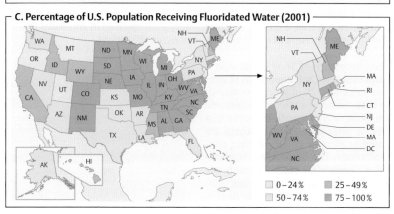

Selenium: Metabolism and Functions

Selenium (Se, 1 µmol ≈79 µg) was not recognized as an essential trace element until 1957. Like sulfur, Se occurs in various oxidation states: in the organic compounds selenomethionine and selenocysteine as Se^{2-}, in selenite (SeO_3^{2-}) as Se^{4+}, and in selenate (SeO_4^{2-}) as Se^{6+}. The only form available to plants is selenate, which is why selenate is used in fertilizer.

It is **absorbed (A)** mainly in the upper small intestine, partially through active transport. Selenomethionine is 100% absorbed. Absorption from a mixed diet can be assumed to be 50–90%. It is not subject to homeostatic control. In blood, Se is found in plasma as well as in the cellular compartment, where concentrations are higher. Most of the total body Se (13–20 mg) occurs in muscle tissue, but concentrations are highest in tissues like liver, kidneys, and spleen. **Excretion** is mainly renal; small amounts are lost through bile (feces), skin, and—especially at high intakes—exhaled as dimethyl selenium. Selenomethionine circulating in the blood is mainly integrated into proteins where it replaces methionine. While it is not known to have a specific function there, it may represent a certain Se pool.

The importance of Se is in the role it plays in specific **selenoproteins** or protein subunits, >20 of which are known to date. Some of those selenoproteins are found only in specific tissues (e.g., a 34 kDa protein in testes); others are found in all cells, but at different concentrations. The best-known is **glutathione peroxidase** (GSH-Px), with one selenocysteine in each of its four subunits. After this enzyme was discovered, the question arose as to how this "abnormal" amino acid is integrated into the proper position of the amino acid sequence. That mechanism **(B)** is now known: a special tRNA (tRNA$_{Sec}$) recognizes the UGA codon, a base triplet on the mRNA, which was once thought to be a stop codon. Through coupling with activated serine and introduction of Se, tRNA$_{Sec}$ is loaded with selenocysteine and introduces the seleno amino acid in the right position.

To date, not all **functions** of Se have been completely elucidated. Glutathione peroxidases reduce peroxides like H_2O_2 or lipid peroxides. So far, the existence of four different variants has been ascertained, each with a different degree of specificity to particular peroxides. In the complex interplay between catalase, superoxide dismutase, GSH-transferase, and antioxidants like vitamin C and E, glutathione peroxidases play important roles in the body's antioxidant protection system. Probably, glutathione peroxidases are also involved in transcription control of immune system cells. The deiodases that activate the thyroid hormone T_3 (see p. 236) are also selenoproteins. In plasma, selenoprotein P is needed for Se transport, on the one hand and is probably itself involved in antioxidant functions, on the other.

A. Metabolism

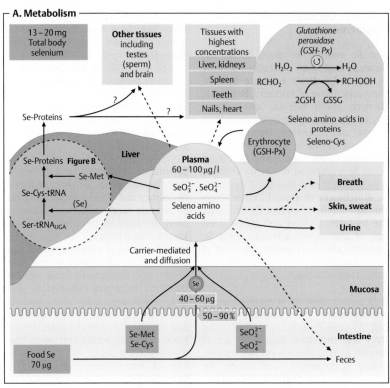

B. Integration of Se-Cys in Proteins (via UGA codon recognition by tRNA_sec)

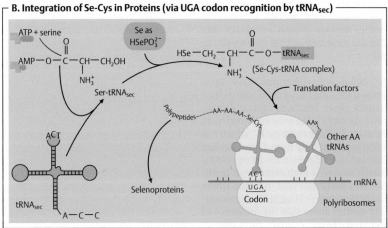

Selenium: Occurrence and Requirements

The Se content of plant **foods** (A) depends largely on soil contents. Most of North America's soils are Se-rich, especially those of northern Nebraska, western South Dakota, and eastern Wyoming. Certain areas of China and Russia, and in Europe, Denmark, Finland, and Germany, have low-Se soils. American wheat contains up to 100 µg/ 100 g Se, compared to German wheat, which usually contains just 2 µg/100 g. Se enrichment of animal fodder alters the Se content of animal foods. Given the intensity of food and animal feed import and export activities, food Se content tables (A) permit at most a rough comparison, but not an absolute calculation of intakes.

It is just as difficult to establish exact **requirements**. The **Adequate Intakes (AI)** (55 µg [0.7 µmol] Se/d or 0.87 µg/kg BW) are, therefore, based on actual intakes and the absence of obvious deficiency symptoms, as well as on the amount necessary for maximum activation of plasma glutathione peroxidase. Se intakes vary greatly around the world. Average intakes in the U.S. and Canada generally appear to exceed the AI.

Se **deficiency symptoms** have been known for a long time from animal husbandry (liver necrosis, cardiac effects, teratogenicity). The only known form in humans is "Keshan Disease," which has been reported only from China. Keshan disease is a dilatative cardiomyopathy, which caused a high number of fatalities in a particular area in China where Se intakes were <11 µg/d. Epidemiological studies show that the incidence of ischemic heart disease increases at plasma levels <60 µg/l; beyond that, there may be a relationship between malignancies and suboptimal Se status. Since these preventive effects—if confirmed—are probably based on the activation of peroxidases, diseases involving increased free radical production appear to be suitable models. For instance, Se supplementation is used successfully in intensive care for severe sepsis and burns.

Selenium's therapeutic range (C) shows that the safe range between marginal deficiency and toxicity is very narrow. Toxicity is rarely observed, however, even in high-Se regions. The only known cases involved an error in the manufacturing of a Se containing supplement. Early toxicity symptoms (selenosis) are nonspecific and include diarrhea, fingernail weakening, hair loss, irritability, itchy skin, metallic taste, nausea and vomiting, tiredness and weakness, as well as a characteristic garlicky odor of breath and sweat from dimethyl selenide.

The **UL** for adults is set at 400 µg (5.1 µmol)/d based on selenosis as the adverse effect.

A. Occurrence and Daily Requirement

50 µg selenium is contained in:

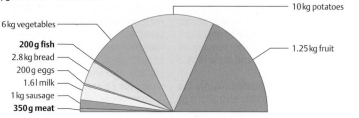

- 6 kg vegetables
- **200 g fish**
- 2.8 kg bread
- 200 g eggs
- 1.6 l milk
- 1 kg sausage
- **350 g meat**
- 10 kg potatoes
- 1.25 kg fruit

B. Adequate Intakes (AI, 2000) and UL

Life Stage and Gender Group	Age	Selenium			UL
		(µg/d)	(µmol)	(µmol/kg)	(µg/d)
Infants	0 – 6 mo	15	0.19	2.1	45
	7 – 12 mo	20	0.25	2.2	60
Children	1 – 3 y	20	0.25		90
	4 – 8 y	30	0.38		150
Adolescents	9 – 13 y	40	0.50		280
Males and females	≥ 14 y	55	0.70		400
Pregnancy	14 – 50 y	60	0.76		400
Lactation	14 – 50 y	70	0.89		400

C. Deficiency and Excess

200 000	Single-dose lethal
70 000	LD for most selenium compounds
∧	
∧	
3500	Upper safety limit for single dose
3000	Intoxication (selenosis) in China
∧	
800	Chronic toxicity sets in
∧	
400	UL for long-term use
250 – 300	Optimal intake for prevention of tumors and CVD
150	Supplementation in case of suboptimal Se status
40 – 100	Estimate of adequate intake
81 – 113	Intake range in North America
55	AI for adults
∧	
20	Lower limit: cardiomyopathy in China at 11 mg

µg/d

Zinc: Metabolism and Functions

Of total body zinc (Zn, 1 μmol ≈65 μg) of 1.5–2.5 g, only traces are found in blood. Most of it is contained in bones, skin, and hair (~70%), with the remainder mainly in liver, kidneys, and muscle (**A**).

Zn homeostasis is regulated mainly via **absorption** (**B**). When concentrations in the lumen are low, active transport occurs, stimulated by Zn deficiency. Inside the mucosa cells, Zn probably induces the transcription of mRNA for several proteins. Due to its high cysteine content, metallothionein has a high metal-binding capacity. Since CRIP (cysteine-rich intestinal protein) has a higher affinity for Zn than metallothionein CRIP is saturated preferentially during periods of low-Zn supply. Both proteins are involved in Zn transport through the cytosol, on the one hand; on the other hand, they represent an intestinal Zn pool.

The **absorption rate of zinc** is dependent on supply as well as on accompanying food components. The inhibiting effect of phytic acid and fiber, which limits Zn bioavailability from grains, is well known. High doses of copper (Cu), iron (Fe), calcium, phosphate, and heavy metals also inhibit Zn absorption. Low-molecular, complex forming molecules like amino acids or citrate enhance absorption. This mechanism probably also accounts for the absorption enhancing effect of animal protein. In plasma, one-third of the Zn is tightly bound to α_2-macroglobulin, the remainder more loosely to albumin.

Excretion occurs mainly through feces via intestinal secretions and sloughed-off intestinal cells. Losses through skin, hair, and sweat are difficult to evaluate.

As early as 1940, a specific **function** of Zn in the activity of erythrocyte carbo-anhydrase was discovered. By now, at least 50 Zn-dependent enzymatic reactions are known in humans. These include enzymes like alcohol dehydrogenase or alkaline phosphatase. The latter is also used as a functional parameter for Zn status. Furthermore, Zn is a component of transcription factors, and has influence on the transcription of DNA in its role as a structural component of histones. Beyond that, Zn may be involved in receptors, like those for growth and thyroid hormone. Insulin is stored inside cells as a Zn-complex, an effect that is used for time-release insulin (delayed release from the complex).

Zn's functions in the **immune system** are partially based on its role as a cofactor of the thymus hormone "thymulin." Thymulin regulates the transformation of thymocytes into active T-lymphocytes. Additionally, it influences the proliferation rate of T-lymphocytes (via DNA synthesis and/or interleukin-2), which pathways explain the reduced activity levels of T-helper and NK-cells during Zn deficiency. In recent times, antioxidant function has also been attributed to Zn. For this purpose, the term "site-specific" antioxidant was coined, since Zn attaches to a specific site on a molecule, preventing its oxidation.

A. Metabolism

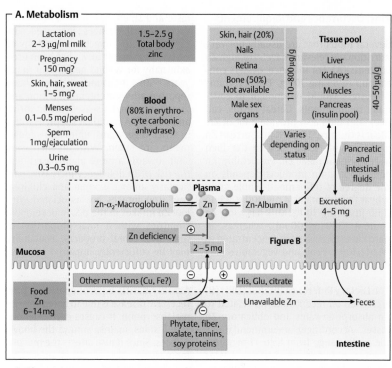

| Lactation 2–3 µg/ml milk |
| Pregnancy 150 mg? |
| Skin, hair, sweat 1–5 mg? |
| Menses 0.1–0.5 mg/period |
| Sperm 1mg/ejaculation |
| Urine 0.3–0.5 mg |

1.5–2.5 g Total body zinc

Blood (80% in erythro-cyte carbonic anhydrase)

| Skin, hair (20%) |
| Nails |
| Retina |
| Bone (50%) Not available |
| Male sex organs |

110–800 µg/g

Tissue pool

| Liver |
| Kidneys |
| Muscles |
| Pancreas (insulin pool) |

40–50 µg/g

Varies depending on status

Pancreatic and intestinal fluids

Plasma

Zn-α₂-Macroglobulin ⇌ Zn ⇌ Zn-Albumin

Zn deficiency ⊕ → 2 – 5 mg

Excretion 4–5 mg

Figure B

Mucosa

Other metal ions (Cu, Fe?) ⊖ ⊕ His, Glu, citrate

Food Zn 6–14 mg → Unavailable Zn → Feces

⊖ Phytate, fiber, oxalate, tannins, soy proteins

Intestine

B. Absorption

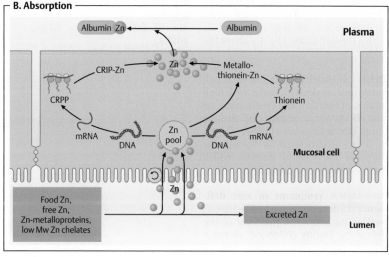

Albumin-Zn ← Albumin **Plasma**

CRIP-Zn → Zn ← Metallo-thionein-Zn

CRPP ← mRNA ← DNA — Zn pool — DNA → mRNA → Thionein

Food Zn, free Zn, Zn-metalloproteins, low Mw Zn chelates → Zn → Excreted Zn

Mucosal cell

Lumen

Zinc: Occurrence and Requirements

Several **foods** that are usually not very nutritionally relevant have very high Zn contents (**A**). For instance, oysters contain up to 85 mg/100 g. Twenty grams of oysters would be enough to cover daily requirements. Cereal germs, calf liver, and nuts also provide a lot of Zn. Meat is the most important source of Zn among staple foods due to the high availability of meat Zn. Predictably, Zn content of grain products depends on the degree of refinement: whole-grain wheat flour contains 4 mg/100 g, white flour just 1 mg/100 g. Milk has a low Zn content (380 µg/100 ml), whereas, in hard cheeses, it is more concentrated to ~4 mg/100 g. Fruit and vegetables play negligible roles with ~200 µg/100 g.

The **Dietary Reference Intakes (DRI)** (**B**) are based on recent findings related to Zn absorption rates and obligatory Zn losses. Accordingly, recommendations for adults range from 8 to 11 mg/d for women and men, respectively. Losses due to lactation should be made up supplementing an additional 6 mg/d. Overt Zn deficiency is uncommon in the U.S., with a median intake slightly above the RDA.

Zn has low **toxicity.** In regions with high nutritional intake, as in areas with high intakes of shellfish and crustaceans, no side effects are to be expected. At high doses, interactions with copper (Cu) set in, a fact that is used for therapeutic purposes in Wilson's disease, which manifests by excess Cu storage.

Pathological symptoms of **zinc deficiency** (**C**) depend on age and gender, as well as duration and intensity of the deficiency. During childhood, retarded growth predominates; later, loss of taste and smell, hair loss, skin lesions, psychological changes, increased susceptibility to infections and poor wound healing set in. Zn has been used externally for wound healing for many years. Zn deficiencies have been reported after parenteral nutrition and due to intestinal diseases (celiac sprue, and others). A marginal supply is likely in strict vegetarians, unless Zn supplements are taken. With an increasing shift towards a more plant-based diet, the risk of Zn deficiency increases, particularly among women and children. Low iron intakes are associated with low Zn intakes in the U.S. In developing countries with a high proportion of high-bran cereal products, availability may be sufficiently impaired to cause deficiencies.

Acrodermatitis enterohepatica, a rare, recessive disease is due to hereditary Zn malabsorption. It causes erythematous skin lesions, mainly around the body's orifices. Since it also affects the mucous membranes, the result is infections, e. g., with *Candida albicans* and severe diarrhea.

The **UL** for Zn is set at 40 mg/d for adults.

A. Occurrence and Daily Requirement

10 mg zinc is contained in:

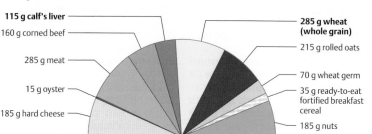

115 g calf's liver
160 g corned beef
285 g meat
15 g oyster
185 g hard cheese

285 g wheat (whole grain)
215 g rolled oats
70 g wheat germ
35 g ready-to-eat fortified breakfast cereal
185 g nuts

B. Daily Reference Intakes (DRI, 2001) and UL

Life Stage and Gender Group	Age	Zinc (mg/d)	UL (mg/d)
Infants	0 – 6 mo	2	4
	7 – 12 mo	3	5
Children	1 – 3 y	3	7
	4 – 8 y	5	12
Boys and girls	9 – 13 y	8	23
Boys	14 – 18 y	11	34
Girls	14 – 18 y	9	34
Males	>18 y	11	40
Females	>18 y	8	40
Pregnancy	14 – 18 y	13	34
	>18 y	11	34
Lactation	14 – 18 y	14	40
	>18 y	12	40

C. Skin Lesions Caused by Zn Deficiency

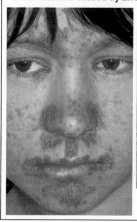
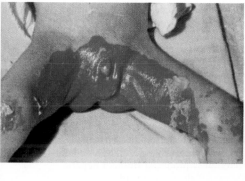

Copper: Metabolism and Functions I

Total body copper (Cu, 1 μmol ≃64 μg) is ~100 mg, of which ~40% is found in bone, ~24% in muscles, ~9% in the liver, and ~6% in the brain.

Considerable amounts from intestinal secretions are regularly added to the Cu supplied by foods (**A**). Approximatly 1–1.5 mg Cu is absorbed each day, with some of that passively absorbed inside the stomach subsequent to gastric acid-induced release from its compounds. The bulk of it, however, is passively absorbed in the small intestine. Absorption rates are largely dependent on accompanying food components (phytate inhibits, amino acids enhance). Zn inhibits absorption, creating an antagonism with Cu on the mucosal side, and induces metallothionein, which binds Cu inside the mucosa cell. On the one hand, this prevents intracellular Cu overload; on the other hand, it interferes with transport to the serosal side. Cu plasma levels are ~0.5–1.5 μg/ml. They are largely independent of nutritional intakes and fasting but nearly double towards the end of pregnancy. The reason for this is unknown. In **blood**, Cu is mostly bound to transcuprein or loosely to albumin; ~10% prevail as low-molecular Cu complexes, mainly Cu-amino acids.

After hepatic uptake, Cu is either integrated into target proteins or released back into the bloodstream as Cu-ceruloplasmin (Cp). Cu-Cp is the **transport form** of Cu between the **liver** and its target tissues. Cellular uptake from the transport proteins probably occurs via a membrane-bound Cu receptor.

Biliary Cu **excretion** is adjusted to maintain Cu homeostasis. Most likely, Cu for excretion is produced through hepatic lysosomal degradation of Cu-metallothionein and Cu-Cp.

In recent years, Cu has become known to be a component of the **endogenous antioxidant system** (**B**). The latter includes CuZn-superoxide dismutase (CuSOD) and cytochrome C oxidase (CCO), which is involved in mitochondrial electron transfer. Reduced CCO activity could lead to incomplete O_2 reduction, resulting in increased superoxide buildup. Lack of CuSOD seems to be at least partially compensated by a mitochondrial manganese-SOD (MnSOD). Cu status can impact the activity of other enzymes even without direct involvement of Cu. Cu deficiency reduces glutathione peroxidase (GSH-Px) mRNA concentrations, as well as mRNA for catalase, a ferric enzyme. Glutathione-S-transferase (GST) and glucose-6-phosphate dehydrogenase (G6PDH) also appear to be affected. The latter could be interpreted as an adaptive reaction to the increased oxidative stress resulting from the Cu deficiency. G6PDH regenerates NADPH, which glutathione reductase (GR) needs to in turn regenerate reduced glutathione (GSH) from its oxidized form (GSSG). Even though the above processes have to date only been identified in animal models, they may, in the future, become extremely important for the pathogenesis of a large variety of diseases.

A. Metabolism

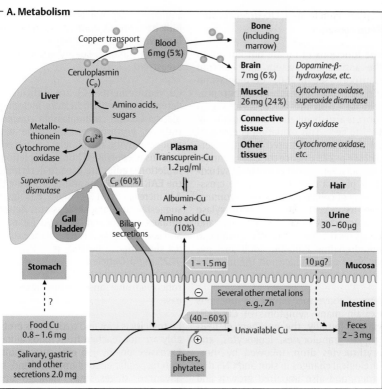

B. Oxidative Stress under Cu Deficiency

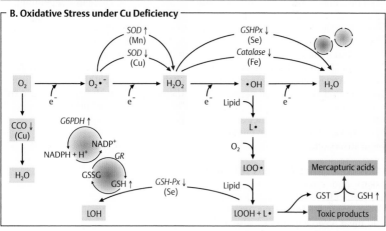

Copper: Functions II, Occurrence, and Requirements

The **functions** of Cu are not limited to the antioxidant system and electron transport (see p. 250). Ceruloplasmin (Cp), the most important transport protein for Cu in the blood, in its Cu-Cp form, is also involved in the oxidation of Fe^{2+} to Fe^{3+}. This oxidation is essential for the binding of stored Fe to transferrin (see p. 228); hence the close connection between Cu and Fe status. Lysyl oxidase plays a central role in the cross-linking of collagen and elastin (connective tissue). Dopamine-β-hydroxylase uses ascorbate as an electron donor and catalyzes the conversion of dopamine to noradrenaline. Probably, additional, not yet verified influences on the immune system occur via interleukin-2.

The above-mentioned functions explain many symptoms of **Cu deficiency**. Initially, the numbers of neutrophil granulocytes, leukocytes, and erythrocytes drop, followed by morphological changes in skin and CNS disorders and also impaired growth and skeletal abnormalities in children. All species also exhibit hypocholesterolemia, but the mechanism is unknown. The effects of Cu deficiency on the vascular system have been known for a long time in animal husbandry: sudden death through aortic rupture—caused by abnormal collagen and elastin synthesis—occurring in apparently healthy animals. Latent Cu deficiency as a cause of cardiovascular disease in humans has been suspected.

Cu is widespread in **foods (B)**. Organ meats and crustaceans are excellent sources. Effectively though, humans derive most Cu from fruit, vegetables, and meat. Whole grains are also a good source but are not widely consumed. Milk has a low Cu content. Neonates are born with a rather large hepatic Cu pool, ensuring their Cu supply while being breast-fed.

Cu **requirements (C)** are difficult to determine. Several indicators, including plasma Cu and ceruloplasmin concentrations, erythrocyte superoxide dismutase activity, and platelet Cu concentrations in controlled human depletion/repletion studies are used to determine the **EAR**. The **DRI** for adults is 0.9 mg/d. An increase to 1.5–3 mg/d has been suggested in recent discussions. **Actual intakes** are 1.5 and 1.0 mg/d for men and women, respectively. Balance studies show that a balance is reached at ~1.25 mg/d. Deficiency symptoms manifest as gastrointestinal diseases, nephrotic syndrome, and possibly heart disease.

Cu **toxicity** is low, and toxic levels probably are not reached from foods alone. Excessive on-the-job exposure results in nonspecific acute symptoms and, in advanced stages, liver damage and hematological changes. Depending on its corrosiveness, water stagnant in copper pipes may dissolve excessive amounts of Cu, which could be dangerous, especially for infants, individuals with Wilson's disease, Indian childhood cirrhosis, or idiopathic copper toxicosis. Usually, public water systems have sufficiently high water pH to prevent such excessive uptake.

The **UL** is set at 10 mg/d for adults.

A. Reactions Catalyzed by Copper Enzymes

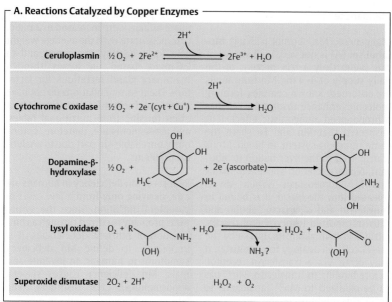

Ceruloplasmin $½ O_2 + 2Fe^{2+} \xrightarrow{2H^+} 2Fe^{3+} + H_2O$

Cytochrome C oxidase $½ O_2 + 2e^-(cyt + Cu^+) \xrightarrow{2H^+} H_2O$

Dopamine-β-hydroxylase $½ O_2 + \underset{H_3C}{\text{(catechol)}} + 2e^- (ascorbate) \longrightarrow$

Lysyl oxidase $O_2 + R\text{–CH(OH)–CH}_2\text{–NH}_2 + H_2O \rightleftharpoons H_2O_2 + R\text{–CH(OH)–CHO} \; (NH_3 ?)$

Superoxide dismutase $2O_2 + 2H^+ \longrightarrow H_2O_2 + O_2$

B. Occurrence

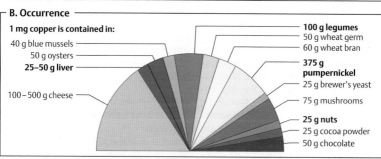

1 mg copper is contained in:

- 40 g blue mussels
- 50 g oysters
- **25–50 g liver**
- 100–500 g cheese
- **100 g legumes**
- 50 g wheat germ
- 60 g wheat bran
- **375 g pumpernickel**
- 25 g brewer's yeast
- 75 g mushrooms
- **25 g nuts**
- 25 g cocoa powder
- 50 g chocolate

C. Recommended Intakes (DRI/AI*, 2002) and UL

Life Stage and Gender Group	Age	DRI/AI* (µg/d)	AI* (µg/kg/d)	UL (mg/d)
Infants	0– 6 mo	200*	30*	No Cu supplements
	7– 12 mo	220*	30*	
Children	1– 3 y	340		1
	4– 8 y	440		3
Adolescents	9– 13 y	700		5
	14– 18 y	890		8
Adults	≥ 19 y	900		10
Pregnancy	14– 50 y	1000		10
Lactation	14– 50 y	1300		10

Manganese

Manganese (Mn, 1 μmol ≈55 μg) **metabolism (A)** is not very well known at this point. Only a few percent of the daily supply of 3–4 mg Mn from foods are absorbed; known complex-forming molecules enhance absorption, Fe^{2+} has a pronounced antagonistic effect. It is suspected that Mn and Fe share the same transport system. In blood, Mn is transported to the liver bound to albumin; biliary excretion appears to maintain Mn homeostasis. When Mn is released into the blood, it is bound to transferrin and α2-macroglobulin and thus transported to peripheral tissues. Little is known about its uptake by the target cells: in analogy to Fe transfer, it may occur via a transferrin receptor. Before binding to transferrin, Mn^{2+} has to be oxidized to Mn^{3+} (analogous to Fe^{2+}); this might occur through ceruloplasmin. Most of the 10–20 mg total body Mn is in the skeleton, in passive storage.

The essential **functions** of Mn are its involvement in a few enzymes and possibly in their activation. Three metalloenzymes are known to have Mn cofactors: Mn-superoxide dismutase, pyruvate carboxylase (gluconeogenesis), and arginase (urea cycle). There are a large number of enzymes in which Mn can be more or less replaced by other metal ions.

Mn is common, particularly in plant **foods (B)**. Excellent sources are whole grains, cereal germs and bran, legumes and brown rice. Meat, fish, and dairy products have rather low Mn contents.

Since **EAR** could not be determined, the **AI** of 2.3 and 1.8 mg/d for men and women, respectively, **(C)** are based on diet studies. Even though there is no evidence of increased requirements during pregnancy and lactation, adequate intakes were increased to 2 mg/d, commensurate with the average weight gain for a healthy pregnancy, and to 2.6 mg/d, based on losses through mammary gland secretions for lactation. The recommendations do not have a very solid scientific basis since Mn is often missing from nutritional tables, and assessments are, therefore, notoriously unreliable—in part due to analytical problems.

Reports of **Mn deficiency** in humans are rare, deriving only from a few cases of parenteral nutrition. Since the symptoms probably occurred through a combination of nutrient deficiencies, it is impossible to define Mn deficiency symptoms in humans. In juvenile animals, Mn deficiency causes skeletal abnormalities, CNS disorders, and altered carbohydrate and fat metabolism. Based thereon, it has been hypothesized that Mn is also involved in epilepsy and insulin resistance. However, there are no practical applications of these hypothetical assumptions at this point.

The **UL** is set at 11 mg/d. No adverse effects have been observed from Western diets.

Even if actual intakes exceed 10 mg/d due to high levels of whole grain consumption, **toxic effects** are not to be expected. In animal experiments, high-level supplementation with Mn led to hematological changes and CNS damage at higher dosages. Similar symptoms have been noted in manganese miners in Chile and India. Daily skin contact or particle inhalation causes twitching resembling the symptoms of Parkinson's disease and/or hallucinations.

A. Metabolism

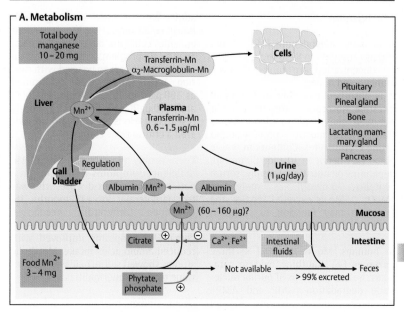

B. Occurrence

3 mg manganese is contained in:

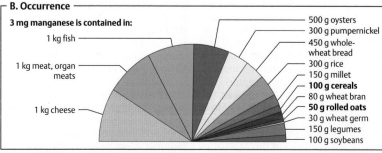

- 1 kg fish
- 1 kg meat, organ meats
- 1 kg cheese
- 500 g oysters
- 300 g pumpernickel
- 450 g whole-wheat bread
- 300 g rice
- 150 g millet
- **100 g cereals**
- 80 g wheat bran
- **50 g rolled oats**
- 30 g wheat germ
- 150 g legumes
- 100 g soybeans

C. Adequate Intakes (AI, 2002) and UL

Life Stage and Gender Group	Age	Manganese (mg/d)	UL (mg/d)	Life Stage and Gender Group	Age	Manganese (mg/d)	UL (mg/d)
Infants	0 – 6 mo	0.003	ND	Men	≥ 19 y	2.3	11
	7 – 12 mo	0.6	ND				
Children	1 – 3 y	1.2	2	Women	≥ 19 y	1.8	11
	4 – 8 y	1.5	3				
Boys	9 – 13 y	1.9	6	Pregnancy	14 – 18 y	2	9
	14 – 18 y	2.2	9		19 – 50 y	2	11
Girls	9 – 13 y	1.6	6	Lactation	14 – 18 y	2.6	9
	14 – 18 y	1.6	9		19 – 50 y	2.6	11

Molybdenum

Total body molybdenum (Mo, 1 µmol ~96 µg) amounts to 8–10 mg. The highest concentrations are found in the liver, kidneys, and bones.

It is absorbed passively in the small intestine. Absorption rates are high but not well quantified. In blood, Mo is transported mostly protein-bound inside erythrocytes. Contents in whole blood vary between 30 and 700 nmol/l, depending on nutritional supply; serum contains ~5 nmol/l as molybdate (MoO_4^{2-}). Mo is excreted renally—the excretion may function to maintain homeostatic balance.

In humans, Mo is involved in three **enzymes** (A). Xanthine oxidase catalyzes the last two steps of purine nucleotide degradation (GMP and AMP). Aldehyde oxidase accepts several heterocyclic substrates and is involved in the degradation of catecholamines. The last step in the degradation of S-containing amino acids is catalyzed by sulfite oxidase. All three enzymes transfer electrons to other cofactors and lastly to electron acceptors like cytochrome C, molecular oxygen, or NAD^+ via their central Mo^{6+} ion. Mo is not bound directly to the enzyme, but to a sulfurous molecule (molybdopterin). To date, the synthesis of this Mo-cofactor (Mo-molybdopterin) has only been researched in bacteria. It is hypothesized that Mo induces a protein that regulates molybdopterin synthesis.

Mo is ubiquitous in **foods** (B). Grain germs, legumes, and organ meats are good Mo sources. The **RDA** for adults is 45 µg/d. An AI for infants has been established at 0.3 µg/kg BW/d. Recent, well-controlled balance studies found no clinical deficiency symptoms in adults with as little as 22 µg Mo/d; however, an impact on Mo-dependent enzymes could not be excluded. Due to analytical problems, the figures in nutrient tables are to be used with caution. **Actual intakes** were determined as 360 µg/d in 1970, 180 µg/d in 1980, and ~80 µg/d in 1987 (U.S.). Poorly researched, Mo is presently not considered a critical trace element.

There is only one reported case of **Mo deficiency symptoms** in humans, in a patient with Crohn's disease, who was fed parenterally for >18 months. He developed tachycardia, headaches, night blindness, vomiting, and finally coma. His symptoms improved with reduced amino acids intake. Metabolic studies showed sulfite oxidase and xanthine oxidase abnormalities.

Other studies related Mo deficiency with cancer, but in each case there was a combination of several trace element deficiencies.
Proof of the essential character of Mo comes from hereditary Mo-enzyme deficiencies. In 1967, postmortem investigation found a sulfite oxidase deficiency in a child which was accompanied by high levels of sulfite and abnormal sulfurous amino acids. Since then, ~20 additional cases have been reported. More frequent is a Mo-cofactor deficiency (~80 known cases), which impacts all three enzymes described above.
The **UL** for adults is 2 mg/d, at which level animals show reproductive and growth impairment.

A. Molybdenum Enzymes

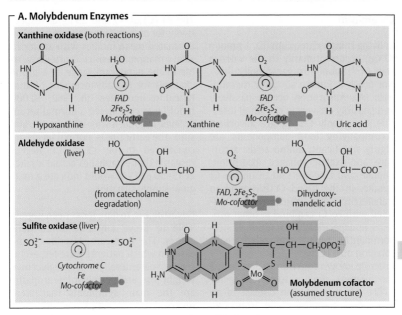

Xanthine oxidase (both reactions)

Hypoxanthine → (FAD, 2Fe₂S₂, Mo-cofactor) → Xanthine → (FAD, 2Fe₂S₂, Mo-cofactor) → Uric acid

Aldehyde oxidase (liver)

(from catecholamine degradation) → (FAD, 2Fe₂S₂, Mo-cofactor) → Dihydroxy-mandelic acid

Sulfite oxidase (liver)

SO_3^{2-} → (Cytochrome C, Fe, Mo-cofactor) → SO_4^{2-}

Molybdenum cofactor (assumed structure)

B. Occurrence

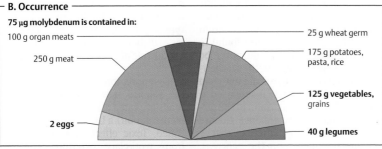

75 μg molybdenum is contained in:

- 100 g organ meats
- 250 g meat
- 2 eggs
- 25 g wheat germ
- 175 g potatoes, pasta, rice
- **125 g vegetables,** grains
- **40 g legumes**

C. Recommended Intakes (DRI/AI*, 2002) and UL

Life Stage and Gender Group	Age	Molybdenum (μg/d)	Molybdenum (μg/kg/d)	UL (μg/d)
Infants	0 – 6 mo	2	0.3*	No supplements
	7 – 12 mo	3	0.3*	
Children	1 – 3 y	17		300
	4 – 8 y	22		600
Adolescents	9 – 13 y	34		1100
	14 – 18 y	43		1700
Adults	≥ 19 y	45		2000
Pregnancy and lactation	14 – 18 y	50		1700
	19 – 50 y	50		1700

Chromium

In living things, chromium (Cr, 1 nmol = 52 ng) occurs primarily in the valence state Cr^{3+}, bound to organic molecules. Not much is known about Cr **metabolism (A)**. Absorption occurs passively and possibly actively in the small intestine. Since only 0.5–3% are absorbed, accompanying food components are highly significant: amino acids, ascorbate, and oxalate enhance absorption; phytate and zinc are said to impair Cr uptake. In the blood Cr is bound to transferrin; when transferrin is saturated with Fe, Cr can bind to other proteins nonspecifically. Excretion is predominantly renal; controlled reabsorption may occur.

Cr's sole known **function** to date is in a (postulated) glucose tolerance factor (GTF), which is said to consist of an octahedral complex made from two nicotinic acid molecules and glutamic acid, glycine, and cysteine. The compound was originally isolated from brewer's yeast, and was later found in liver and plasma, but could never be purified. Experiments with synthetically produced complexes did not yield the expected results. GTF is supposed to enhance the effects of insulin in the target cells and thereby enhance glucose uptake. It was also hypothesized that Cr has direct influence on the pancreas. Final proof of the existence of GTF and of the significance of Cr for its activities is still pending, even though Cr appears to improve glucose tolerance.

Cr occurs in **foods (B)** in both organic and inorganic forms. Good sources are liver and kidneys, but also muscle meat, whole grains, and vegetables.

The **AI (C)** of 35 and 25 µg/d, respectively, for men and women, are based on estimated mean intakes with an added safety margin. Cr, which is often available in the nanogram range, is a prime example for the advancement of analytical technologies: in 1962, 10 000 nmol/l was considered a normal serum Cr level. In 1968, it was ~450 nmol/l, and since the early 1980s, normal levels are considered to be <3 nmol/l. Recent research that establishes actual intakes at 15–50 µg Cr/d would indicate a marginal supply situation.

Nevertheless, to date it has been impossible to prove any nutritional **deficiency**. The literature describes three cases in which patients were fed exclusively parenterally. Hyperglycemia, weight loss, and peripheral neuropathy are the main symptoms that were reversed by Cr supplementation. Cr deficiency was subsequently discussed as a positive factor in the etiology of type 1 diabetes. Supplementation studies in diabetics gave mixed results leaving the role of Cr in diabetes unresolved.

Since reports about **toxic effects** of Cr in the valence states typically found in foods are rare (result of excessive supplementation), a **UL** has not been established. Toxic effects are known only from workplace exposure. The extremely reactive hexavalent Cr^{6+} forms during stainless-steel production and leather processing, where it may be inhaled or ingested. Besides acute symptoms like dermatitis, it may contribute to an increased risk of lung cancer.

A. Metabolism

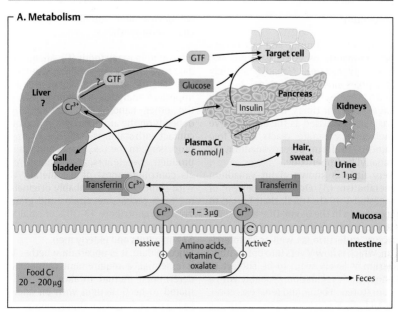

B. Occurrence

100 µg chromium is contained in:

150 – 200 g spices

300 g beef

200 – 500 g beef liver

300 – 1000 g cheese

300 g wheat bran

80 g wheat germ
200 g whole-grain bread

300 g corn germ oil

500 g white beans

400 g vegetables, fruit

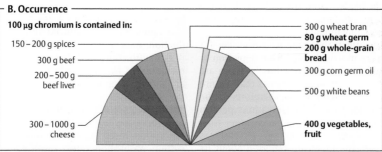

C. Adequate Intakes (AI, 2002)

Life Stage and Gender Group	Age	Chromium (µg/d)	(ng/d)	Life Stage and Gender Group	Age	Chromium (µg/d)	(ng/d)
Infants	0 – 6 mo	0.2	~ 29	Men	19 – 50 y	35	
	7 – 12 mo	5.5	~ 611		≥ 50 y	30	
Children	1 – 3 y	11		Women	19 – 50 y	25	
	4 – 8 y	15			≥ 50 y	20	
Boys	9 – 13 y	25		Pregnancy	14 – 18 y	29	
	14 – 18 y	35			19 – 50 y	30	
Girls	9 – 13 y	21		Lactation	14 – 18 y	44	
	14 – 18 y	24			19 – 50 y	45	

Vanadium

Vanadium (V, 1 nmol $\approx$51 ng) occurs predominantly as VO^{2+} (vanadyl) and VO_4^{3-} (vanadate). Vanadyl strongly resembles ions like Ca^{2+}, Mg^{2+}, or Fe^{2+}, and competes with them for binding sites. In recent times, the peroxo form has been discussed as the actual active molecule: vanadate reacts with free radicals to form peroxovanadium or vanadyl hydroperoxide.

Very little is known about vanadium **metabolism (A)**. Only a few percent of ingested V is absorbed, then bound to transferrin in the blood. Due to its similarity to Fe, binding probably also occurs to ferritin, as well as lactoferritin, which is how V gets into breast milk. Serum V levels seem to be subject to only a static regulation, probably with a pool stored in bone, and renal excretion. Total body V is estimated to be ~100 µg. The highest concentrations are found in hair and lungs, with most of the latter probably inhaled.

The **effects** that have been described for V are mostly derived from depletion or overdose studies in animals. There are no known human enzymes that require V as a cofactor. It can, therefore, not be excluded that all observations pertain to pharmacological effects rather than to an essential function. As early as 1979, the literature reported about its importance for the bone growth in chickens. A possible explanation would be nonspecific inhibition of phosphotyrosyl protein phosphatase (**B**): osteoblast activity is stimulated by growth factors that cause phosphorylation of tyrosine R-groups in specific proteins through a membrane-bound tyrosyl kinase. The antagonistic reaction is catalyzed by the same phosphatase that is inhibited by V and fluoride. V is also supposed to mimic insulin effects in adipocytes and inhibit endogenous cholesterol synthesis.

V is found in many **foods (C)**. Analytical data vary greatly and are highly unreliable. On the one hand, this is due to imperfect analytical methods, and on the other hand, V content greatly depends on the airborne uptake and on contact with stainless-steel, e. g., during processing. In the U.S., grains and grain products, sweeteners, and infant cereals contribute most of the dietary V, with some of that V probably originating from processing. Grains and grain products contribute 13–30 % of total V to the adult U.S. diet and beverages 26–57 % in adults and elderly men.

Since to date, it is uncertain whether V is essential, a requirement cannot be determined. **Actual intakes** are estimated to be 6–18 µg/d with an additional mean 9 µg from supplements.

In animals, V deficiency leads to elevated abortion rates, reduced milk production, retarded growth, edema, thyroid malfunction, and disturbed lipid metabolism. No deficiency symptoms are known in humans.

Toxic effects are known to occur due to workplace exposure. Respiratory absorption rates far exceed digestive system absorption rates, resulting in much higher blood levels. Beyond acute symptoms like inflammation of the respiratory tract and skin lesions, spasms and gastrointestinal disturbances were observed in humans in a long-term trial with oral supplementation in mg ranges. In vitro experiments showed that V inhibits various ATPases and other enzymes at high dosages.

The **UL** for V is set at 1.8 mg of elemental V/d. Data are insufficient to establish any other recommendations.

A. Metabolism

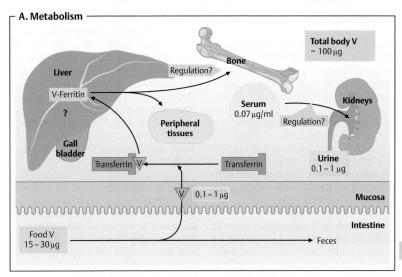

Total body V
~ 100 µg

Liver

V-Ferritin

?

Gall bladder

Bone

Regulation?

Peripheral tissues

Serum 0.07 µg/ml

Regulation?

Kidneys

Urine 0.1 – 1 µg

Transferrin V

Transferrin

V 0.1 – 1 µg

Mucosa

Intestine

Food V 15 – 30 µg

Feces

B. Bone Metabolism

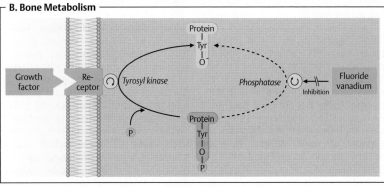

Growth factor

Receptor

Tyrosyl kinase

Protein Tyr O⁻

Phosphatase

Fluoride vanadium

Inhibition

Protein Tyr O P

P

C. Occurrence

30 µg vanadium is contained in:

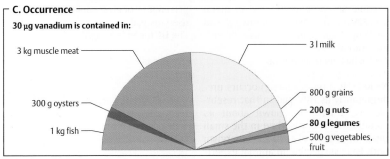

3 kg muscle meat

3 l milk

300 g oysters

800 g grains

200 g nuts

80 g legumes

500 g vegetables, fruit

1 kg fish

Tin and Nickel

Since **tin** (Sn, 1 µmol $\approx$ 119 µg) occurs as Sn^{2+} and Sn^{4+}, theoretically it can be assumed that it participates in the body's redox systems and/or is significant for the tertiary structure of proteins.

Sn **absorption** (A) depends on the dosage as well as the form in which it is ingested. Foods contribute 1–3 mg Sn/d (excluding canned foods), mostly in organic complexes. Those are said to be absorbed relatively well, whereas inorganic Sn is poorly used.

Even though Sn is widespread in **foods**, excessive amounts may be ingested if it is leached into foods from unlacquered tin cans or tin dishes. This is particularly common in case of sour fruit juices or low pH preserves.

Sn was added to the list of essential trace elements when its growth-enhancing effect was discovered in rats. It may be involved in gastrin, which regulates gastric HCl production. To date, its essentiality has not been confirmed in humans. Sn deficiency symptoms have not been reported for any species. Reports of **toxic effects**, however, abound. In one documented case, 24-hour storage of orange juice in a tin pot caused reversible intestinal symptoms. Organic Sn compounds used in metal processing, the plastics industry, and pest control are common causes of non-nutritional toxicity.

No **UL** has been set for Sn.

Nickel (Ni, 1 µmol $\approx$ 59 µg) occurs predominantly as Ni^{2+} and in that resembles Fe^{2+}. Little is known about its metabolism. It is absorbed in the small intestine at a rate of 1–10 %. A synergism with Fe is suspected. In animal experiments, Ni deficiency disturbs Fe metabolism and blood building. Ni has never been shown to be part of the human enzyme system. Since there are no reports about Ni deficiency in humans, its essentiality remains controversial.

Requirements can only be extrapolated from animal experiments and are estimated at ~50 µg/d. The **actual intakes** of 79–105 µg/d (including a mean of 5 µg from supplements) far exceed hypothetical needs.

Ni has gained a reputation for its **toxicity**, which causes acute asthma-like symptoms. While such toxicity is not known to be caused by dietary intakes, exposure may occur during production and processing of dried batteries, metal alloys, etc., through inhalation of volatile Ni compounds.

More common is **Ni allergy**, which usually manifests as contact eczema (B). Because of early ear piercing, women are more commonly affected than men (~1 in 8 women to 1 in 20 men). In ~50 % of sensitized persons, oral provocation causes eczema, either generalized or restricted to the hands. In these cases, it is advisable to avoid **Ni-rich foods** (C). These include cocoa, chocolate, legumes (including soy), tea, oats, and nuts. Ni can also be released from stainless-steel cookware at acidic pH; enamel or glass cookware should be used instead.

The **UL** for Ni is 1 mg/d.

A. Tin in Foods

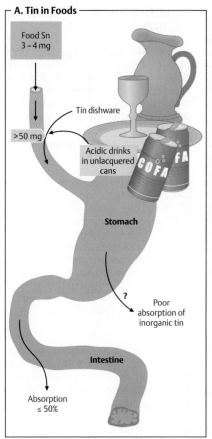

Food Sn
3 – 4 mg

Tin dishware

>50 mg

Acidic drinks
in unlacquered
cans

COFA

Stomach

? Poor
absorption of
inorganic tin

Intestine

Absorption
≤ 50%

B. Nickel Allergy

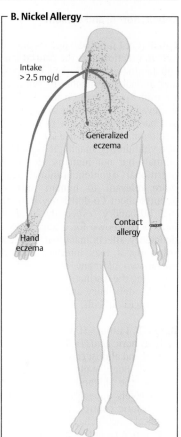

Intake
> 2.5 mg/d

Generalized
eczema

Hand
eczema

Contact
allergy

C. Occurence of Nickel

50 µg nickel is contained in:

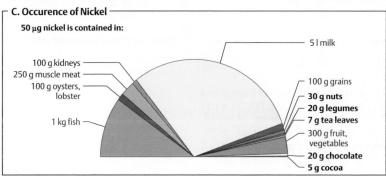

5 l milk

100 g kidneys
250 g muscle meat
100 g oysters,
lobster

1 kg fish

100 g grains

30 g nuts
20 g legumes
7 g tea leaves

300 g fruit,
vegetables

20 g chocolate
5 g cocoa

Cobalt, Boron, and Lithium

Cobalt (Co, 1 µmol $\approx$59 µg) has only one known function: it is the central ion in cobalamin (vitamin B_{12}). Since humans and animals are unable to synthesize vitamin B_{12}, human Co metabolism is irrelevant. Only certain algae, yeasts, and bacteria (**A**) are able to synthesize it. Intestinal bacteria use Co to synthesize vitamin B_{12}, making it available to animals but not humans. Hence, the nutritional Co content in animal foods is more relevant to human nutrition. Reports about Co deficiency from animal husbandry (especially in sheep) have been known for a long time. Co deficiency affects many bacteria. Consequently, it may interfere with the breakdown of many other nutrients, rendering the distinction between vitamin B_{12} deficiency and other nutrient imbalances difficult.

Boron (B, 1 µmol $\approx$11 µg) prevails in the body as boric acid (H_3BO_3). Absorption is rapid and almost complete; excretion is renal. Bone, nails, hair, and teeth exhibit the highest concentrations. Blood levels appear to be subject to homeostatic control. To date, no biochemical function has been ascertained for boron. A recent hypothesis assumes involvement of B in membrane transport processes. Deficiency symptoms are known only from two experimental studies: increased activity of erythrocyte superoxide dismutase supports the concept of B's involvement in membrane-bound redox processes.

The median adult intake of dietary and supplemental B in the U.S. is ~1.0–1.4 mg B/d (supplements 0.14 mg). Plant foods (**B**) like tomatoes, pears, apples, and soy are particularly rich in B (up to 12 mg/100 g).

The **UL** for B is set at 20 mg/d, based on data from animal research.

Lithium (Li, 1 µmol $\approx$3 µg) has been used in the treatment of psychiatric disorders for several decades and has, therefore, been more thoroughly researched than other trace elements. Its absorption occurs passively in the upper small intestine, excretion is primarily renal in adults. Nothing is known about lithium's physiological functions.

In animal experiments, Li deficiency causes low birth weight, increased abortion rates, altered enzyme activity, and behavioral disorders.

No deficiency symptoms have ever been described in humans; hence the essentiality of lithium is controversial. Animal foods tend to have higher Li contents (**C**), making eggs, milk, and meat possible important sources. Actual intakes range between 0 and >3000 µg/d.

Epidemiological research indicates that suicide rates are lower in areas with higher Li intakes (mostly from drinking water). Pharmacological Li dosages (~200 mg Li/d) are far higher than any potential nutritional intakes. At such high dosages, blood Li levels have to be monitored to avoid toxic effects like vomiting, diarrhea, tremors and seizures (in extreme cases).

No **DRI** or **UL** have been set for Li.

A. Cobalt

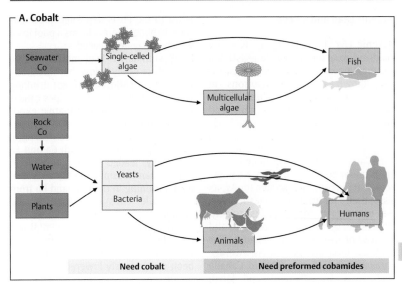

Need cobalt | Need preformed cobamides

B. Occurrence of Boron

2 mg boron is contained in:

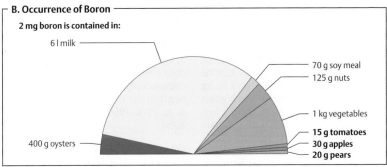

6 l milk

70 g soy meal
125 g nuts

1 kg vegetables

15 g tomatoes
30 g apples
20 g pears

400 g oysters

C. Occurrence of Lithium

500 µg lithium is contained in:

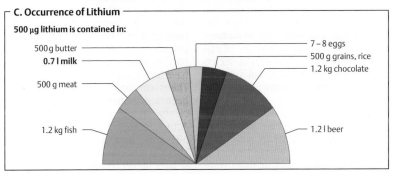

500 g butter
0.7 l milk

500 g meat

1.2 kg fish

7 – 8 eggs
500 g grains, rice
1.2 kg chocolate

1.2 l beer

Arsenic Lead and Silicon

Arsenic (As, 1 μmol ≈75 μg) is easily oxidized to arsenic trioxide (As_2O_3), a tasteless powder that has been historically known as the "King of poisons." In unexposed people, the highest arsenic contents are found in skin, nails, and hair, which can be used to assess long-term loads. In the 1970s, one research team observed decreased reproduction rates and growth impairment in animals under arsenic depletion. No physiological functions are known for As; its essentiality for humans is questionable. As content in foods varies widely, depending on soils, air As content, and the use of As-containing biocides. Fish and sea food are rich in As. Average intakes in the U.S. are ~33 μg/d, Canada ~48.5 μg/d, UK ~89 μg/d, and Japan ~300 μg/d (reflecting higher seafood consumption). Extrapolations from animal experiments (**A**) would result in a 12–25 μg/d "requirement."

The threshold of As **toxicity** is difficult to determine: careful estimates assume safe, long-term intakes up to 1 μg/kg BW/d; according to WHO, the highest tolerable dose is ~3.5 mg/d. The U.S. EPA oral **Reference Dose (RfD)**, an estimate of the daily exposure to humans that is likely to be without appreciable risk of deleterious effects during a lifetime, is 0.1–0.8 μg/kg/d, which translates into 7–56 μg/d for a typical 70 kg adult. The current U.S. EPA limit, the **Maximum Contaminant Level (MCL)**, is 10 μg/l (lowered from 50 μg/l in 2001), which is exceeded in ground-water in substantial parts of the U.S., particularly in the Southwest.

Lead (Pb, 1 μmol ≈207 μg) is an additional example of elements with questionable essentiality, whose toxicity is commonly known (**B**). Due to its similarity to Ca, Pb is deposited preferentially in bone; there it forms a pool from which it may be released.

Adult cumulative lead intakes of 50–60 μg/d are safely below that threshold. Exposure of children through drinking water from Pb-containing pipes can be more critical where cumulative exposure from water (70 μg), food (100 μg) and air (18 μg) can exceed 190 μg/d, especially if combined with Ca and Fe deficiency, leaded paint (common in older urban housing—the top source of lead poisoning in the U.S.) and Pb from automobile emissions close to the ground.

In 1970, a blood level of 40 μg Pb/dl was considered evidence of poisoning. Since then, the permissible threshold has been continuously lowered to 10 μg/dl in 2001. Yet, in some inner-city populations, 30–60% of 1–8-year-olds were found to exceed the most recent new threshold. A recent study estimates that nationwide, 2.2% of children 1–5 years of age have blood levels >10 μg/dl. Children's blood Pb levels have decreased continuously since monitoring first began in the 1970s (13.4 million >10 μg/dl in 1976–1980 to 434 000 in 1999–2000).

Silicon (Si, 1 μmol ≈28 μg) naturally occurs as silicon oxide (SiO_2) or silicate (SiO_4^{4-}), is important for connective tissue and the skeleton. In foods, Si occurs predominantly bound to organic compounds (e.g., pectin) from where it is hard to absorb; silicic acid monomers have better availability.

The essentiality of Si for humans has not been ascertained, nor have any deficiency symptoms been described. Actual intakes are estimated at 20–50 mg/d. There are no reliable data about Si contents in foods; plants tend to have higher contents.

A. Arsenic

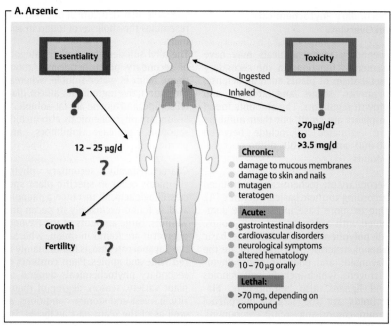

B. Lead

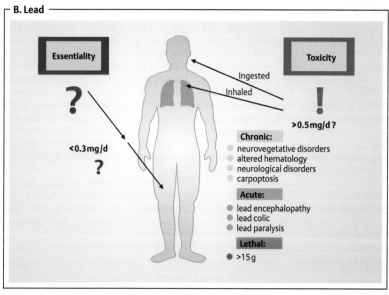

Secondary Phytochemicals: An Overview

Secondary phytochemicals may have numerous functions in the secondary metabolism of plants such as defense, pigments, scents and aromas, and growth regulators. The amounts found in plants are small, but their numbers are estimated to include between 60 000 and 100 000 different compounds.

Secondary phytochemicals are grouped according to their basic structures (**A**). One or more base units can be combined with a large variety of R groups. All **polyphenols** have the same basic phenol structure. Among them are the flavonoids and phenolic acids. Phytoestrogens, which include isoflavonoids and lignans, also belong here. **Flavonoids** are the largest polyphenol group, comprising ~6500 compounds. Anthocyans, a flavonoid subcategory, are again subdivided into nonglycosylated anthocyanidins (aglycones) and glycosylated anthocyanins. Some anthocyanins are used as food colorants under category E163.

Carotenoids consist of eight isoprenoid subunits and are therefore tetraterpenes. We distinguish between oxygen-free carotenes (α- and β-carotene, lycopene) and oxygen-containing xanthophylls.

Myrosinase-mediated degradation of **glucosinolates** may result in the active forms: isothiocyanates, thiocyanates, and/or indoles.

Monoterpenes contain two isoprene subunits. They are the main constituents of etheric oils.

Isoflavonoids, lignans, and coumestans are **phytoestrogens**.

The molecular structure of **phytosterols** resembles the cholesterol found in animals.

The allyl sulfides are another category of secondary phytochemicals. Among them, alliin is water-soluble, whereas the main active ingredients, allicin, diallyl sulfide, and ajoene are fat-soluble.

Secondary phytochemicals also include saponins, protease inhibitors, and phytic acid.

Characteristically, secondary phytochemicals occur in **specific** plant species. Ellagic acid, for instance, a phenolic acid, is found exclusively in pecan and walnuts. Large amounts of the flavonol quercetin are found in onion, whereas the flavanol catechin, is found mainly in red wine and apples. Plant **contents** of secondary phytochemicals depend on plant variety, season, degree of maturity, harvest and storage conditions, as well as of the plant part analyzed. For instance, glucosinolate content in wild broccoli exceeds that of cultivated broccoli by a factor of 1000. **Processing** also has a major impact. Only carotenes and soy saponins are heat-resistant. Phenolic acids and flavonoids are found only in the outer layers. Consequently, juices, for example, have much lower contents. Terpenes and phenolic acids are susceptible to oxidation; glucosinolates are degraded within two weeks during fermentation. Refined soy oil contains only a third of the phytosterols of native oil.

Bioavailability varies, as well: anthocyans, lignans, esterified phenolic acids, phytosterins, and saponins have low bioavailability, whereas that of carotenes (especially when heated), glucosinolates, sulfides and terpenes is high.

A. Secondary Phytochemicals

Group: typical representatives	Basic structure	Occurrence in foods
Anthocyans: Cyanidin Delphinidin	Anthocyanidin 	Red, blue, and purple colored fruit and vegetables, their juices and wines Red and black legumes
Carotenoids: α- and β-Carotene Lycopene Lutein Zeaxanthin		Carotene in orange, red, yellow fruit and vegetables Xanthophylls in green leafy vegetables
Flavonoids: Flavonoles: quercetin Flavanoles: catechin Flavanones: hesperidin Flavones: luteolin	Flavonoles 	Many kinds of fruit and vegetables, mainly in the outer layer, e.g., onions, cabbage, apples, red wine
Glucosinolates		Cabbage, mustard, cress, horseradish
Monoterpenes	D-Limonene 	Orange and grapefruit juice, citrus peel, ginger
Phenolic acids: Hydroxycinnamonic acid: caffeic acid, ferulic acids, Hydroxybenzoic acid: gallic acid	Hydroxycinnamonic acids 	Many kinds of fruit and vegetables, mainly in the outer layer Coffee, whole grains, bran, potatoes with skin
Phytoestrogens: Isoflavones: genistein Lignans: secoisolariciresinol Coumestans	Isoflavones 	Isoflavones in soy, clover, lignans in whole grain, oil seed, flax seed
Phytosterins: β-Sitosterin Stigmasterin Sitosanol	Isoflavones 	In oily plant parts Grains, nuts, seeds Virgin plant oils
Saponins: Glycyrrhizin	Basic triterpene structure 	Licorice, legumes, spinach, asparagus, oats
Sulfides: Alliin, allicin, diallyl sulfide Diallyldisulfide: ajoene		Garlic, onions, scallions, shallots, leek

Secondary Phytochemicals: Effects and Activities

The use of plants for healing has been documented since antiquity. In recent history, more emphasis was placed on the negative effects of various phytochemicals, like cyanide, protease inhibitors, or phytic acid. Based on intensive research conducted in recent years, secondary phytochemicals are gaining popularity as health-enhancing phytonutrients. As an example, phytic acid used to be known only for its negative effect as a complexing agent, preventing mineral absorption; recent reports emphasize its blood glucose stabilizing and possible anticancer effects.

Secondary phytochemicals can have a broad range of **effects (A)**. Many findings, however, are based on in vitro and animal studies. To date, human studies remain the exception.

A major aspect of the discussion of all secondary phytochemicals is their **interference with carcinogenesis (B)**, with a wide range of proposed mechanisms. In the initiation phase, the formation of procarcinogens may be prevented (B1). Some carcinogens are present in the body, but require activation by phase I enzymes. Phase II enzymes, in turn, can deactivate activated carcinogens. Secondary phytochemicals may act by inhibiting phase I and activating phase II enzymes (B2). They can also directly bind activated carcinogens (B3). Free radical scavengers can prevent damage to DNA (B4). All secondary phytochemicals have been reported to have anticarcinogenic activities during the tumor promotion phase (B5). These include: binding of tumor promoters, increasing the rate of apoptosis, inhibition of various phases of the cell cycle, thereby preventing cell proliferation, inhibition of growth factors, enhancing the activity of tumor-killing immune cells, or regulating effects on cell signaling via gap junctions.

The **antioxidant** effects of secondary phytochemicals are not limited to protecting DNA; they also prevent the oxidation of lipids, like cell membranes and LDL particles. Via the prostaglandin metabolism, secondary phytochemicals can have **antithrombotic** and **anti-inflammatory** effects. The **cholesterol-lowering effect** of phytosterols may be based on their metabolic competition with cholesterol. Saponins can form insoluble complexes with cholesterol, and have an inhibitory effect on primary bile acids.

Many results of in vitro studies could not be reproduced in intervention studies. However, epidemiological studies show a clear correlation between high fruit and vegetable intakes and low incidence of cardiovascular disease and many forms of cancer. Some individual substances may just represent indicators of a high fruit/high vegetable nutrition. Therefore, the "5 A Day" rule is still the best recommendation for an optimal intake of secondary phytochemicals.

Estimated **intakes** of secondary phytochemicals range between 1 and 1.5 g/d. Vegetarian and traditional Asian nutrition, for example, provide significantly higher amounts.

A. Possible Effects of Secondary Phytochemicals

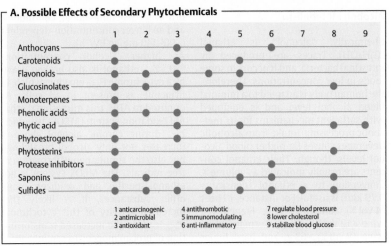

1 anticarcinogenic   4 antithrombotic   7 regulate blood pressure
2 antimicrobial   5 immunomodulating 8 lower cholesterol
3 antioxidant   6 anti-inflammatory 9 stabilize blood glucose

B. Possible Interference with Carcinogenesis

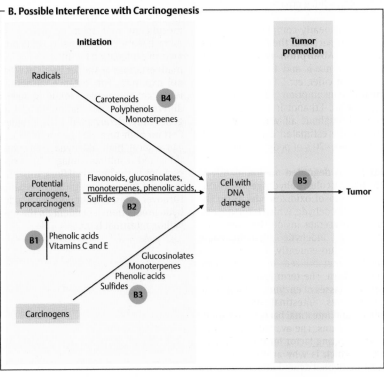

Alcohol: Metabolism

Chemically, "alcohol" is ethanol (C_2H_5OH). Traces are produced by intestinal bacteria, and it occurs in some foods in low concentrations. Therefore, the human body is adapted to a minimal blood alcohol level and is equipped with sufficient mechanisms for its metabolic processing. Intake from **alcoholic beverages** causes far higher blood alcohol levels, though. Their ethanol contents are usually indicated as volume %. Conversion to g ethanol (density = 0.79 kg/l) is useful. For instance, 1 l beer (4 vol%) contains ~32 g, French red wine (12 vol%) ~95 g, German white wine (8 vol%) ~63 g, and hard liquor (40 vol%) ~360 g ethanol.

Ethanol is nearly completely absorbed in the stomach and the proximal intestine (**A**). **Absorption** is faster on an empty stomach and from hot drinks (grog, hot cider, etc.). Prior or simultaneous consumption of food slows absorption. Ethanol is rapidly distributed throughout all watery compartments, the estimated distribution volume being ~70 % of body weight.

Ethanol is **degraded** predominantly in the liver. **Alcohol dehydrogenase** (ADH) in the cytosol oxidizes ethanol to the toxic acetaldehyde, which is further oxidized to acetate inside the mitochondria by aldehyde dehydrogenase (ALDH). Subsequently, the acetate is further metabolized in intermediate metabolism. The term ADH designates several classes of enzymes that occur in hepatocytes, intestinal mucosa, and buccal and intestinal bacteria in various constellations. The availability of NAD^+ is the limiting factor for the ADH reactions, which is why at concentrations >0.2 ‰, alcohol degradation turns into a

0th order reaction—linear, continuous, and no longer concentration-dependent (~90–140 mg/kg BW/h).

At higher alcohol concentrations (>0.5 ‰), ethanol is also broken down by a cytochrome P_{450} enzyme, which, in principle, is present in all cells. As opposed to ADH, this microsomal ethanol oxidation system (**MEOS**) is inducible: during chronic alcohol abuse it increases not only alcohol breakdown but also the simultaneous formation of free radicals. The MEOS system is not ethanol-specific and oxidizes many other substances. It is likely that increased activity of this cytochrome P_{450} leads to the increased transformation of procarcinogens to carcinogens.

The discovery of **ADH and ALDH polymorphisms** and their occurrence in extra-hepatic compartments could provide an explanation for differing clinical manifestations at similar levels of ethanol exposure. For instance, alcoholics with carcinomas were found to have a different ADH constellation, indicating genetically determined risk profiles. Certain high-turnover gastric ADH can cause local high aldehyde concentrations and resulting damage. The same pertains to the intestinal flora: different bacterial species have different ethanol turnover rates, making intestinal aldehyde production dependent on the prevailing intestinal flora.

A. Metabolism

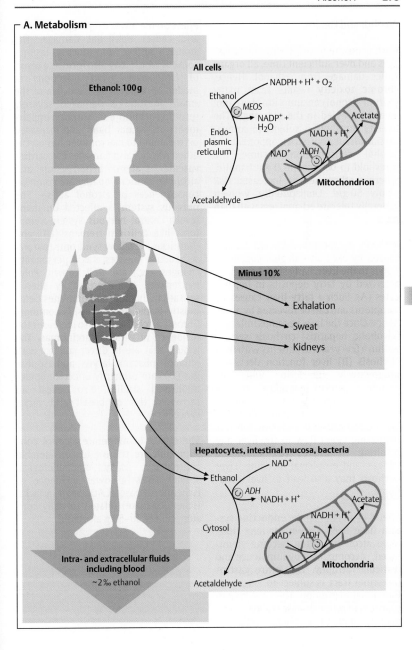

Alcohol and Health

With exposure to sufficiently high dosages and over sufficient time, all organs suffer damage from ethanol. Hence, **chronic toxicity** results from many years of alcohol consumption at ethanol levels expressed in the g/d range. The toxicity threshold is subject to controversial discussion: strict opponents of alcohol consumption assume the threshold to be close to 0 g ethanol/d, whereas others see no increased risk below 50 g/d. Undisputedly, women generally tolerate ethanol less well than men.

Probably the most well-known damage caused by excessive alcohol consumption is to the **liver**. Early stages are characterized by fatty deposits in hepatocytes (**A**). Such a **fatty liver** causes no symptoms and can be reversed by abstinence. Once the liver becomes inflamed (alcoholic hepatitis) cirrhosis sets in within a few years. In patients with **liver cirrhosis** (**B**) liver function decreases progressively, interfering with bile secretion (icterus: jaundice), protein synthesis (tendency towards hemorrhage, edema, etc.), and blood flow. The latter effect causes portal hypertension, restricting blood flow to the liver and resulting in ascites (**C**), esophageal varices, and esophageal bleeding. Liver cirrhosis may also lead to liver carcinoma.

Effects of alcohol on the **endocrine system** have been known for long time. Male alcoholics often become "feminized," accompanied by impotence and testicular atrophy. The entire **gastrointestinal tract** is subject to long-term functional disruption. The well-known gastric acid reflux disease (GERD) is frequently due to alcohol's inhibiting effect on the lower esophagal sphincter and causes epithelial damage. The stomach suffers from mucosal lesions, some of which may also form as a result of *Heliobacter pylori* infections in moderate drinkers. The mucosa of the small intestine is damaged severely resulting in multiple absorption impairments on the one hand, and increased permeability to macromolecules on the other. Alcohol also damages the **cardiovascular system**: hypertension and alcoholic cardiomyopathy are common consequences of alcohol abuse. The **nervous system** is affected on many levels: central nervous system symptoms like delirium tremens (DT) and Wernicke-Korsakow syndrome (paralysis of ocular muscles, ataxia, personality changes, etc.) are well known. Polyneuropathy, characterized by altered sensation, tingling, and numbness, etc., mostly in the extremities, is common. Chronic alcohol abuse also increases the incidence of various **carcinomas**. The tissues that are in direct contact with ethanol—pharynx, larynx, and esophagus (**D**)—are primarily affected. Epidemiological studies also reveal an increased risk of breast and rectal cancers.

The effects of **moderate alcohol consumption** are subject to considerable controversy. Many epidemiological studies show a lower incidence of ischemic disease (CAD, heart attacks, ischemic stroke) related to daily consumption of 30–50 g alcohol/d.

A. Fatty Liver

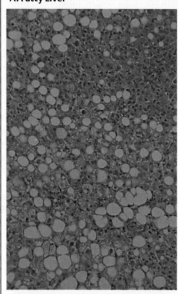

B. Liver Cirrhosis

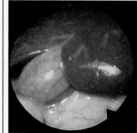

Normal liver

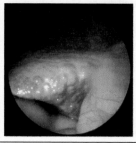

Cirrhotic liver

C. Ascites

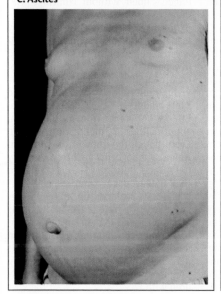

D. Esophagal Carcinoma

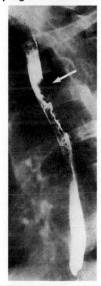

Alcohol and Nutrition

Overall alcohol consumption the U.S. is well-documented through tax records. While alcohol tax rates vary by state, they provide considerable revenue to state and federal governments (total $11.5 billion in 1996). On the flip-side are the economic costs of alcohol consumption, (medical treatment, hospitalization, loss of productivity, loss to society from premature deaths). These were estimated to be $148 billion in 1992.

After the end of prohibition (1935), **alcohol consumption** increased slowly, peaking in the 1980s (10.4 l of pure ethanol/year, on average, for anyone above 15) and has since fallen by 20 % back to 1970s levels (8.3 l/year or 22.7 g/d and person) (**A**). Present consumption rates are similar to those in Canada. Fifteen million Americans are "alcoholics"; an additional 31.9 million are binge drinkers (≥5 drinks on the same occasion on ≥1 day during the past month) and 11 million drinkers are under 21.

Beer makes up ~56 % of all alcohol consumed, wine ~15 %, and spirits ~29 % (**B**). Compared to European figures, U.S. spirits and wine consumption is similar to that of Central and Eastern Europe; Western Europeans consume more wine and fewer spirits.

Most **alcoholics** are of normal weight or overweight and probably suffer from multiple nutrient deficiencies. This becomes evident from a simple calculation: with a caloric content of 7 kcal/g, several bottles of beer can easily amount to 50 % or more of daily energy requirements—the nutrients from the corresponding amount of nutrient-dense foods are therefore missing. Additionally, excessive alcohol consumption leads to impaired absorption and altered metabolism. **Nutrient defi**ciencies (e. g., magnesium, zinc, potassium) are the rule (**C**). Among the vitamins, the B-complex is most commonly deficient. Impairment of the central and peripheral nervous systems is related to a lack of vitamins B_1 and B_6. Macrocytosis (enlarged erythrocytes) is mainly associated with folic acid deficiency and is common among alcoholics. Up to 50 % of cirrhotic alcoholics have vitamin A deficiency, caused in part by increased retinol oxidation. The combined effects of malabsorption and reduced exposure to sunlight cause vitamin D deficiency. Increased free radical production, caused, in part, by the preferential use of the MEOS, may lead to increased use of vitamin E, causing deficiency when combined with marginal intakes.

It should be noted that all the above-mentioned results were observed in people with clinically apparent alcohol-related impairments. Whether moderate alcohol consumption has similar effects—albeit without clinical consequences—is unknown.

Exposure to alcohol in the womb may lead to **Fetal Alcohol Syndrome** (FAS). It is estimated to occur in 2.0 out of 1000 live births in the U.S. and the cost of treatment of infants, children, and surviving adults with FAS was an estimated $1.9 billion in 1992. **Fetal Alcohol Effects** (FAE) range from morphological abnormalities to mental impairment. Even though the number of women in America who drink before pregnancy (69 %) and during (48 %) is similar to that in European countries and Australia/New Zealand (69 and 49 %, respectively), the rate of FAS in the U.S. is 20 times higher than in any other country ("**American paradox**"). The reason for this high incidence is unknown. Four percent of "heavy" drinkers during pregnancy in the U.S. give birth to children with FAS.

A. Alcoholic Drinks

U.S.	Canada	France	Italy	Spain	Germany	China	Japan	Alcohol per capita/year (l)
4.6	4.2	2.1	1.2	3.1	6.1	1.0	6.0	Beer
1.3	2.2	6.3	5.9	4.5	2.5	4.4	2.0 (incl. sake)	Wine
2.4	1.2	2.4	0.6	2.5	2.0	0.1	0.75	Spirits
7.3	**7.6**	**10.8**	**7.7**	**10.1**	**10.6**	**5.5**	**8.75**	**Total**

B. Women Reporting ≥ 7 Drinks/Week or ≥ 5 Drinks During Previous Month (18 – 44 y)

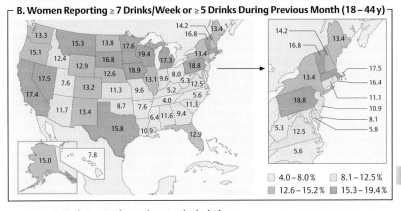

4.0 – 8.0 %   8.1 – 12.5 %
12.6 – 15.2 %   15.3 – 19.4 %

C. Vitamin Deficiencies from Chronic Alcohol Abuse

Vitamin	Incidence	Causes	Clinical consequences
A, carotenoids	10 – 50 %	Diminished intake, impaired metabolization azoospermia	Night blindness,
D	10 – 50 %	Diminished intake, increased catabolism, malabsorption	Osteomalacia, increased colon cancer risk
E	?	Malabsorption, increased catabolism	CVD
K	10 %	Impaired metabolism coagulation, osteoporosis	Impaired blood
C	50 %	Reduced intake	Pre-scurvy, cataract risk
B_1	20 – 70 %	Inhibition of active transport	Wernicke-Korsakoff syndrome
B_2	20 – 40 %	Reduced intake	Glossitis, stomatitis
B_6	> 50 %	Unclear (impaired hepatic metabolization)	CNS damage
B_{12}	< 10 %	Malabsorption	CNS damage
Folic acid	20 – 70 %	Reduced intake, impaired absorption, hydrolysis, transport and metabolism	Macrocytosis, CVD risk, teratogenicity

Herbs and Spices

Herbs and spices are by definition plant components suited for human consumption due to their natural content of flavor and fragrance-providing compounds. They are used mostly dried and processed (e.g., ground), also fresh or deep-frozen, and are increasingly available as spice aroma extracts.

Herbs and spices have been used for millennia to enhance food **flavor** and **fragrance** and formerly for preservation purposes since many of them have antimicrobial effects. The oldest records of spice use date from 2000 BC, from Babylonia. U.S. spice imports exceed $370 million per year, with capsicum peppers (including paprika) >$60 million followed by sesame seeds with >$43 million.

With the exception of larger portions of fresh herbs, herbs and spices generally do not supply nutrients to humans. Unquestionably, though, they do influence our nutritional choices. A well-prepared, deliciously flavored meal "makes our mouth water"; is this reaction due to conditioning of our brains or is it elicited by the actual compounds in the herbs and spices?

Juniper berries (A) can be used to exemplify how difficult it is to answer this question. Different books on herbs and spices describe their flavor and use in rather different ways—apparently, perceptions are subjective and influenced by regional use and traditions. Chemical analysis reveals that juniper berries may contain hundreds of substances. The flavor is usually attributed to etheric oils, which are mixtures of many different compounds.

There is abundant literature about the **effects** of these complex herbs and spices on the digestive, excretory, and circulatory system. For instance, chili peppers are said to affect saliva secretion, mustard and paprika bile secretions, and turmeric and mint bile formation. The lay literature claims that juniper berries "enhance appetite," are "diaphoretic," and "diuretic." Mostly, such claims are not scientifically proven but based on traditional use. Such firmly established beliefs make scientific studies very difficult. Any spice that has to be tasted and/or smelled in order to exert its effects automatically evokes thoughts associated with that specific taste and/or smell. Therefore, it is impossible to distinguish between pharmacological effects and conditioning. Only a few substances have been more thoroughly researched. Capsaicin from chili peppers and paprika has vasodilatory effects, which may cause sweating in sensitive people. The compounds in garlic (e.g., allicin) and onions are being investigated for their protective properties. Carnosol and carnosolic acid, the two main active ingredients of rosemary, are potent antioxidants and have shown anticarcinogenic and antiviral effects in vitro. Turmeric (*Curcuma longa*), to which curry owes its yellow color, was shown to have antibacterial, antiviral, anticancer, antispasmodic, fungicidal, anti-inflammatory, and antioxidant properties.

A. Juniper Berries

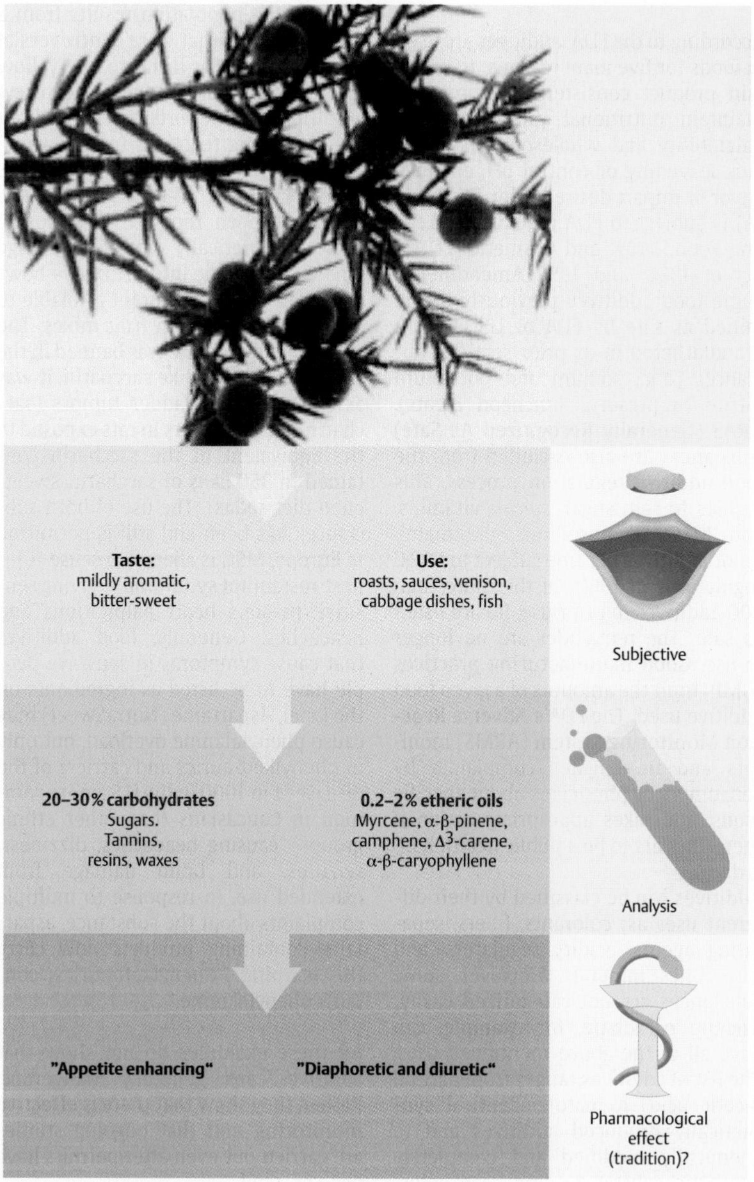

Taste:
mildly aromatic,
bitter-sweet

Use:
roasts, sauces, venison,
cabbage dishes, fish

Subjective

20–30% carbohydrates
Sugars.
Tannins,
resins, waxes

0.2–2% etheric oils
Myrcene, α-β-pinene,
camphene, Δ3-carene,
α-β-caryophyllene

Analysis

"Appetite enhancing"

"Diaphoretic and diuretic"

Pharmacological
effect
(tradition)?

Additives: An Overview

According to the FDA, additives are used in foods for five main reasons: to maintain product consistency, improve or maintain nutritional value, maintain palatability and wholesomeness, provide leavening or control pH, enhance flavor or impart desired color. Their use (**A**) is subject to FDA regulations (Federal Food, Drug, and Cosmetic [FD&C] Act of 1938, and 1958 Amendment). Some food additives previously determined as safe by FDA or USDA were grandfathered in as prior-section substances (e. g., sodium and potassium nitrite to preserve luncheon meats). **GRAS** (**G**enerally **R**ecognized **A**s **S**afe) substances are also excluded from the food additive regulation process. This applies to salt, sugar, spices, vitamins, and MSG (monosodium glutamate). Color additives became subject to FD&C regulations in 1960. Of the more than 200 additives in prior use, 90 are listed as safe. The remainder are no longer in use. **Good manufacturing practices** (**GMP**) limit the amounts of a given food additive used. The FDA's **Adverse Reaction Monitoring System** (**ARMS**) monitors and investigates complaints by consumers or physicians about specific foods, and takes appropriate action if there appears to be a public health hazard.

Additives can be classified by their different uses as: colorants, fillers, separating agents, acidity regulators, and sometimes minerals. However, some substances are not categorized easily: calcium carbonate, for example, can have all of the above-mentioned uses. The list of additives ranges from natural (acetic acid) to nature-identical synthetically produced additives and to chemically modified and completely synthetic substances (e. g., azo colorants). The poor image of additives in parts of the population results from a few substances that were **controversial** at some point. For instance, the yellow colorant tatrazine repeatedly drew attention after reports emerged about pseudoallergic reactions to it in acetyl salicylic acid (aspirin)-sensitive persons in 1959. Similar reactions to benzoic acid have been reported. Erythrosine could theoretically introduce large amounts of iodine into the body—however, it is the only colorant available to color cherries (red) in fruit mixes. The sweetener cyclamate was banned in the U.S. in 1970 since, like saccharin, it was associated with bladder tumors (saccharin caused tumors in rats exposed to the equivalent of the saccharin contained in 350 cans of saccharin-sweetened diet sodas). The use of both substances has been and still is permitted in Europe. MSG is alleged to cause "Chinese restaurant syndrome"—giving sensitive persons heart palpitations and headaches. Generally, food additives that cause symptoms in sensitive people have to be listed as ingredients on the label. Aspartame (NutraSweet) may cause phenylalanine overload, but only in phenylketonurics and carriers of the disease (1 in 1000 in the U.S., more common in Caucasians than other ethnic groups), causing headaches, dizziness, seizures, and brain damage from extended use. In response to multiple complaints about the substance, aspartame-containing products now carry this warning: "Phenylketonurics: contains phenylalanine."

All these examples do not show that additives are generally dangerous. Rather, they show that there is **effective monitoring** and that ongoing studies are carried out even after permits have been granted.

A. Additives

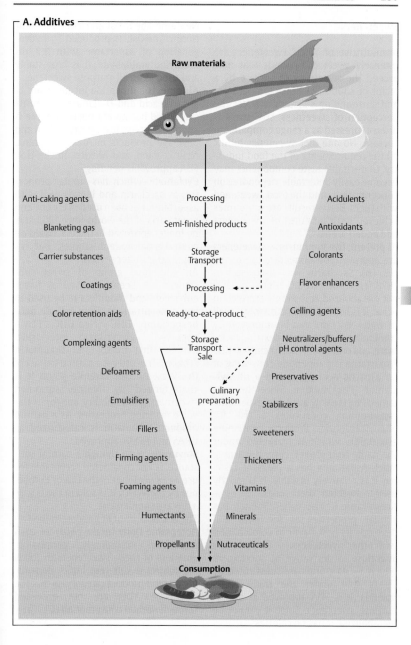

Sweeteners

Nonnutritive or "diet" sweeteners are intensely sweet compounds that may exceed the sweetness of sucrose by a factor of ≤3000 (**A**). Since temperature and surrounding substances affect the perception of sweetness, sweetness is often expressed as a range compared to sucrose. No one diet sweetener fulfills all the requirements of the food industry. Undesirable taste components may become easily detectable, depending on concentrations and the food sweetened with them. Better results are sometimes achieved with mixtures of sweeteners and added aromas.

At present, five nonnutritive sweeteners are approved for alimentary use in the U.S. (**B**). **Saccharin** was discovered in 1878. It is absorbed quickly, but since it is not metabolized, it is simply excreted in urine. It is heat-stable and dissolves well in water. Its taste can be improved by combining it with maltodextrin, cyclamate, and other flavor enhancing agents.

Aspartame is a dipeptide consisting of an aspartic acid (Asp) and a phenylalanine (Phe) subunit. Since the contained Phe is easily available, aspartame consumption constitutes a risk for phenylketonurics. Products containing aspartame, which is marketed under the name Nutrasweet, carry a warning label. Aspartame has a pleasant taste, but it is relatively instable. It is mostly used to sweeten "diet" sodas.

Acesulfame K, also called Sunnet, has similar properties as saccharin and develops its best flavor in combination with other sweeteners.

Sucralose, a derivative of sucrose, in which 3–OH groups are substituted by Cl, is sold under the trade name Splenda. It is FDA approved as an all-purpose sweetener. Since it cannot be metabolized, it has no calories.

Neotame, the latest and sweetest addition to the list, is produced by hydrogenation of aspartame with 3,3 dimethylbutyraldehyde. It is heat-stable and used as an all-purpose sweetener.

Alitame, is a dipeptide formed from L-aspartic acid and D-alanine. It is heat-stable and has no aftertaste. Alitame is approved for use in a variety of food and beverage products in Australia, China, New Zealand, and Mexico. In the U.S., FDA approval is pending.

Cyclamate, which has similar properties as saccharin and blends well with aspartame, has been used in Europe and other parts of the world since 1963. It is no longer approved in the U.S. based on controversial rodent studies, but re-approval is under review.

An additional group of sweet substances has been approved as flavor enhancers and modifiers to be used in low concentrations. They include **neohesperidine DHC** (Neo-DHC, FEMA approved), glycyrrhizin, stevioside, maltol, ethyl maltol and **thaumatin** (Thalin). The latter is a natural extract of the West African katemfe plant. It is characterized by intense, sustained sweetness, good stability, and for its flavor-enhancing properties. As a natural product, thaumatin is categorized as **GRAS** and FEMA-approved.

Stevioside, even though a natural substance, is not considered acceptable for use as a sweetener in the U.S. or Europe, nor by the WHO. It is sold in the U.S. as a dietary supplement.

The U.S. Government has determined an **Acceptable Daily Intake** (**ADI**) for each sweetener. Accordingly, permissible amounts of these sweeteners in foods are subject to different limits, depending on their product category, so that the respective ADIs are not exceeded through normal consumption (**C**).

A. Relative Sweetness of Diet Sweeteners

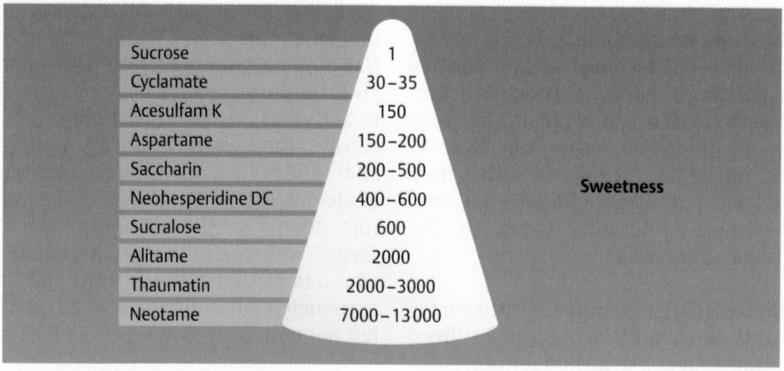

Sucrose	1
Cyclamate	30–35
Acesulfam K	150
Aspartame	150–200
Saccharin	200–500
Neohesperidine DC	400–600
Sucralose	600
Alitame	2000
Thaumatin	2000–3000
Neotame	7000–13000

Sweetness

B. Compounds Approved for Use as Sweeteners in the U.S.

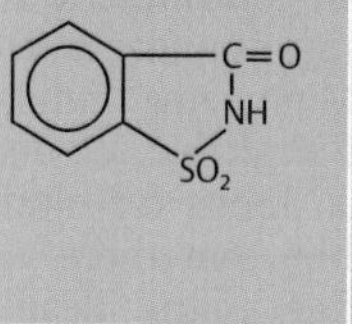

Saccharin

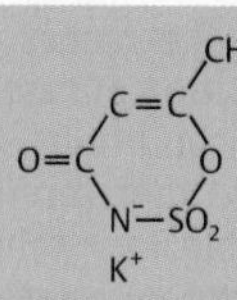

Acesulfame K

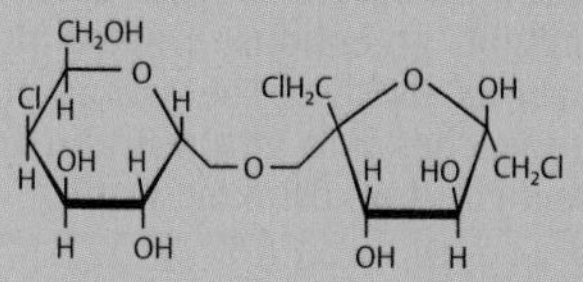

Neotame

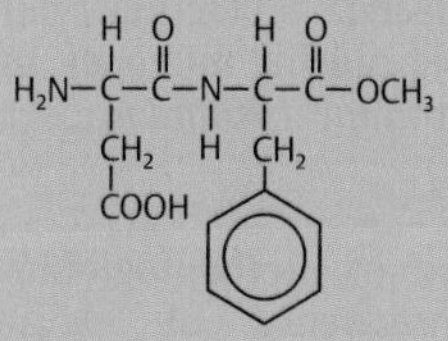

Aspartame

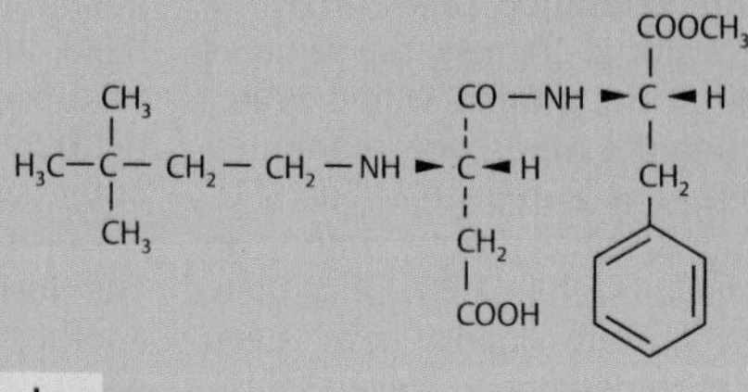

Sucralose

C. Toxicity

Daily ADI Values (WHO/U.S.*)	Sweeteners								
(mg/kg body weight)	15	50*	11	5	15	18	ND	ND	Unlimited
Sugar equivalents (mg/kg BW)	125	700	300	180					
	Acesulfame K	Aspartame	Cyclamate	Saccharin	Sucralose	Neotame	Neohesperidine DC	Alitame	Thaumatin

Contaminants I: Nitrate/Nitrite

The term "contaminant" is used here in the sense of residues and impurities originating either from food production (from agriculture to packaging) or from the environment (water, air). Nitrate and nitrite are exceptions in that they are also permitted additives and are, therefore, sometimes added to the product purposely.

Nitrate (NO_3^-) is a source of nitrogen for plants and therefore used as fertilizer. Certain plants like Boston lettuce, spinach, and radishes can store large amounts of nitrate (≥ 7 g/kg), especially when conditions are not favorable (lack of sunlight, greenhouse). If too much fertilizer is used at the wrong time, nitrate leeches into groundwater from where it gets into drinking water.

Other sources of nitrate are meat products and cheeses, for which nitrate is used as a preservative. In the U.S., the EPA's Oral Reference Dose (RfD) for drinking water is 10 mg/l, the same as the EU limit for ground water. Water nitrate contents have been monitored since 1992. The European Union (EU) limited permissible nitrate content in lettuce and spinach in 1997. Since then, consumer nitrate loads have been reduced somewhat. Nevertheless, under unfavorable conditions, nitrate intakes can still reach 400 mg/d on occasion, which is >50% above the Acceptable Daily Intake (ADI) suggested by the WHO. On average, organically grown plants tend to have lower nitrate content, but since factors like time of harvest and growth location are also significant, the lower contents are within the range of natural variation.

Nitrite content (NO_2^-) in plant foods is negligible. Nitrite is used for the curing of meat products (limit 200 ppm $NaNO_2$/g). Nitrite preserves meats and gives them a lasting red color by turning to NO, which binds to myoglobin.

Nitrite reacts with secondary amines and amides in foods to form carcinogenic nitrosamines/-amides. The old rule "don't grill cheese over cured meats" is obsolete, though; measurable amounts of nitrosamines form only in extremely high-amine fish (e.g., tuna), but not with ham or other cured meats.

Since ingested nitrate is reduced to nitrite during the digestive passage (A), both substances can contribute to the formation of carcinogens under favorable conditions. Minimizing intakes would therefore be desirable. We may be able to establish limits for nitrate content in vegetables, but there will never be nitrate-free plants. Regulations on the addition of nitrite to meat products are a compromise between potential carcinogenicity, on the one hand, and effective protection against food poisoning-causing microbes, particularly Clostridium botulinum on the other hand.

The formation of methemoglobin is another consequence of elevated nitrate/nitrite intakes. Nitrite oxidizes Fe^{2+} to Fe^{3+}, preventing the attachment of O_2. In infants, the reductase which reduces Fe^{3+} back to Fe^{2+} has very low activity; hence, infants are particularly sensitive to nitrate/nitrite.

The user can take preventive measures to reduce nitrate/nitrite intakes: consume cured meats only occasionally and purchase seasonal (or frozen) instead of hothouse vegetables.

A. Nitrate/Nitrite Metabolism

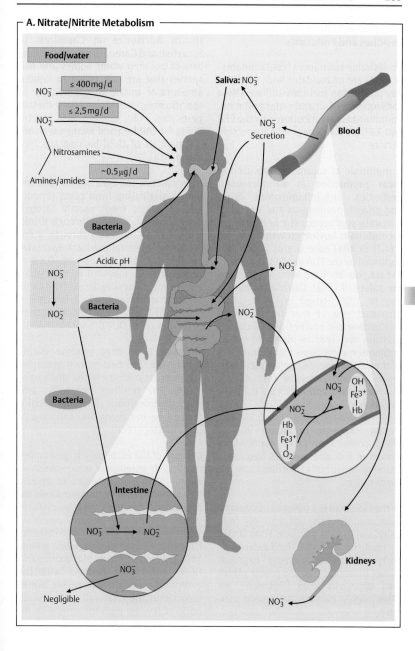

Food/water

NO_3^- ≤ 400 mg/d

NO_2^- ≤ 2,5 mg/d

Nitrosamines

Amines/amides   ~0.5 μg/d

Saliva: NO_3^-

NO_3^-
Secretion

Blood

Bacteria

NO_3^-
↓
NO_2^-

Acidic pH

NO_3^-

Bacteria

NO_2^-

Bacteria

NO_3^-

NO_2^-

$\begin{array}{c} OH \\ | \\ Fe^{3+} \\ | \\ Hb \end{array}$

$\begin{array}{c} Hb \\ | \\ Fe^{3+} \\ | \\ O_2 \end{array}$

Intestine

$NO_3^- \rightarrow NO_2^-$

NO_3^-

Negligible

Kidneys

NO_3^-

Contaminants II:
Residues and Pollutants

Undesirable substances (contaminants) in foods are unavoidable with modern-day production methods and are also a consequence of air and water pollution. Contaminants are monitored by the EPA and USDA Food Safety and Inspection Service.

A multitude of substances are used in **meat production** as antimicrobials, pesticides, anti-inflammatory drugs and growth promotants and to stimulate milk production. The best know is **recombinant bovine growth hormone** (**rBGH** or **rBST**) the use of which was approved by the FDA in 1993. Outside of the U.S., doubts have been raised about the safety of rBGH. Canada banned its use in 1999, based on findings of increased risk of mastitis, infertility, and lameness in bovines. More frequent mastitis may lead to increased use of antibiotics, a problem that contributes to the development of antibiotics resistance. Among excessive contaminant residues found, antibiotics are the most common.

Human exposure to **dioxin**—90% of which comes from foods, mainly fatty tissues of fish and meat—is frequently found to be within a toxicologically relevant range.

In the U.S., **lead** is a ubiquitous contaminant, mainly of the water supply, from paint and leaded gasoline. Food intake accounts for 10–15% of lead exposure. Forty percent of **mercury** exposure comes from coal-burning power plants. Fish, especially from freshwater, are often highly contaminated with mercury.

All states in the U.S. and Canada have **Health Advisories on Chemicals in Sportfish and Game**. These contain long lists of polluted water bodies and fish species that are safe to eat in limited amounts or unsafe to eat because of specific toxic pollutants (heavy metals, pesticides, PCBs, dioxin), with stricter limits for children and women who are pregnant or of child-bearing age (see also p. 316).

Heavy metals and **agricultural contaminants** originating from plant production pass into foods mostly through crops, but also directly through drinking water or indirectly through accumulation in animal products. Excessive pesticide residue is found in ~0.8% of domestic fruit, followed by vegetables and grains. Generally, levels tend to be higher in imported produce, which also frequently contains compounds banned in the U.S. (e.g., DDT).

Pollutant loads may increase during **processing**. The best-known examples are charcoal grilling and the smoking of meats. The resulting polycyclic, aromatic hydrocarbons (PAH) are considered to be mutagens and carcinogens (e.g., benzopyrene).

Because of the extremely large number of all such potentially toxic "contaminants" (**A**) in foods, consumers are easily swayed to believe that our foods are "poisoned." Scientific risk assessment yields a different picture: problems with nutritional choices and hygiene have much larger impact, while pollutants and contaminants play a comparatively minor role perhaps with the exception of certain fish species, due to bioaccumulation. Overall, risks should be kept low by monitoring and minimizing residues and contaminants.

A. Sources of Food Contaminants

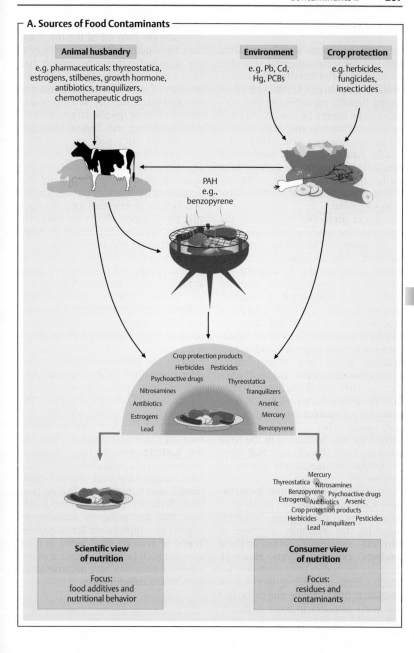

Pre- and Probiotics

Pre- and probiotics supplementation aims to achieve the same goal: changing the balance of the intestinal flora—particularly in the large intestine—by introducing friendly microbes (**A**). This balance can be altered by directly affecting existing microbes as well as by displacing undesirable ones. Beyond the quantitative aspect, improving adhesion of beneficial microbes to the surface of the epithelial cells and reducing adhesion of potentially pathogenic microbes have been suggested.

The use of **prebiotics** is based on the principle that offering larger amounts of substrate to beneficial microbes increases their numbers. Such substances must be able to traverse the stomach and upper small intestine without being hydrolyzed or absorbed. They have to reach the colon intact to provide a fermentable substrate for lactobacilli, eubacteria, and/or bifidobacteria. Several oligosaccharides, particularly inulin and other fructooligosaccharides have these characteristics. Their specificity lies in the fact that the desired bacteria have a β-fructosidase that enables them to break β-(1,2) bonds. Other soluble fibers (e.g., pectin) are also fermented in the large intestine but enhance microbial overproduction nonspecifically across all species.

Experiments with fructooligosaccharides have shown that the numbers of bifidobacteria rise rapidly, whereas clostridia, for example, decrease in numbers—apparently confirming these products' expected effects. However, there are no studies to confirm positive health effects of the long-term use of prebiotics; this might be due to the fact that their amounts in most foods are rather low.

Probiotics are used in an attempt to influence the balance of the intestinal flora by supplementing live microbes. The principle is not new: yogurt has been used for the treatment and prophylaxis of gastrointestinal infections for more than a century. What is new is the selection of specific strains for targeted probiotics use. Several goals can be achieved with such supplementation: optimizing resistance to acids and digestive enzymes in the stomach and upper small intestine, improving the duration of the digestive passage (adhesion factors), or selection for other, specific, physiological effects. For the latter purpose, *Lactobacillus reuteri* is used. This bacterium produces a mixture of compounds that impairs the growth of bacteria, fungi, and protozoa. Presently available studies indicate that probiotics might improve immunological defense, prevent intestinal infections, and inhibit colonic carcinogenesis. Final proof of these positive effects is pending.

Most of the above-mentioned studies were performed with "normal" fermented milk products, not supplements. As a result of the studies, the consumption of fermented—but not heat-treated—products can be recommended. Since heat treatment kills the live bacteria, remarks like: "Contains live cultures of *L. acidophilus*," are found only on products that are not heat-treated after fermentation. To date, positive effects of especially tailored probiotics that are presently available as yogurts or supplements are unproven. There is also no final word yet on whether such targeted alteration of the intestinal flora may have negative long-term health consequences.

A. Effects

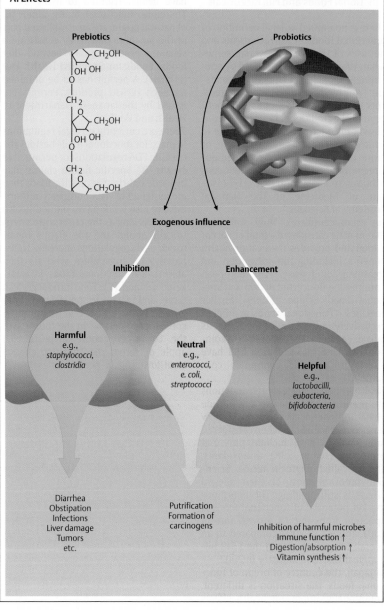

Functional Foods and Nutraceuticals

There is no unified or legal definition of **functional foods** or **nutraceuticals** and the uses of these terms overlap somewhat. Working definitions used by government agencies for "functional foods" are: "Any modified food or food ingredients that may provide a health benefit beyond the traditional nutrients it contains" or "Functional foods are those in which the concentrations of one or more ingredients have been manipulated or modified to enhance their contribution to a healthful diet." (US Institute of Medicine of the National Academy of Sciences.)

For "nutraceuticals": "Any substance that may be considered a food or part of a food and provides medical or health benefits, including the prevention and treatment of disease." The European Commission Concerted Action on Functional Food Science (1999) further specifies: "Functional foods ar offered exclusively in the form of foods, not as pills or capsules. They should be a component of normal nutrition and have effects in amounts commonly consumed."

Health-enhancing/preventive functions are presently attributed to a multitude of natural chemicals in food (**A**), now termed nutraceuticals when considered individually. These include pre- and probiotics (see p. 288), antioxidants, and so-called phytochemicals. Scientific proof of most of their alleged effects is still pending. The enormous market potential of functional foods is apparent from the 7% growth rate in 2001, and 9% in 2002 compared to an overall 3% growth rate in the $518 billion/year U.S. food industry in 2002.

In Japan, the country of origin of functional foods, the situation is different. Traditionally, important health effects have been attributed to many foods. Therefore, functional foods, albeit all of natural origin, are an established part of the Japanese diet. They constitute a separate product group beyond diet foods: **Foods for Specified Health Use (FOSHU)**. A permit has to be obtained for each FOSHU product. Permits are issued by the Japanese Department of Health and Welfare.

There are currently no legal regulations in place for functional foods besides the existing FDA regulations for permissible claims (**B**). Specific health claims may be made only for the specific foods they are assigned to. The European authorities are also working on unified health claims. As long as the criteria are scientifically sound and the claims monitored, such regulations increase transparency for consumers, who are then able to use functional foods in a targeted fashion (**C**). Food producers can target and market to specific consumer groups. In the end, it will be up to the consumer to decide: in the future, will the consumer choose a pectin-rich apple or rather the "healthy, cholesterol-lowering, hi-pectin applesauce?"

A. Foods of the Future?

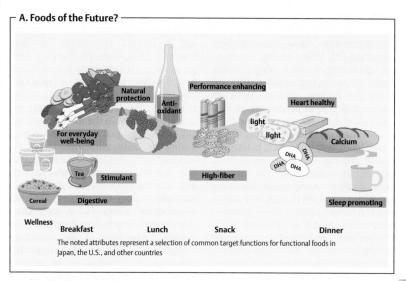

The noted attributes represent a selection of common target functions for functional foods in Japan, the U.S., and other countries

B. Health Claims in the U.S.

Permitted	Not permitted
Calcium/osteoporosis	Fiber/cancer
Folic acid/neural tube defects	Fiber/CVD
Fat/cancer	Antioxidants/cancer
Fat/CVD	Zinc/immunity
Sodium/hypertension	Omega-3 fatty acids/CVD
Fiber in foods/cancer	
Fiber in foods/CVD	
Antioxidants in foods/cancer	

C. Development of Health Claims

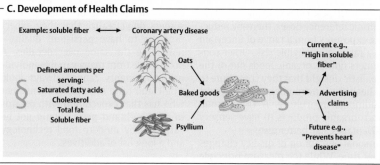

Quality Defined

For the consumer, "quality" is extremely important (**A**). When asking the question pertaining to food groups, staple foods like meats, vegetables, or fruit are given the highest priority. With an increased degree of **processing**, quality becomes less important, only one-third of consumers consider the quality of processed foods very important. In terms of quality criteria, freshness comes first, followed by taste, origin, and brand-name. Reality, however, contradicts the above ranking: even though only one in four consumers claims to attach importance to the brand, brand-name products are most prominently represented on store shelves. An even larger discrepancy appears when it comes to money: price ranks No. 1 among purchase criteria. Hence, quality is a subjective term. It encompasses sensory parameters as well as arguments related to belief systems, suitability, and perceived healthiness (**B**). Different people have different criteria. For instance, some buy "**organic**" foods because of perceived lower contents of pesticides and contaminants—an expectation that is not always met by reality. However, one recent American study on children's exposure to organophosphate (OP) pesticides yielded the conclusion that consuming organic products may reduce exposure levels for various OP pesticides to below the EPA's chronic reference doses, there-by reducing exposures from a range of uncertain to a range of negligible risk. Other consumers opt for organic foods out of the (realistic) insight that they contribute to a healthier environment and support traditional agriculture. A third group finds organic products to have sensory advantages, like better taste.

Personal perception of quality **changes** over time. While the pleasure principle prevails during youth, rational arguments gain the upper hand as people age. "Awareness" of nutrients' roles, the fear of nutrition-related diseases, and sometimes, existing disease, contribute to a different perception of "quality." Last but not least, those aspects of the scientific and technological progress that are reflected in the media continually shape the "quality" concept. While during the 1950s, white bread and lots of meat were considered healthy, and fiber useless "roughage," more recent nutritional knowledge has shifted the emphasis to fiber-rich whole grains and whole-grain products. Where that "awareness" is put into practice, it is mostly in the form of fiber-enriched cereals and baked goods. Unfortunately, whole grains continue to be mostly neglected, except maybe in Chinese restaurants in big cities. Right now, a similar shift is occurring regarding fatty acids: polyunsaturated fatty acids, touted for decades as ideal, are replaced more and more by monounsaturated fatty acids (see p. 114). In the U.S., for the past 30 years, fats were considered unhealthy, and low-fat was the doctrine; now, the fad is low-carb, high protein, and sometimes high-fat.

The **individual character of the quality profile** leads to an extremely large and varied range of foods in the market. Manufacturers have their own ideas about the meaning of "quality." Consumers don't realize that they expect products to have persistent quality—remaining the same over decades. A pizza made from many variable individual components cannot always look, smell, and taste the same. A consumer who has that expectation with regards to a name-brand pizza should not be surprised by modern food technology and a long list of additives.

A. The Importance of "Quality"

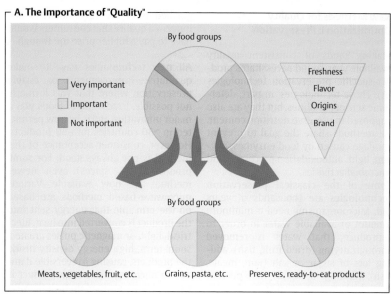

By food groups

- Very important
- Important
- Not important

Freshness
Flavor
Origins
Brand

By food groups

Meats, vegetables, fruit, etc.   Grains, pasta, etc.   Preserves, ready-to-eat products

B. What Is Quality?

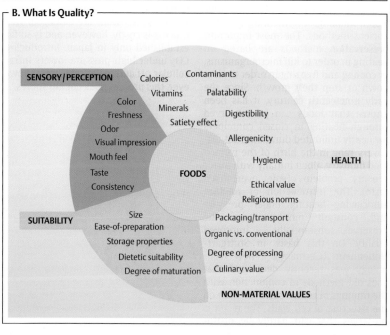

SENSORY / PERCEPTION

Calories   Contaminants
Vitamins   Palatability
Color   Minerals
Freshness   Digestibility
Odor   Satiety effect
Visual impression   Allergenicity
Mouth feel
Taste   Hygiene   **HEALTH**
Consistency   **FOODS**
Ethical value
Religious norms
Size
Ease-of-preparation   Packaging/transport
Storage properties   Organic vs. conventional
Dietetic suitability   Degree of processing
Degree of maturation   Culinary value

SUITABILITY

NON-MATERIAL VALUES

New Methods for Quality Optimization I: Preservation

Making foods of consistent quality available year-round necessitates product-specific preservation technologies (**A**). Those technologies, in part, determine sensory qualities, but they are also supposed to preserve nutrition content. All methods share the goal to prevent spoilage caused by food enzymes, oxygen, light, autooxidation processes, and microbial activities.

Some of the **classical preservation technologies** are thousands of years old. Microorganisms need a minimum amount of available water in order to reproduce; that water is removed through drying (dried fruit, fish), adding lots of sugar or salt (jam, meats, fish). Pickling in liquids that prevent microbial growth (vinegar, alcohol), using oil to displace oxygen and/or water, smoking, or fermenting are other ancient methods. The most important preservation methods are based on heating in order to kill microorganisms, or cooling and freezing in order to slow down or stop their growth. Since the early nineteenth century, it has been known that foods can be preserved through heating in closed containers for nearly unlimited duration. That discovery rang in the birth of the canned food industry, albeit initially with major sensory problems (soft, overcooked taste). The introduction of rotation autoclaving—heating under pressure and constant movement of the preserves—substantially improved quality. On this basis, in Stuttgart-Hohenheim (Germany), a new technology was recently developed that uses old methods in conjunction with the findings of recent basic research on the structure of cell walls. The result is preserves that can hardly be distinguished from the raw materials any longer—a quality that consumers would have to pay a higher price for, though.

All **new technologies** have to make qualitative improvements or enable preservation where that was formerly not possible. Irradiation of foods was a major innovation and is by now permitted in >30 countries for ~50 products. However, consumer acceptance of this method is not always good. For some products (e.g., spices) even newer methods are now available. Various microwave-based methods are based on the principle that energy sent into the product is converted into heat. Electrical, light, or magnetic pulses create a short-term, high energy density inside the products, causing irreversible damage to microorganisms. If a product is exposed to pressure of up to 1000 MPa, large molecules like enzymes, DNA, and microbial cell walls are damaged. This process is costly, however, and is so far established only in Japan. Introducing CO_2 under high-pressure lowers intracellular pH and make cells burst; however, this process does not kill spores.

A. Preservation Methods

New Methods for Quality Optimization II: Genetic Modification

An example of possible quality optimization through genetic modification (GM) is the **Flavr-Savr tomato** that was introduced in the U.S. in 1994. First, the gene that encodes the maturation enzyme polygalacturonase (PG) in tomatoes had to be identified and located. Restriction endonucleases (**A**) were used to cut the complementary DNA strands at specific sites. The same enzymes were then used to cut a plasmid that also carries an antibiotics resistance gene as a marker. By mixing the linear plasmid with the DNA fragments, the fragments were integrated into the plasmids. This process is called gene **cloning**.

The resulting ring-shaped plasmids are introduced into bacteria (**transformation**), which are subsequently grown on growth media, and successfully transformed plasmids are selected by exposure to the respective antibiotic. The surviving bacteria contain plasmids that contain and express the target DNA. Labeled gene probes, the DNA sequence of which is complementary to a part of the cloned sequence, can be used for further selection.

The soil bacterium *Agrobacterium tumefaciens* used to be the only vehicle available for the transfer of such recombinant genes into higher plants. The bacterium produces a so-called Ti plasmid, which integrates into the plant cell chromosomes of dicots. Protoplast transformation is used instead for monocots like rice and cereals. It was recently discovered that by applying the DNA to be transformed to tiny gold or tungsten balls, the DNA can be shot into cells (gene gun) without destroying them; some portion of that DNA is integrated into chromosomes.

In case of the tomato, an inverted copy of the PG-encoding gene was inserted next to the existing normal gene. **Transcription** of both genes results in two complementary RNA strands that join each other, preventing translation. Since the PG enzyme is now missing, the tomato remains firm. The initial goal was to be able to harvest the engineered tomatoes when ripe, making artificial ripening with ethylene unnecessary. The engineered tomatoes could have ripened on the stem, making them far superior in flavor and aroma to commonly available conventional tomatoes. It turned out however, that the skin of the engineered tomatoes is not sufficiently stable when mechanically harvested. Therefore, the **Flavr-Savr tomato** is now used mainly for tomato preserves and tomato paste.

In the U.S., no labeling is required for genetically modified foods. GM foods are considered by the FDA as **GRAS**, which limits the testing required before approval. In the EU, GM foods must be labeled according to the **Novel Food Regulation** of 1997. The **Flavr-Savr tomato** would fall under these regulations even though, unlike most GM foods, it contains no genes from a different species. At this point in time, many GM plant varieties have been approved by the FDA. Approximately 34 % of corn and ~55 % of soy harvested in the U.S. are GM, and 70 %–80 % of all foods found in supermarkets are GM or contain GM components (2002). Most GM varieties in the U.S. are engineered to prevent harvest losses and reduce farm labor costs through either pest (Bt corn, soy, etc.) or herbicide (e.g., glyphosate) resistance, not to improve food characteristics for the consumer.

A. Genetic Engineering

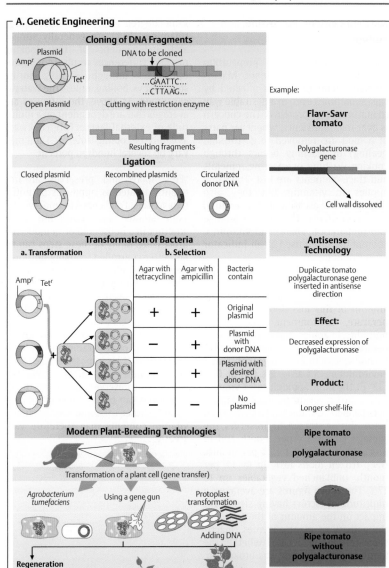

Cloning of DNA Fragments

Plasmid
Amp^r
Tet^r

DNA to be cloned

...GAATTC...
...CTTAAG...

Open Plasmid

Cutting with restriction enzyme

Resulting fragments

Ligation

Closed plasmid

Recombined plasmids

Circularized donor DNA

Transformation of Bacteria

a. Transformation

Amp^r Tet^r

b. Selection

	Agar with tetracycline	Agar with ampicillin	Bacteria contain
	+	+	Original plasmid
	−	+	Plasmid with donor DNA
	−	+	Plasmid with desired donor DNA
	−	−	No plasmid

Modern Plant-Breeding Technologies

Transformation of a plant cell (gene transfer)

Agrobacterium tumefaciens   Using a gene gun   Protoplast transformation

Adding DNA

Regeneration

Transformed cell   Callus culture   Regenerated transgenic plant

Example:

Flavr-Savr tomato

Polygalacturonase gene

Cell wall dissolved

Antisense Technology

Duplicate tomato polygalacturonase gene inserted in antisense direction

Effect:

Decreased expression of polygalacturonase

Product:

Longer shelf-life

Ripe tomato with polygalacturonase

Ripe tomato without polygalacturonase

Nutrient Content, Processing, and Storage

Storage, processing, and preparation alter food nutrient contents. Macronutrients tend to be less affected by this, sometimes even in a desirable way (denaturation of proteins). The concern is over micronutrients: whenever parts of a food are removed (e.g., through peeling) or leaching occurs through cooking, washing, or watering, minerals and trace elements are lost. The same applies to vitamins but they also degrade. Since ascorbic acid (vitamin C) is very sensitive to the effects of storage and preparation, changes in **vitamin C** content are often used as an **indicator** for nutrient losses.

Food **storage** always causes vitamin C loss (**A**). During normal storage, the amount of this loss depends on temperature, environment, and relative humidity. In apples stored at room temperature, all vitamin C is lost within several weeks. In CA storage (controlled environment, 5 % CO_2, 2 % O_2) at 0 °C (32° F), the same apples lose 0 % vitamin C over the same time period. Even products labeled "durable" suffer vitamin C losses during storage. In **preserves**, the average loss is 1 % per month and in precooked foods up to 5 % per month. **Deep-frozen** foods lose up to 3 % per month, unblanched vegetables up to 17 %. The above figures are averages, a multitude of factors having significant impact on the amount of the loss: pH, the activity of plant enzymes (inactivated through blanching), whether the food remains intact or was broken up, cut, etc.

Vitamin losses during **preparation** (**B**) are mainly dependent on the preparation time. If foods are cooked to the same degree each time, losses (e.g., thiamine ~10 %) are generally similar and independent of the cooking method. Differences result from potential losses through leaching during steaming vs. boiling, unless the water is consumed. As above, these figures are averages that are dependent on a multitude of external factors (pH, cookware as catalysts, cooling time, etc.) and may vary by several hundred percent.

"Fresh foods" and "preserves" are frequently treated as opposites by nutrition writers. Foods have to undergo the same storage and processing steps, whether in a household or in industrial processing. Many of these steps can be far better controlled (cooking until just done) in an industrial setting than by a cook, no matter how perfect. On the other hand, even the industry cannot make the tomato jump right from the field into the can. The time of harvest is fixed—losses through intermediate storage are preprogrammed. A direct comparison (**C**) is impossible due to the large number of factors. Whether "fresh" or preserved foods are used, conditions can be favorable or unfavorable in either case, and the remaining vitamin contents may therefore vary greatly.

A. Vitamin C Losses During Storage

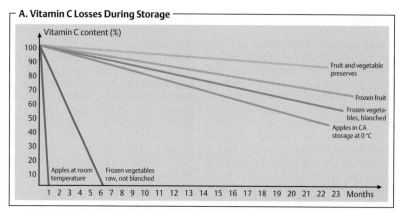

B. Thiamin Loss in Vegetables during Preparation

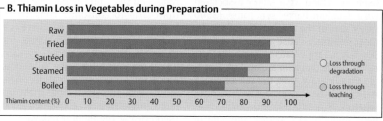

C. "Preserves" vs. "Fresh"

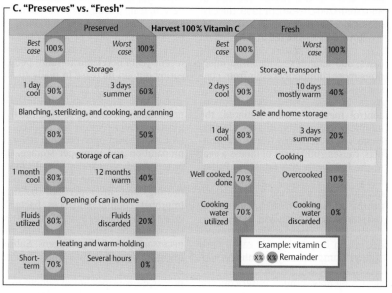

Hygiene

Microorganisms have been and will always be the main food safety concern. According to CDC statistics, in 1999, 25% of Americans were sickened by **food-borne illness**, 0.1% were hospitalized, with 5000 **fatalities**. *Campylobacter jejuni* recently overtook *Salmonella* as the **most common cause of food-borne illness** in the U.S. Ninety percent of chicken tested by the USDA was found to be infected with *C. jejuni,* which is becoming increasingly fluoroquinolone resistant. *C. jejuni* has also been identified as a factor associated with Guillain-Barre syndrome (3500 cases/year in the U.S. and Canada)—the most common cause of acute paralysis—but it rarely causes death. Both *C. jejuni* and *Salmonella* are also transmitted through raw milk, the sale of which is illegal in the U.S. (except within states where it is produced) and Canada (Canada and the U.S. permit the sale of unpasteurized cheese). In 1999, the cost of *Salmonella*-related illness to the U.S. economy was estimated at $2.3 billion (1.4 million reported salmonellosis cases, 600 fatalities). *Salmonella* infections most commonly result from consumption of contaminated poultry and meat. In 1992, when the salmonella control measures were initiated, the numbers were even higher. *Listeria monocytogenes,* mostly from milk products, causes 2000 cases of illness a year in the U.S., with 20% fatalities. Pathogenic *E. coli* (0157: H7 and 0111:H8), mostly found in ground beef, cause 60 deaths annually. These pathogenic *E. coli* strains cause hemolytic uremic syndrome (HUS). They secrete nephrotoxins, which may ultimately cause renal failure. Comparatively, botulism, with less than 60 cases per year (13% fatalities) is by now a much lesser concern, probably due to increased propagation of knowledge about proper canning methods.

YOPIs (young, old, pregnant, and immunocompromised), about 20% of the U.S. population, are at greatest risk from food-borne illness. Known immunosuppressive factors (age, nutritional status, medications, HIV, etc.) allow otherwise harmless germs to become problems. It has also been hypothesized that improved hygiene causes the overall population to become more sensitive to food-borne illness.

Nearly all steps on the passage of food from farm to consumer constitutes a **hygiene risk potential (A)**. There is no guarantee of uncontaminated raw materials, hence the necessary safety has to be ensured during subsequent processing and preparation. Since industrially processed foods make up a large proportion of consumed foods, theoretically, the highest risk would be here. In reality, though, they are a minor source. **Improper food handling** is responsible for 95% of food-borne illness. Increase in food-borne illness in recent years is related to more people eating out, an increase in ready-to-eat foods (with fewer preservatives), the global food supply, and off-site food preparation. According to CDC, the five most common reasons for food-borne illness are: improper cooling, advance preparation and improper storage, infected food preparation staff, inadequate hand washing, inadequate preheating, and improper hot holding. Improper cooling enhances bacterial growth; improper heating of eggs, poultry, raw milk, meat, etc. prevents the necessary killing of pathogens. Subsequent storage of food or keeping it warm allows even a few remaining germs to propagate, causing clinical symptoms.

A. Potential Risks

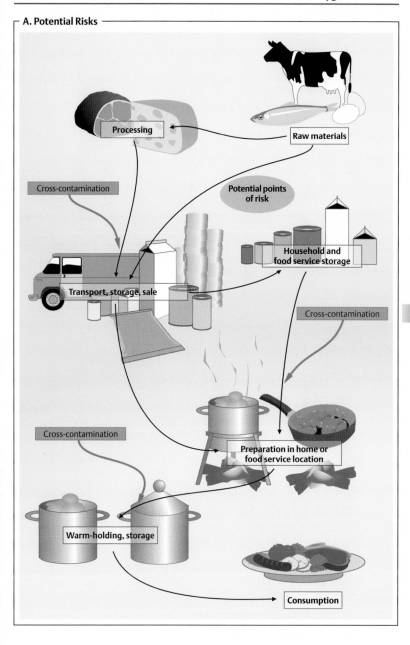

Applied and
Medical Nutrition

Nutrition for Healthy People I

The authorities of many countries issue **nutritional guidelines** aimed at keeping the population healthy. Such recommendations are made available by government agencies as well as private organizations. The industry, for purposes of nutritional marketing and advertising, generally tends to pick up on the official guidelines. In spite of these efforts, alarming reports about **nutrition-related diseases** abound. The combined total cost of the three most common nutrition-related diseases (diabetes, CVD, cancer) was $656 billion in the U.S. in 2000 (**A**). Many diseases have additional hereditary components. That means that the above-mentioned costs could never be reduced to zero, even with optimal nutrition. Nevertheless, there is great potential to reduce the incidence of several major diseases through a change in eating habits and activity levels.

In the Western industrial nations, there is a distinct discrepancy between nutritional recommendations and actual consumption in terms of nutrient, as well as caloric, intakes. Undisputedly, the hygiene standard of foods is high, and protein and caloric intakes are more than adequate, if not often excessive. A comparison of ideal with actual consumption patterns (**B**), however, shows imbalances, in particular, with regard to carbohydrate and fat choices. Analysis of carbohydrate intakes reveals an excess of mono- and disaccharides at the expense of complex carbohydrates, including insufficient fiber intakes (actual: 12 g/d, ideal: 36 g/d). Ideal intakes also do not include energy intake from alcoholic beverages. Actual caloric intakes result increasingly from consumption of animal protein, simple sugars, fat, and alcohol, resulting in a selection of high calorie foods with low **nutrient density**. Nutrient density of food is defined as:

Nutrient content
(μg or mg or g/100 g)
Caloric content
(kcal or kJ or MJ/100 g)

Nutritional patterns have changed dramatically in the U.S. in the past 30 years (**C**). Compared to the guidelines, actual consumption of foods with low nutrient density, like baked goods, sugar and sugary foods, alcohol, as well as fatty meat, meat products, and fatty cheeses, is high, while high nutrient density foods like whole-grain bread and cereals, vegetables other than high-glycemic index preparations of potatoes and iceberg lettuce, fruit, and low-fat dairy are consumed less frequently than recommended. In risk groups like the elderly or pregnant women in particular, this may cause a marginal supply of certain minerals (e. g., Ca, Fe, or iodine) and vitamins (e. g., folic acid) in spite of adequate or even excessive caloric intakes.

A. The Cost of Nutrition-Related Illness

Disease	Number of people affected	Deaths per year	Medical cost (billions)	Productivity loss (billions)	Total cost (billions)
Diabetes	>17 million 29 million projected for 2050	>200 000	91.8	39.8	132
Heart disease and stroke	61 million	950 000	209.3	142.5	351.8
Cancer	>1.3 million new cases projected for 2003	555 600	60.9	110.7	171.6
Obesity and overweight	~186 million (>64%)	300 000	61	56	117

B. Actual Consumption

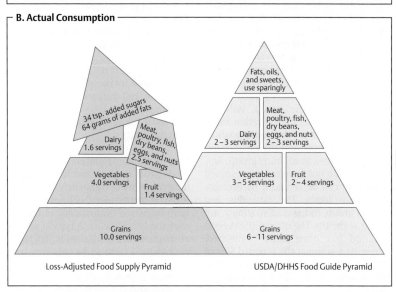

Loss-Adjusted Food Supply Pyramid

USDA/DHHS Food Guide Pyramid

C. Changes in U.S. per Capita Food Consumption, 1970–1997

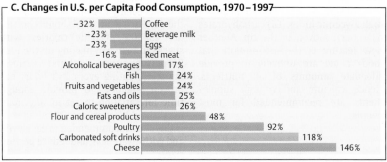

Nutrition for Healthy People II

Since the recommended intakes are abstract numbers for individual nutrients and energy, consumers find it difficult to translate them into appropriate food choices and amounts. This has led to attempts to facilitate the transfer of the scientific findings into easy to understand guidelines for daily nutrition.

The USDA **Food Pyramid** exemplifies this effort (**A**). Recommended amounts of servings to be consumed have been assigned to five **food groups**. Foods rich in complex carbohydrates (bread, cereals, rice and pasta group) represent the base of the pyramid. The second, major basis of proper nutrition should be the fruit and vegetable group, with an emphasis on vegetables. Protein foods are represented by the milk, yoghurt and cheese group, and the meat, poultry, fish, dry beans and nuts group. Animal foods do not have to be consumed daily, and can be replaced by protein-rich plant foods. The fats, oils and sweets group, to be used sparingly, are found at the tip. The official USDA Food Pyramid has often been challenged. Recently, a group at the Harvard School of Public Health published an alternative pyramid (**B**) in which plant oils are placed at the base of the pyramid, next to whole grains, whereas red meat and high **glycemic index** (**GI**) carbohydrates have been moved to the tip. Another new feature is the assumption that foods alone are unlikely to provide adequate amounts of all nutrients. Hence, calcium and vitamin supplements are recommended for most people.

The Dietary Guidelines for Americans: Aim... Build... Choose... for Good Health
Aim for Fitness
- Aim for a healthy weight
- Be physically active each day

Build a Healthy Base
- Let the Pyramid guide your food choices
- Choose a variety of grains daily, especially whole grains
- Choose a variety of fruits and vegetables daily
- Keep food safe to eat

Choose Sensibly
- Choose a diet that is low in saturated fat and cholesterol and moderate in total fat
- Choose beverages and foods to moderate your intake of sugars
- Choose and prepare foods with less salt
- If you drink alcoholic beverages, do so in moderation

Beyond recommendations about which foods to eat and how much, recommendations on meal frequencies and serving sizes can be useful (**C**). Serving sizes have increased dramatically in the U.S. over the last 20 years. A typical serving of spaghetti in a restaurant is 50% larger now than it used to be. Muffins have doubled in size. Soft drink sizes have often more than doubled.

Recommended meal frequencies are 5–6 meals evenly distributed throughout the day. Each main meal should contribute 25–30% of daily calories, with snacks in between making up the rest. For personnel working shifts (e. g., nursing staff), eating every 2–3 hours has proven effective. To provide enough time for satiation to set in, any main meal should last at least 20 minutes. It is therefore recommended to eat slowly and with awareness, and reduce portion sizes.

A. The USDA Food Pyramid

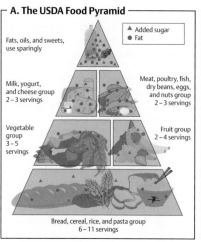

▲ Added sugar
● Fat

Fats, oils, and sweets, use sparingly

Milk, yogurt, and cheese group
2 – 3 servings

Meat, poultry, fish, dry beans, eggs, and nuts group
2 – 3 servings

Vegetable group
3 – 5 servings

Fruit group
2 – 4 servings

Bread, cereal, rice, and pasta group
6 – 11 servings

B. Harvard Public Health Food Pyramid

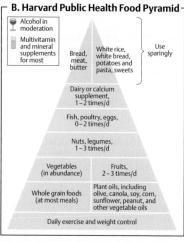

Alcohol in moderation

Multivitamin and mineral supplements for most

Bread, meat, butter | White rice, white bread, potatoes and pasta, sweets — Use sparingly

Dairy or calcium supplement, 1 – 2 times/d

Fish, poultry, eggs, 0 – 2 times/d

Nuts, legumes, 1 – 3 times/d

Vegetables (in abundance) | Fruits, 2 – 3 times/d

Whole grain foods (at most meals) | Plant oils, including olive, canola, soy, corn, sunflower, peanut, and other vegetable oils

Daily exercise and weight control

C. Food Groups

Food group	Major nutrients	Intake recommendations	Notes
Breads, cereal, rice, and pasta	Complex carbohydrates Fiber Plant protein B vitamins Potassium	Rice or pasta (75 – 90 g dry weight) or 4 – 5 medium potatoes, (or equivalent in other starchy roots) plus 200 g of baked flour products (bread etc.) daily	Grains whole, where possible
Vegetables	Carbohydrates Fiber Vitamins Minerals	As many as possible	In season, where possible
Fruits	Carbohydrates Vitamin C Potassium Fiber	250 – 300 g (2 – 3 servings/pieces)	
Milk, yogurt, and cheese	Protein Calcium Vitamin A Vitamin D B vitamins	0.25 l low-fat milk/d plus 60 g cheese	
Meat, poultry, fish, eggs, beans, nuts	Protein Fat Magnesium Iron Iodine Zinc B vitamins	340 g of ocean fish/week plus 450 g of meat or poultry, up to 3 eggs (including egg in processed foods)	Choose variety, prefer lean cuts, use meat sparingly Eat nuts in moderate amounts
Fats, oils, and sweets	Essential fatty acids Fat-soluble vitamins		Use plant oils preferentially, use animal fats sparingly Count hidden fats and avoid hydrogenated fats in dressing, snacks etc. Avoid simple sugars in condiments, soft drinks, candy, baked goods, etc.
Fluids	Water Minerals	~ 2.5 l fluids/d: water, mineral water, fruit and vegetable juices, tea and coffee	

Vegetarianism

"As long as humans kill animals, they will also kill other humans." This statement made by the Greek philosopher Pythagoras (570–500 BCE) was at the foundation of a movement which has since been called vegetarianism (Latin, vegetus = spry, vigorous).

Reasons (A) for the renunciation of animal products have changed over time. In ancient Greece and Rome, the resistance movement against widespread hedonism predominated; later, various religious and ethical aspects came into play. Nowadays, "health" factors have come to the fore. Terms like cholesterol, purine, hormones in animal husbandry, etc., have created a fertile ground for a general mistrust of animal products. However, humans are not vegetarians by nature. Our bodies (teeth, digestive system) are adapted to a mixed nutrition.

All **vegetarian** types of nutrition (**B**) renounce meat and fish. Ovo-lacto-vegetarians consume eggs and dairy products but lacto-vegetarians avoid eggs as well. Up to that level, the same basic tenets of nutritional physiology as to mixed nutrition apply: if nutritional variety and balance is maintained, nutrient deficiencies are rare. Since, in effect, relatively high-calorie foods (meat, sausage) are replaced by larger amounts of nutrient-rich products (vegetables, whole grains), micro-nutrient supply is often improved.

Strict vegetarians or vegans do not consume any animal products. This eliminates dairy products as a source of protein, Ca, vitamin B_{12}, among others. Nevertheless, even vegans rarely have overt, clinical deficiency symptoms (in a few cases, children of vegan mothers have had B_{12} deficiency symptoms), but blood tests (iron, B_{12}, homocysteine levels, etc.) tend to reveal a marginal supply. Strictly vegetarian nutrition usually becomes dangerous when a lack of knowledge is paired with increased nutrient requirements. The risk of inadequate supply is elevated during pregnancy and lactation, as well as during childhood—nonspecific general symptoms are rarely interpreted as related to individual nutrition.

So-called "pudding vegetarians" are a particular category. They renounce animal products but do not otherwise change their (often unbalanced) nutritional habits—an unhealthy phenomenon that is often observed in youngsters.

If raw foods are used exclusively, nutritional deficiencies may result since many protein containing foods (e.g., legumes) are excluded.

Classic vegetarians tend to be well-informed—the nutrition of most vegetarians is closer to the official nutritional recommendations than that of the average citizen. Also, they tend to practice health-awareness beyond nutrition (lots of exercise, no alcohol, no nicotine)—all factors which certainly influence the positive results seen in studies of vegetarians.

The original lacto-vegetarian diet has found many imitators. Provided with a snazzy name and an attractive promise (e.g., fit, miracle, weight loss), a "fad diet" is easily created, which may, however, lag behind the quality of the original.

A. Motives

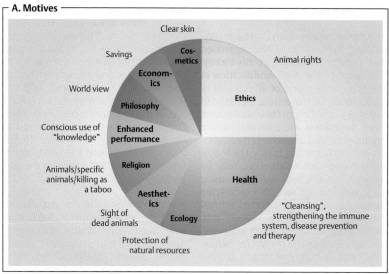

B. Forms of Vegetarianism

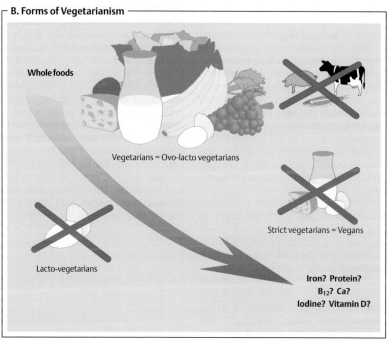

Separation Nutrition

The American physician Dr. Hay is considered the founder of the separation diet concept. According to his theory, first published in 1907, **acidification** of the body is the cause of all diseases of civilization. Consequently, he divided foods (**A**) according to their alkalinizing (fruit, vegetables, etc.), neutral (whole grains, etc.), and acidifying (meat, etc.) properties. According to Hay, the body's proper acid-base balance can only be achieved/maintained by consuming 80 % alkalinizing and 20 % acidifying foods. He completely rejected refined foods like white flour, refined oils, white sugar, etc. They were considered acidifying, while the respective "whole food" was at least categorized as neutral.

In his book *A New Health Era*, published in 1933, Hay presented his theory of the chemical **laws of digestion**. According to him, the human body is unable to digest and process carbohydrates and proteins simultaneously. Therefore, they may not be consumed together, but may be consumed together with neutral foods (**B**). This means that, for instance, meats with vegetables may be consumed at lunch and potatoes with vegetables for dinner. For adults, one "concentrated" meal per day is enough; children over six months are allowed two.

A number of "new diets" are based on the separation diet. One of these became very popular in 1985, with the publication of the book *Fit for Life*. Well anchored in the tradition of American marketing specialists, the Diamonds recognized that several ingredients were needed for success: a large, defined target group (overweight) and a couple of strange rules of behavior that would upset the daily routine, as well as the science. Thus, they introduced the theory of natural body cycles. According to them, eating and digestion of foods occurs between noon and 8:00 pm, absorption and further metabolization between 8:00 pm and 4:00 am, while metabolic wastes and excrement are eliminated until noon. Also, foods should have a similar composition as the human body: ~70 % water. Hence, fruits are considered the most important foods. "Distilled water" is the only permitted drink.

From a nutrition physiologist's standpoint, the separation diet is easy to evaluate: there is no acidification due to nutrition, nor is our digestive system geared towards individualized nutrients. The frequently used phrase "formation of toxins through undigested foods" has no scientific foundation. However, the separation diet is rich in fiber, is low-calorie and low-fat, and is rich in fruit and vegetables. This is likely to cause preventive and even sometimes therapeutic success, which, however, owes nothing to the separation principle. The "miracle cures" reported by its advocates (including remission in cancer patients) are anecdotal and impossible to prove. Variations on the separation diet, like for instance the "Fit for Life" concept, aren't worthy of further discussion. They usually serve only to maximize profits and thereafter quickly disappear from the market.

A. The Acid – Base Balance According to Hay

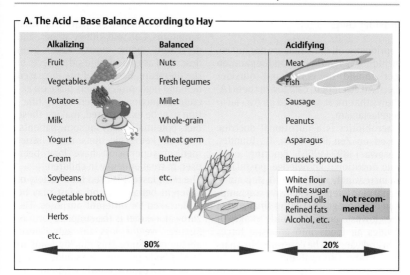

Alkalizing	Balanced	Acidifying
Fruit	Nuts	Meat
Vegetables	Fresh legumes	Fish
Potatoes	Millet	Sausage
Milk	Whole-grain	Peanuts
Yogurt	Wheat germ	Asparagus
Cream	Butter	Brussels sprouts
Soybeans	etc.	
Vegetable broth		White flour
Herbs		White sugar
etc.		Refined oils **Not recommended**
		Refined fats
		Alcohol, etc.

80% — 20%

B. The Separation Diet According to Hay

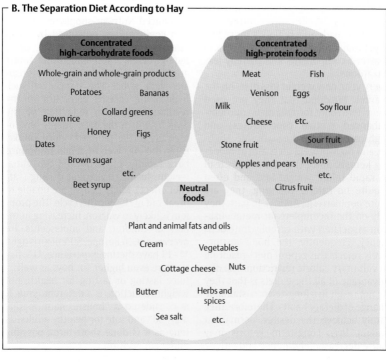

Concentrated high-carbohydrate foods

Whole-grain and whole-grain products

Potatoes   Bananas

Brown rice   Collard greens

Honey   Figs

Dates

Brown sugar

etc.

Beet syrup

Concentrated high-protein foods

Meat   Fish

Venison   Eggs

Milk   Soy flour

Cheese   etc.

Stone fruit   Sour fruit

Apples and pears   Melons

etc.

Citrus fruit

Neutral foods

Plant and animal fats and oils

Cream   Vegetables

Cottage cheese   Nuts

Butter   Herbs and spices

Sea salt   etc.

Outsider Diets

In principle, all diets that are not mixed, including vegetarianism and separation diet should be considered outsider diets. An attempt to categorize them (**A**) shows that most are based on ovo-lacto vegetarianism.

Macrobiotics is a nutritional doctrine based on Zen Buddhism. Its founder, Ohsawa (1893–1966), ignoring available nutritional knowledge, postulated an increasingly restrictive 10-step nutritional plan (step 7 = exclusive consumption of whole grains) with a final goal of the lowest possible fluid intake. It divides all foods into opposite forces (yin and yang), to be consumed in a particular ratio. Ohsawa's diet caused huge nutrient deficiencies and long-term growth retardation in children, and several deaths. Modifications introduced by Kushi made macrobiotics more like vegetarian nutrition with small fish and seaweed components and thereby less hazardous.

Every year, new **weight loss** diets hit the market. Provided that they are used short-term only, formula diets (nutrient-enhanced protein concentrates) and high-carbohydrate diets are safe. High-fat and high-protein diets aim at inducing **ketosis**. Since they sometimes lead to rapid initial weight-loss and often require no calorie counting, they are quite popular (e. g., Atkins). In part, they rely on the incomplete fat metabolization associated with carbohydrate deficiency. Frequently, the body instinctively rejects this type of diet—resulting in voluntary caloric restriction. The disadvantage of all these diets is that they do not result in a long-term, sustainable change of dietary habits. Therefore, they rarely achieve the desired permanent weight loss. Long-term ketosis may cause decreased endurance and fatigue as well as unspecific gastrointestinal symptoms. Gall and kidney stones, and decreased bone mass have been described as undesirable side-effects in the literature. Because of the increased demand high-protein diets place on excretory function, impaired kidney function may be exacerbated, making these diets potentially risky for some patients. Extreme ketogenic diets under strict medical supervision have long been used to treat epilepsy in children.

The term **fasting** is used for a variety of different behaviors, and a fast may be undertaken for different purposes. The zero calorie diet is the simplest form of fasting: weight loss through caloric abstinence. Since this quickly leads to loss of body proteins (lean body mass), as well as a drop in **basal metabolic rate** (**BMR**), the so-called modified fast was introduced. Nutrient-supplemented protein concentrates, enhanced by small amounts of carbohydrates to avoid hypoglycemia (400–600 kcal/d total), are consumed. Initial weight loss is usually very good. The danger of such hypocaloric (crash) diets lies in the resulting long-term reduction of the BMR by which the body adapts physiologically to the reduced caloric intake. After dieting, weight tends to bounce back rapidly, often beyond the initial weight, leading to repeat dieting (ratchet effect). Many people are unable to break out of this vicious cycle. The problem is likely to worsen. Increasing numbers of children and adolescents are overweight. In Europe, 50 % of girls aged 11–13 have dieting experience; U.S. figures are even higher, for boys as well.

Juice fasting or fasting for health, not weight reduction, is a different issue. It is considered a "holistic naturopathic method" and safe for healthy adults, as long as it is done short-term, possibly under supervision.

A. Diets by Main Characteristics

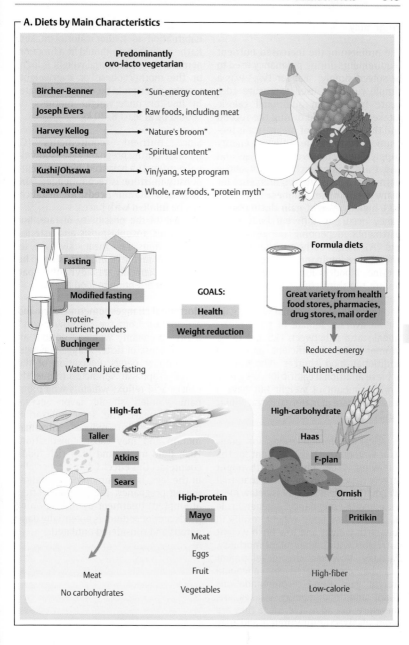

Predominantly ovo-lacto vegetarian

Bircher-Benner → "Sun-energy content"

Joseph Evers → Raw foods, including meat

Harvey Kellog → "Nature's broom"

Rudolph Steiner → "Spiritual content"

Kushi/Ohsawa → Yin/yang, step program

Paavo Airola → Whole, raw foods, "protein myth"

Fasting

Modified fasting

Protein-nutrient powders

Buchinger

Water and juice fasting

GOALS:

Health

Weight reduction

Formula diets

Great variety from health food stores, pharmacies, drug stores, mail order

Reduced-energy

Nutrient-enriched

High-fat

Taller

Atkins

Sears

Meat

No carbohydrates

High-protein

Mayo

Meat

Eggs

Fruit

Vegetables

High-carbohydrate

Haas

F-plan

Ornish

Pritikin

High-fiber

Low-calorie

Pregnancy

The problem of the increased nutrient requirements during pregnancy used to be solved simply: "Eat for Two" was a simple rule that used to ensure adequate intakes. An additional caloric intake of 300 kcal/d during the second and third trimester of pregnancy is recommended to assure sufficient energy supply. Energy needs during the second and third trimesters are ~15% above normal, whereas the requirements for many vitamins and minerals are 20–50% higher. **Weight gain** during pregnancy occurs in different body compartments, depending on gestational age (**A**). While early on, the increase affects predominantly maternal and uterine blood volumes, weight gain during the third trimester occurs predominantly in the fetus, maternal fat, and tissue fluids. A normal weight gain for an average female of good nutritional status is between 11.5 and 18 kg. Women with insufficient access to additional food sources who cannot achieve additional caloric intakes gain a similar amount of weight but have a lesser increase in maternal extracellular fluids and fatty deposits.

Practical recommendations for pregnant women must also account for the following: The **child's birthweight** largely depends on the initial maternal weight (**B**). "Ideal" weight is below ideal for a healthy pregnancy. A general rule of thumb: low body weight results in low birth weight and low birth weight correlates with higher infant mortality. Partially, however, this development can be compensated by adequate weight gain. Blind recommendations about additional energy intakes are, therefore, not advisable, since they are often incorrectly interpreted and may lead to overweight—mostly through habituation to higher caloric intakes. Rather, weight gain should be a function of initial weight: if initial weight is high, or the mother obese or overweight, weight gain should be rather moderate. In low or underweight mothers, it should be at least 8–10 kg.

Since **nutrient requirements** (**C**) increase during pregnancy (see individual nutrients), a balanced, high nutrient-density nutrition is recommended. The increased vitamin needs, for instance, can be fulfilled with juices.

Because of the possibility of rare, but dangerous, toxoplasmosis and listeriosis infections, raw meat, raw eggs, as well as all raw milk products should be avoided. Generally, it is advisable to pay particular attention to food hygiene.

Hormonal changes sometimes demand a deviation from the "healthy norm." Many pregnant women notice an altered sense of taste, strange cravings, and hunger pangs. Relaxation of the lower esophagal sphincter frequently causes acid reflux; which is why pregnant women should favor several smaller meals. The same relaxation mechanism also reduces intestinal motion and may cause constipation. High fluid intake and fiber-rich foods counteract this effect. Edema, especially in the legs, is a common phenomenon during pregnancy. The previous (often attempted) treatment by restriction of fluids and/or sodium is potentially dangerous and considered outdated.

A. Weight: Compartments

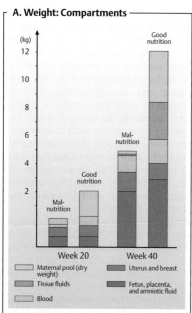

(kg)

Good nutrition

Good nutrition

Mal-nutrition

Mal-nutrition

Good nutrition

Week 20

Week 40

Maternal pool (dry weight)

Tissue fluids

Blood

Uterus and breast

Fetus, placenta, and amniotic fluid

B. Initial Weight

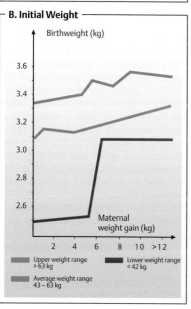

Birthweight (kg)

3.6

3.4

3.2

3.0

2.8

2.6

Maternal weight gain (kg)

2   4   6   8   10   >12

Upper weight range > 63 kg

Average weight range 43 – 63 kg

Lower weight range < 42 kg

C. Nutrition

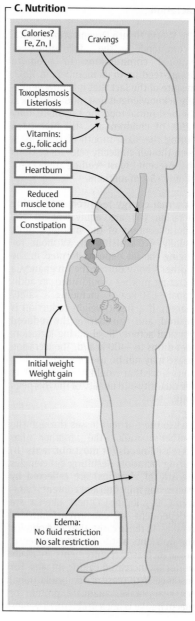

Calories? Fe, Zn, I

Cravings

Toxoplasmosis Listeriosis

Vitamins: e.g., folic acid

Heartburn

Reduced muscle tone

Constipation

Initial weight Weight gain

Edema: No fluid restriction No salt restriction

Lactation

The World Health Organization (WHO) recommended the formation of national **commissions to promote breast-feeding** to its members in 1992. In spite of the fact that it is now generally acknowledged that mother's milk is the best initial food for a neonate, only ~29% of children are still breast-fed during the sixth month of their lives, even though clinically relevant reasons that prevent breast-feeding are present in only ~5% of mothers.

Maternal **energy requirements** during lactation (**A**) are equivalent to the caloric content of the mother's milk, usually ~70 kcal/100 ml. Without reducing the fat deposits formed in the mother's body during the pregnancy, a lactating mother would need an additional ~650 kcal/d, including a safety margin. If a slight weight reduction is desired, and considering the reduced physical activity level during lactation, that drops to ~400 kcal/d. The lactation phase may not be used for weight loss diets since that would negatively affect the quantity and quality of the mother's milk.

Due to the nutrient losses through the mother's milk, the mother has increased **needs for most nutrients (B)** during lactation. Resulting deficiencies (mostly of vitamins) are reflected by decreasing milk nutrient contents (vitamin C, B_{12}, iodine). Others, like Ca, are independent of concurrent nutrient intakes. In these cases, the child obtains the nutrients at the mother's expense. Some increased requirements are made up for by increased caloric intakes. For instance, in the case of a daily additional 650 kcal intake, adequate protein or niacin intake is not a problem. However, even elevated caloric intakes do not always guarantee adequate intakes of nutrients that were already marginal before the pregnancy (e.g., iodine). Since mothers can normally be expected to be well motivated during pregnancy and lactation, these periods should be used for nutritional education. In reality, however, there is frequently no room for such "preventive" measures, especially in women receiving inadequate or no prenatal care (24% of pregnant women on average in the U.S., 43% in Utah), where often not even supplements are used to provide the missing nutrients.

Residues of bioaccumulating chemicals found in mother's milk (PCBs, DDT, dioxins, flame retardants, etc.) have led to concerns about breast-feeding. At this point, the contents in mother's milk are usually low enough so that the advantages of breast-feeding during the first 4–6 months of life usually outweigh the potential risks from these residues (see, however, p. 286). Unfortunately, one of the major sources of such chemicals in breast milk is fish. The FDA considers the consumption of up to 375 g of other fish/week as safe for children, women of childbearing age, pregnant, and lactating women. With the exception of large predators like shark, swordfish, king mackerel, tuna, or tilefish, where methyl mercury is the concern, and which the above groups are advised to avoid completely, ocean fish tend to have lower contents than freshwater fish.

Illicit drug use (amphetamines, cocaine, heroin, and marijuana), smoking, and alcohol abuse by the mother represent additional risk factors for the nursing infant (see p. 274).

A. Energy Needs

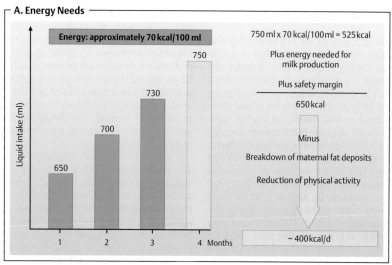

Energy: approximately 70 kcal/100 ml

750 ml x 70 kcal/100ml = 525 kcal

Plus energy needed for milk production

Plus safety margin

650 kcal

Minus

Breakdown of maternal fat deposits

Reduction of physical activity

~ 400 kcal/d

Liquid intake (ml)

650 — 1
700 — 2
730 — 3
750 — 4 Months

B. Nutrient Requirements

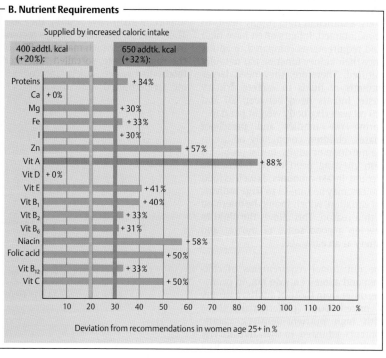

Supplied by increased caloric intake

400 addtl. kcal (+20%):   650 addtk. kcal (+32%):

Proteins + 34%
Ca + 0%
Mg + 30%
Fe + 33%
I + 30%
Zn + 57%
Vit A + 88%
Vit D + 0%
Vit E + 41%
Vit B₁ + 40%
Vit B₂ + 33%
Vit B₆ + 31%
Niacin + 58%
Folic acid + 50%
Vit B₁₂ + 33%
Vit C + 50%

10 20 30 40 50 60 70 80 90 100 110 120 %

Deviation from recommendations in women age 25+ in %

From Neonate to Adolescent

The first year of life can be divided into three sections with regard to nutrition (**A**). During the first four months, the infant is fed exclusively with mother's milk or infant milk preparations. During the fifth month, one begins to add some pureed normal foods, increasing their amounts until the ninth month. Starting with the 10th month, pureed foods can be slowly replaced by regular foods and the child slowly introduced to normal family foods. At the end of the first year, the child will be able to tolerate most foods. Some hard to digest foods like legumes or certain cabbages, and very hard to digest foods like nuts and fatty foods are unsuitable for children of that age. Foods should not be excessively salty or spicy. When introducing solid foods, a sufficient fluid supply needs to be maintained. Infants often have high fluid requirements compared to adults since their kidney function has not fully matured. Therefore, they need larger amounts of fluids to excrete urinary waste. Infants need between 80 and 120 ml water/kg body weight per day.

During the toddler and preschool phases, children completely adjust to the nutrition of adults. Initial problems with chewing need to be taken into account. Intake amounts, as well as food choices, may be subject to large individual variation, which should be tolerated within reason. This allows the child to develop a good sense of hunger and satiety at an early age.

The nutritional requirements of children and adolescents do not, in principle, differ from those of adults: a variety of mixed foods (preferentially those with high nutrient-density); caloric contents adjusted to age and activity level; sufficient fluid intake; balanced meal distribution. During childhood and adolescence, these recommendations are to be adjusted somewhat to individual preferences. The child's preferences, for instance for sweets, should be permitted within reason. One-sided nutrition, however, should not be tolerated. The parental role model is of great importance during childhood and youth, even if it is not accepted immediately.

The practical application of the nutritional recommendations for children and adolescents is shown in the "Optimized Mixed Nutrition" (**B**). It provides sufficient nutrients for growth, development, and health and also has preventative functions. It should be taken into account that to a child of that age, how foods taste is seemingly more important than how healthy they are. Therefore, in addition to the recommended foods, which make up >80% of the caloric intake, so-called "tolerated foods" like sweets, cakes, and cookies, etc. are permitted.

A. Nutrition Schedule for the 1st Year of Life

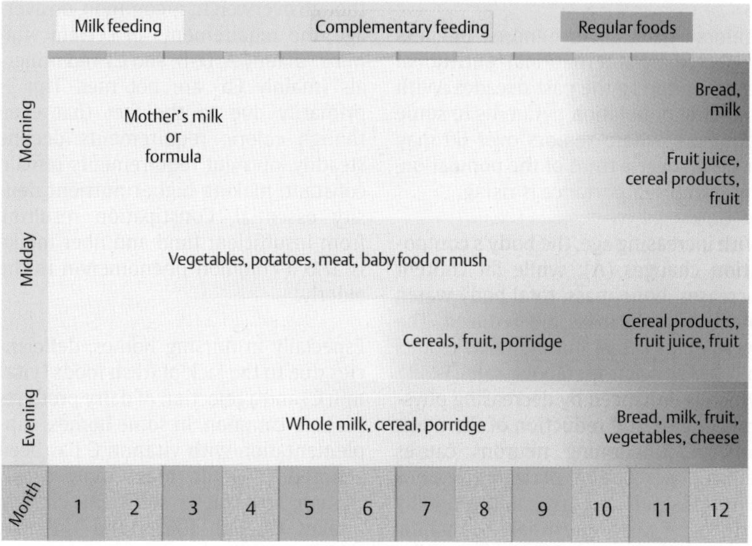

| Milk feeding | Complementary feeding | Regular foods |

Morning
Mother's milk
or
formula

Bread,
milk

Fruit juice,
cereal products,
fruit

Midday
Vegetables, potatoes, meat, baby food or mush

Evening

Cereals, fruit, porridge

Cereal products,
fruit juice, fruit

Whole milk, cereal, porridge

Bread, milk, fruit,
vegetables, cheese

Month | 1 | 2 | 3 | 4 | 5 | 6 | 7 | 8 | 9 | 10 | 11 | 12 |

B. Optimized Mixed Nutrition

Plenty	Units	Children 4–6 y	Adolescents 13–14 y
Fluids	ml/d	800	1000
Bread, cereals (rolled or flakes)	g/d	170	280
Pasta, rice, potatoes, grains	g/d	130	200
Vegetables	g/d	200	280
Fruit	g/d	200	280

Moderately			
Milk, milk products	ml (g)/d	350	430
Meat, sausage (lean)	g/d	40	70
Fish	g/week	100	200
Eggs	each/week	2	2–3

Sparingly			
Butter, oil, margarine	g/d	25	35

Occasionally tolerated			
High-sugar	g/d	<40	<70
High-fat	g/d	<10	<15

Seniors

Seniors have been more or less neglected by international nutritional research during the past decades. With changing population pyramids in some countries, where seniors over 60 may make up over a third of the population, this group's importance is rising.

With increasing age, the **body's composition** changes (**A**): while fat content increases, bone mass, total body water, and lean body mass are reduced. The decrease of active muscle mass results in a lower basal metabolic rate (BMR), which is enhanced by decreasing physical activity. The reduction of the numbers of functioning neurons causes reduced perception of thirst, lessens sense of smell and taste, and generally reduces gastrointestinal function. Decreased glucose tolerance predisposes the aging to the development of diabetes mellitus.

Besides these **physiological changes**, a multitude of additional factors influence the nutrition of the elderly. Upon questioning, "difficulty chewing" and "lack of appetite" are cited as reasons for insufficient food intake. Continuously rising life expectancy is partially due to long-term, multi-drug medication of most seniors. Drug interactions with foods are hard to predict. There are numerous reports about appetite reduction induced by excessive tranquilizer use. Moreover, many degenerative diseases decrease appetite and/or absorption, or create problems with utilization. Even this obviously incomplete list shows that more attention needs to be paid to seniors' nutritional needs.

The few existing nutritional studies of seniors show that their nutritional intakes are often marginal (**B**). Even though overweight is common, on average, the requirements of certain vitamins (mainly A, D, B, and C) and minerals (mainly Ca) are not met. This is primarily due to the fact that even though caloric requirements decline steadily, nutrient requirements remain constant, making higher nutrient density essential. Constipation resulting from insufficient fluid and fiber intake is also a common phenomenon in the elderly.

Especially in nursing homes, deficiencies due to the lack of fresh foods (vitamin C) and a rejection of dairy products (Ca) are common. In some homes, supplementation with vitamin C has been adopted. It would make more sense, though, to achieve sufficient vitamin intakes through juices and the like, which would also improve immune function. More than 50% of hospital inpatients are underweight. Malnutrition represents an additional risk factor for seniors, since a malnourished person has no reserves in case of increased need during illness and recovery. Regardless of this, nutritional therapy and prevention are rarely used. A study of elderly and hospital patients in the U.S. showed that more than a third of the over 65-year-olds had protein energy malnutrition, most of them undiagnosed.

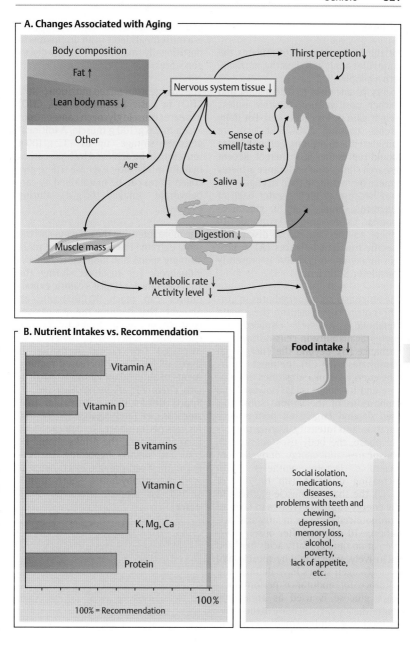

A. Changes Associated with Aging

Body composition

Fat ↑

Lean body mass ↓

Other

Age

Nervous system tissue ↓

Thirst perception ↓

Sense of smell/taste ↓

Saliva ↓

Muscle mass ↓

Digestion ↓

Metabolic rate ↓
Activity level ↓

Food intake ↓

Social isolation, medications, diseases, problems with teeth and chewing, depression, memory loss, alcohol, poverty, lack of appetite, etc.

B. Nutrient Intakes vs. Recommendation

Vitamin A

Vitamin D

B vitamins

Vitamin C

K, Mg, Ca

Protein

100 %

100% = Recommendation

Athletes

For the basic nutrition of athletes the same rules apply as to healthy, normally active people.

Energy balance has to be constant and neither positive nor negative unless weight gain or loss is desired. For daily intense training 200–2500 kcal are considered a minimum. Carbohydrates should represent ~60% thereof. Recent research shows that endurance athletes require more protein than strength athletes because of their greater need of glucogenic amino acids for gluconeogenesis. Other authors continue to adhere to the concept of **discipline-specific nutrient balances** (A). A protein intake of 1.5 g/kg BW is presently considered sufficient.

The emphasis on carbohydrates in athletic nutrition is based on the known metabolic processes required for energy availability in cells during performance (**B**). Beyond the energy-rich phosphates (ATP, CP), the most important energy supply substrates are glucose and free fatty acids. However, the proportions of the various substrates used depend largely on performance duration and intensity. During the initial phase, the body uses energy-rich phosphates and energy derived from anaerobic lactate synthesis. With increasing **duration** (up to 70% of V_{max}), the share of muscle glycogen in the energy supply decreases in favor of a pronounced increase in fatty acid oxidation, ~10 minutes after onset. However, at no time are fatty acids oxidized exclusively, which is why muscle and liver glycogen stores have definite significance for endurance performance. Since glucose is used as an energy source during each increase of the activity level (e.g., an intermediate spurt in endurance sports, 80–100% of V_{max}), it is a must for athletes in all disciplines to nutritionally maximize muscle glycogen stores.

The change from mixed nutrition (~40% CHO) to basic nutrition (~55% CHO) increases muscle glycogen content from ~1.7 g to 2.6 g/100 g muscle. Additional glycogen storage (up to ~3.2 g/100 g muscle) can be achieved by high-carbohydrate intake after exercise. These glycogen stores can be maintained by carbohydrate intake (65 g/d) during exercise.

The more intensive the exertion and the more extreme the conditions, the more strongly sports nutrition has to be individualized. For instance, during the Tour de France, a cyclist's caloric expenditures can reach 10 000 kcal/d—an amount that requires the use of concentrates or even infusions. Under such conditions, reperfusion ischemia or increased free radical formation is likely, which is why increased requirements of antioxidant vitamins (particularly vitamin E) are being discussed.

Sports drinks play a particular role, since proper fluid balance is essential for top performance. To achieve rapid fluid absorption, the drinks should be cool and slightly hypotonic. Furthermore, they can provide electrolytes as well as carbohydrates. Sports drinks should be sipped (frequent small doses).

A. Athletics – Discipline-Specific Nutrient Ratios

	Training	Precompetition	Competition	Regeneration	
Strength sports e.g., weightlifting, throwing	55	65	60	55	%CHO
	15	15	20	20	%F
	30	20	20	25	%P
Strength and endurance sports e.g., rowing, bodybuilding	55–60	60	60	57.5	%CHO
	25	25	22.5	25	%F
	15–20	15	17.5	17.5	%P
Speed and game sports e.g., gymnastics, tennis	60	65	65	57.5	%CHO
	22.5–25	22.5–25	25	25	%F
	15–17.5	10–12.5	10	17.5	%P
Endurance sports e.g., running, swimming	62	70	62	57.5	%CHO
	25.5	20	25.5	27.5	%F
	12.5	10	12.5	15	%P

% CHO = % carbohydrates   % F = % fat   % P = % proteins

B. Energy Sources during Performance

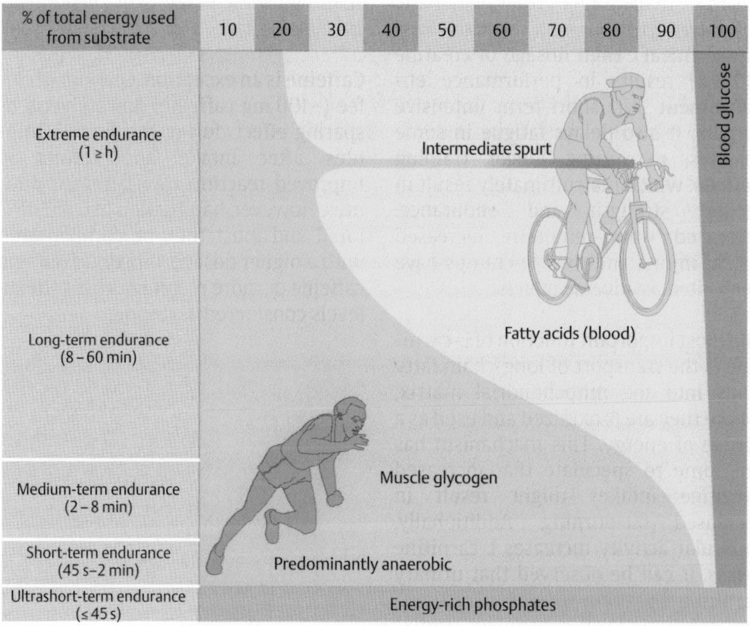

% of total energy used from substrate	10	20	30	40	50	60	70	80	90	100

Extreme endurance (1 ≥ h)

Intermediate spurt

Long-term endurance (8–60 min)

Fatty acids (blood)

Medium-term endurance (2–8 min)

Muscle glycogen

Short-term endurance (45 s–2 min)

Predominantly anaerobic

Ultrashort-term endurance (≤ 45 s)

Energy-rich phosphates

Blood glucose

Ergogenic Aids

Ergogenic aids are intended to enhance athletic performance. They include pharmaceuticals like anabolics. However, performance-enhancing foods are more attractive to the average sports enthusiast since they are freely available and have the image of the "healthy, natural nutrient, free of side-effects."

Creatine is one of the oldest known ergogenic aids. Its creatine monophosphate form (**B**) is an easily available energy source for muscles that is used up within ~10 seconds during intense effort. When creatine monophosphate is aromatized (without enzymatic involvement) the product is creatinine, a non-recyclable compound that has to be excreted renally. The daily loss of ~2–4 g creatine/d, through renal excretion, has to be made up for either by hepatic *de novo* synthesis or through food intake (meat). High dosage of creatine (30 g/d) results in performance enhancement for short-term intensive activity. It also delays fatigue in some athletes, permitting longer training periods, which may ultimately result in greater strength and endurance. Increased water-retention, increased risk of injury, and muscle cramps have been cited as adverse effects.

The most important function of **L-carnitine** is the transport of long-chain fatty acids into the mitochondrial matrix, where they are β-oxidized and used as a source of energy. This mechanism has led some to speculate that increased carnitine intakes might result in increased fat-burning. Additionally, muscular activity increases L-carnitine losses. It can be observed that urinary carnitine excretion increases with rising exertion. Well-controlled studies have shown, however, that carnitine supplements have no effect on performance or fatty acid oxidation. Apparently, the body's own synthesis and/or intake from food (meat) are sufficient.

Taurine is mainly added to sports drinks. Modern designer sports drinks contain up to 400 mg taurine/100 ml; ~200 mg/d are consumed with foods. Taurine has been ascribed poorly researched developmental functions in the nervous system as well as neurotransmitter functions. It is supposed to improve mood, concentration, and psychomotor performance. Scientific proof, however, is lacking to date.

There is also no scientific proof to date for the ergogenic effects of any other substances (branched-chain amino acids, β-hydroxy-β-methyl butyrate, coenzyme Q10, conjugated linolenic acids) for which claims of such effects have been made.

Caffeine is an exception. One cup of coffee (~100 mg caffeine) has a glycogen-sparing effect during the first 15 minutes after intake and results in improved reaction time after 30 minutes. However, habituation to caffeine is rapid and must then be compensated with a higher dosage. Intakes of 600 mg caffeine or more result in urine caffeine levels considered as doping.

A. Strength and Performance Through Individual Substances

Metabolic Products
- Creatine
- Orotic acid
- α-Lipoic acid
- L-carnitine
- Q10
- Pyruvate
- Hydroxy citrate (HCA)
- Hydroxy methyl butyrate (HMB)

Amino acids
- Taurine
- Arginine
- Aspartate
- Branched chain amino acid (BCCA)

Enzymes and Phytochemicals
- Caffeine
- Papaine
- Flavonoids
- Bromelain

Lipids / Vitamins, Minerals
- Lecithine
- Conjugated linoleic acid (CLA)
- Medium-chain triglycerides
- Vitamin C, zinc, selenium

Endurance Athlete

B. Creatine

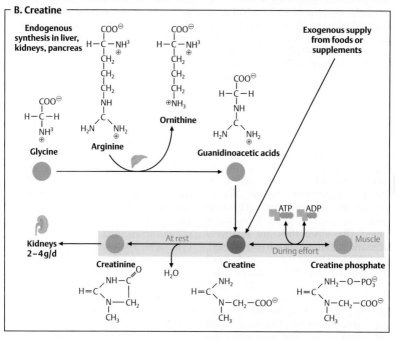

Endogenous synthesis in liver, kidneys, pancreas

Exogenous supply from foods or supplements

Glycine   Arginine   Ornithine   Guanidinoacetic acids

ATP   ADP

Kidneys 2–4 g/d   At rest   During effort   Muscle

Creatinine H_2O Creatine   Creatine phosphate

C. L-Carnitine

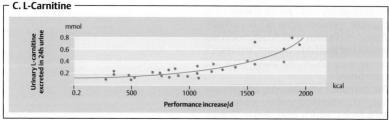

Urinary L-carnitine excreted in 24h urine (mmol)

Performance increase/d (kcal)

Drugs and Diet I

Interaction between medications and foods may occur at various levels.

Rates of gastric emptying, stomach pH, complex formation, and intestinal motility are influenced by foods and, in turn, affect the **absorption rates of medicines**. Other factors that are influenced by foods also play important roles. For instance, fatty meals delay normal gastric emptying. Usually, the consequence is delayed absorption of digested nutrients. On the other hand, it may cause other medications to be better dissolved and therefore more quickly absorbed in the intestine. The answer to the question: "Before, during, or after the meal?" therefore depends on the medication and the desired effect.

The drug paracetamol (**A**) exemplifies how drug intake after a meal can greatly delay a drug's effect. For a patient in pain, an immediate effect is desired. It therefore makes sense to take analgesics on an empty stomach. This also applies to enteric-coated, form-stable tablets (**B**). Since they are relatively large and pass the stomach undissolved, they do not leave the stomach until after the food has left. If such tablets are taken several times a day, they may accumulate in the stomach.

Solubility as well as degradation are often pH-dependent. Incoming foods alter stomach pH. This may affect the **bioavailability of medications**. For example, penicillamine (**C**) is partially degraded if taken with foods, reducing by half the available amount, expressed as the area under the curve (AUC) of absorption.

The antibiotic griseofulvin, on the contrary (**D**), is better dissolved when taken with foods, which may, depending on the food's fat content, double its bioavailability.

Complex formation may also impact a drug's bioavailability. When tetracyclines or ferrous salts are taken with milk and/or dairy products, they form very low-solubility Ca compounds, reducing the drugs' availability.

Tannin-rich black tea forms complexes with alkaline, nitrogenous neuroleptics and antidepressants.

The fiber in oat bran reduces the bioavailability of antidepressants and HMG-CoA reductase inhibitors (lipid-lowering drugs), whereas guar gum affects the bioavailability of penicillin.

Generally, **intake recommendations** should be observed, but are often misunderstood. "Before meals" means one hour before a meal. "After meals" means within a reasonable period after a meal (~0.5–1 hour).

Body position and fluid intake also play major roles: many medications damage mucous membranes, in rare cases leading to esophageal or gastric ulcers. These include many antibiotics and chemotherapeutics, but also acetylsalicylic acid. Therefore, medications are best taken while standing upright. To minimize the time they can affect the mucosa, recommended fluid intakes must be strictly observed.

A. Delayed Absorption

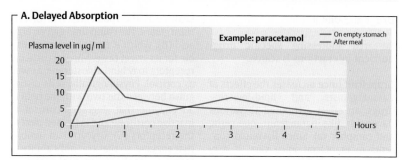

Example: paracetamol — On empty stomach / — After meal

Plasma level in μg/ml

B. Enteric-Coated Tablets

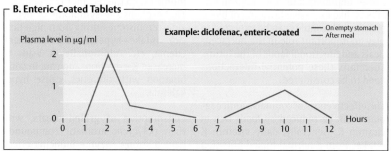

Example: diclofenac, enteric-coated — On empty stomach / — After meal

Plasma level in μg/ml

C. Reduced Bioavailability

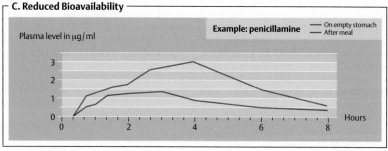

Example: penicillamine — On empty stomach / — After meal

Plasma level in μg/ml

D. Enhanced Bioavailability

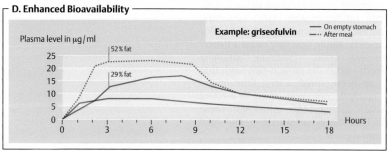

Example: griseofulvin — On empty stomach / --- After meal

Plasma level in μg/ml

52% fat

29% fat

Drugs and Diet II

Research addressing **specific drug-nutrient interactions** is scarce.

Grapefruit juice increases the effects of Ca-antagonists and lipid-lowering drugs, an effect attributed to various flavonoids like narangenin, quercetin, and camphor oil. Since flavonoid contents in grapefruit juice vary, it may cause unpredictable and undesirable effects, like excessive lowering of blood pressure. Flavonoids can be expected to play an important role in the nutraceuticals and functional foods of the future. Therefore, these potential interactions need to be considered.

The effectiveness of coumarin anticoagulants can be reduced by foods rich in vitamin K. Generally, daily **vitamin K** intakes from a normal mixed nutrition should vary by at most ± 250 µg, making the recommendation to avoid foods rich in vitamin K unnecessary. Persons, however, who consume seasonally high amounts of vegetables (e. g., growers, gardeners) need to heed this warning.

Tyramine is a biogenic amine with vasoconstricting properties. Tyramine forms when food-decomposing bacteria decarboxylate the amino acid tyrosine (**A**). After absorption, tyramine is degraded by monoamine oxidase. Certain antidepressants (MAO inhibitors) inhibit this enzyme, leading to a build-up of tyramine that may cause a hypertensive crisis. Tyramine-containing foods—generally protein-rich foods that have been stored a long time or are slightly decomposed—must be avoided when taking MAO inhibitors. These include meats, yeast extract, and aged hard cheeses.

Licorice is the root extract of *Glycyrrhiza glabra*. The compound glycyrrhizic acid (**B**), which it contains, is responsible for its sweet taste. Mineral corticoid receptors may bind aldosterone, as well as cortisol. Physiologically, cells distinguish between the two with the help of an enzyme that degrades cortisol to inactive cortisone and is located next to the receptors (**C**). Glycyrrhizin inhibits that enzyme, so that cortisol's ability to interact with the receptor is kept intact. This explains the symptoms of hyperaldosteronism resulting from high licorice intake—hypertension, dizziness, edema, etc. Additionally, it leads to increased K excretion, and can, in combination with diuretics, cause hypokalemia.

Consumption of grilled meats, with their polycyclic aromatic compounds, have a strong enzyme-inducing effect. This leads to more rapid break down of medications, preventing them from reaching sufficient blood levels. This effect has been shown, for instance, for theophylline, which is used in asthma therapy.

A. MAO Inhibitors

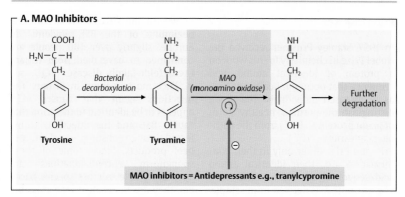

Tyrosine — *Bacterial decarboxylation* → Tyramine — *MAO (**m**ono**a**mino **o**xidase)* → Further degradation

⊖

MAO inhibitors = Antidepressants e.g., tranylcypromine

B. Licorice

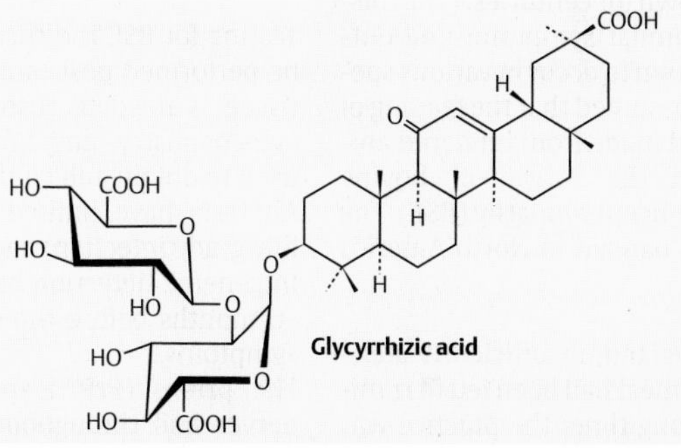

Glycyrrhizic acid

C. Licorice's Mechanism of Action

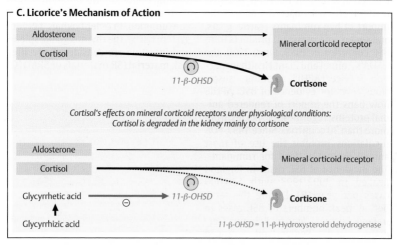

Aldosterone → Mineral corticoid receptor

Cortisol → Mineral corticoid receptor

11-β-OHSD → Cortisone

Cortisol's effects on mineral corticoid receptors under physiological conditions: Cortisol is degraded in the kidney mainly to cortisone

Aldosterone → Mineral corticoid receptor

Cortisol → Mineral corticoid receptor

Glycyrrhetic acid ⊖ → *11-β-OHSD* → Cortisone

Glycyrrhizic acid

11-β-OHSD = 11-β-Hydroxysteroid dehydrogenase

Prion Diseases

In 1997, Stanley Prusiner received the Nobel Prize in chemistry for his work on a protein of identical amino acid sequence that occurs in healthy as well as in diseased individuals. Today, we distinguish the normal, "healthy" form of **prion protein** C (PrP^C) from the pathological variety (PrP^{SC}).

PrP^C and PrP^{SC} differ only in their conformation, i. e., their identical amino acid sequences are folded differently. The attribute ^{SC} is derived from scrapie, a deadly disease of goats and sheep that has been known for centuries. Prion diseases with similar symptoms and outcome are known to occur in various species (**A**). It is assumed that the feeding of infected meal made from rendered animals caused the spread of **bovine spongiform encephalopathy** (**BSE**). The practice was banned in North America in 1997.

Mainly in England, insufficiently sterilized animal meal had been fed to ruminants for a long time; the practice was banned in Britain in 1988 and in the EU in 1994. The U.S. enacted a ban on the import of live ruminants (cattle, goats, and sheep) and ruminant products from BSE countries in 1989. Since 1990, the USDA's Animal and Plant Health Inspection Service (APHIS) monitors suspicious cows for evidence of BSE. APHIS now bans the import of rendered animal proteins, regardless of species, from more than 30 countries. Since 1997, FDA regulations prohibit the use of most animal protein as feed for ruminants. The incidence of BSE cases in England peaked in 1992/1993 with >36 000 cases per year (**B**). During the same period, peak numbers of BSE cases in Ireland, Portugal, France, Belgium, Germany, and Switzerland, ranged between 1 and 170 cases/year. Since the beginning of the BSE epidemic in Europe, slightly over 100 people are confirmed to have died from variant **Creutzfeldt-Jakob disease** (**vCJD**, see p. 332), most of them in Britain. The infectious agent that causes vCJD appears to be identical to the prion that causes BSE and the infections transferred through consumption of infected beef products. Since some of these spongiform encephalopathies are apparently able to cross species barriers, they are now called **transmissible spongiform encephalopathies** (**TSE**).

Testing for BSE is difficult and can only be performed post mortem since brain tissue is needed. Histology, immunocytochemistry, and Western blots are used to obtain and confirm a diagnosis. All tests have limited sensitivity and low grade infection may go undetected. In general, detection becomes possible ~6 months before the onset of clinical symptoms.

The prions (PrP^{SC}) spread along the nerves and throughout the lymphatic system. Consequently, different animal parts carry different levels of risk from consumption. In older bovines, nervous system tissue, the thymus gland, spleen, and intestine are considered **specified risk material (SR materials or SRM)** (**C**).

A. Prion Diseases in Animals

Disease	Host	Origin and occurrence	Typical symptoms
Scrapie	Sheep, goats	Infection of (genetically) susceptible animals, sporadic (?)	Ataxia, scratching, chronic wasting
Transmissible mink encephalopathy (TME)	Mink	Infections through contaminated animal meal (?)	Ataxia, scratching, itching, metabolic wasting
Bovine spongiform encephalopathy (BSE)	Bovines	Infections through contaminated animal meal (scrapie or BSE), maternal transfer (?)	Ataxia, loss of coordination, rubbing
Feline spongiform encephalopathy (FSE)	Pet cats, zoo felines	Infections through contaminated beef	Chronic wasting, rubbing, ataxia,
Exotic ungulate encephalopathy	Antelopes, cheetahs, pumas, bison	Infection through contaminated animal meal	Loss of coordination, ataxia, falling
Chronic wasting disease (CWD)	Mule deer, white-tailed deer, elk, black-tailed deer	Unknown origins; U.S. only; up to 15% of natural game population infected	Metabolic wasting, itching, loss of coordination

B. BSE and vCJD Cases in Great Britain

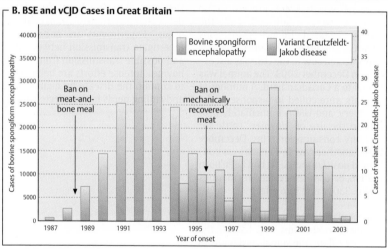

C. SR-Material in Cattle

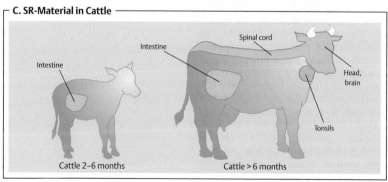

Prion Diseases in the U.S.

With the exception of one person who had lived in England during the peak of the epidemic, no cases of **variant Creutzfeldt-Jakob disease (vCJD)** have been detected in the U.S. to date (**A**). U.S. efforts to prevent the emergence of **bovine spongiform encephalopathy (BSE)** are coordinated with Canada and Mexico. In May 2003, the Canadian inspection program discovered one BSE-infected cow. In the subsequent control effort, a total 2800 animals, none of which were proven to be infected, were eradicated and the rapidly instated import restrictions from Canada lifted thereafter. The first BSE-infected cow in the U.S. was discovered in December 2003. The animal was traced to a Canadian herd. A number of animals were culled in response to the discovery, and USDA immediately prohibited the use of "downer" cattle for human consumption. In December 2004, another cow in Canada was confirmed positive for BSE. It had been born in 1996, before the new feed regulations (see p. 330) came into effect.

Since it was shown that slaughtering by air-injection-stunning, and halving the carcasses along the spinal cord tends to contaminate blood and muscle meat with **specified risk materials (SRM)**, the tissues that are most likely to contain prions, i. e., mainly nervous system, tonsils, thymus, and intestinal tissue, slaughtering methods have been modified in many places, including the U.S. and Europe. It has been proposed to ban the use of **advanced meat recovery (AMR)** products containing SRM. AMR products containing certain specific SRM (vertebral column, dorsal root ganglia, skull or head), and mechanically separated beef are now banned from the human food supply.

Chronic wasting disease (CWD) is a TSE found only in North America in captive and wild deer and elk (14 U.S. states, Canada) (**B**). In some herds, up to 15 % of the animals are infected. According to the CDC: "It is generally prudent to avoid consuming food derived from any animal with evidence of a TSE. To date, there is no evidence that CWD has been transmitted or can be transmitted to humans under natural conditions. However, there is not yet strong evidence that such transmissions could not occur." Experiments are underway to investigate transmission between deer and possible transmission from deer to bovines. Intense efforts are being made to contain the disease by quarantining and culling herds in the affected areas.

A. Prion Diseases in the U.S.

Year	Referrals	Prion D. Total	Sporadic	Familial	Iatrogenic	vCJD
1997	104	60	54	6	0	0
1998	94	51	44	6	1	0
1999	114	74	65	9	0	0
2000	169	111	97	12	2	0
2001	247	154	138	16	0	0
2002	265[1]	151	127[1]	22	1	1[2]
2003	284[3]	191[4]	142	45	1	0
Total	**1277**	**792**	**667**	**116**	**5**	**1**

[1] Includes 2 inconclusive
[2] Acquired in United Kingdom; living
[3] Includes 1 inconclusive
[4] Includes 3 type unknown

B. Chronic Wasting Disease in North America

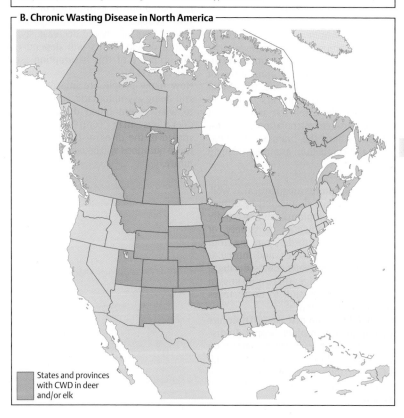

States and provinces with CWD in deer and/or elk

Creutzfeldt-Jakob Disease (CJD and vCJD)

After passing through the intestinal lining, ingested PrPsc probably reaches the Peyer's patches via the bloodstream (**A**). This is where follicular dendritic cells (FDC), which are found in the patches as well as other lymphatic organs, get infected. Maturation of these FDC is induced by lymphotoxin β, secreted by B cells. Thus lymphotoxin β is essential for the further spread of prion infections. Ultimately, the prions reach the CNS via the peripheral nervous system, spinal chord, and possibly directly via the vagus nerve, as well.

In analogy to animal prion diseases like bovine spongiform encephalopathy (BSE), e. g., humans show similar **histological changes** of the brain after an incubation period of one to several years (**B**)—large numbers of florid plaques in the cerebellar and cerebral cortex, nerve cell vacuolation and astrocytosis, where the brain stem, thalamus, and cerebellum are most strongly affected.

Clinical symptoms are identical as well. The first stage is dominated by diffuse neurological symptoms, later by rapidly progressing dementia. A variety of neuromuscular disorders ranging from tetraparesis to seizures, and muscular atrophy set in. Death comes during a comatose final stage; there is no known treatment. Progression to death takes between 4 to 8 months.

Creutzfeldt-Jacob disease (CJD) occurs predominantly in older people. To distinguish the new variant caused by PrP^{sc} from this exceedingly rare (0.5–1.0 cases per million people) disease, the variant is called **vCJD** or **nvCJD** (new variant CJD).

In the past, ~20–30 cases of CJD annually were registered annually in England. Since the early nineties, this number has doubled. Whether the numbers reflect an actual increase in the case load or increased awareness on behalf of physicians and pathologists cannot ultimately be ascertained.

By the end of 2000, an additional 70 confirmed cases of vCJD were added to this load, with still increasing tendencies (**C**). vCJD occurs predominantly in younger people; the first victim in England was just 19 years old.

The BSE case load peaked in 1992/93. Since then, the numbers have been falling. Based on the assumption of a 5–8 year incubation period, the vCJD case load in England should decrease soon. Future developments will depend on the accuracy of this assumption (see also Fig. 331 B).

How many people are infected while still being asymptomatic, whether and to what extent blood donations and operations may contribute to the spread of the disease—the answers to those questions will be borne out by the future.

A. How Prions Spread Inside the Body

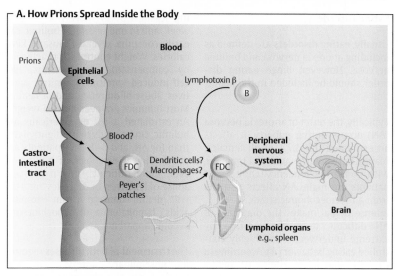

B. CJD and vCJD in Great Britain

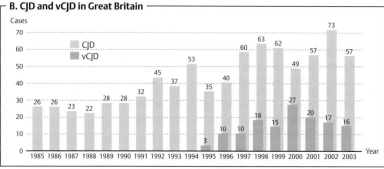

C. BSE, CJD, and vCJD Histology

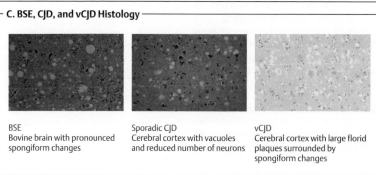

BSE
Bovine brain with pronounced spongiform changes

Sporadic CJD
Cerebral cortex with vacuoles and reduced number of neurons

vCJD
Cerebral cortex with large florid plaques surrounded by spongiform changes

Eating Disorders

Usually, eating disorders are defined as including anorexia nervosa and bulimia nervosa. However, binge eating disorder should be included in the definition.

Typically, the onset of **anorexia nervosa** (AN) occurs during puberty. It affects an estimated 0.5–3.7 % of all females, mainly between the ages of 13 and 35, with increasing tendency. Only 5 % of patients are male. AN affects patients from all socioeconomic strata.
Intense denial makes the diagnosis of AN difficult. It is characterized by extreme underweight and highly controlled eating behavior (**A**). According to the WHO diagnostic criteria (**B**), underweight means 15 % below normal weight, which in this age group is a BMI <17.5. This underweight is controlled and self-induced. Self-image is intensely distorted. Even in states of extreme emaciation, the perception of fatness and the urge to lose weight persists. Lack of energy and nutrients lead to a variety of clinical symptoms, ranging from the classic amenorrhea—often disguised by estrogen therapy to prevent osteoporosis—to dry skin, low heart frequency, and hypotension. Lab tests reveal the classical markers of malnutrition, hypoalbuminemia and metabolic acidosis. Sometimes, vitamin deficiencies are so extreme that classical symptoms become apparent. Even with treatment over a course of 20 years >15 % of patients die.

Bulimia nervosa (BN) is characterized by binging attacks. It shares with AN the loss of control over eating behavior (**B**). Bulimics, too, are obsessed with being slim. The loss of control causes a constant struggle for the bulimic. Binge eating sessions occur more than once a week, and in one session, a bulimic can easily consume several thousand kilocalories. Weight control (**C**) is achieved by compensatory mechanisms, like self-induced vomiting (purging), laxatives, abuse of diuretics, and/or fasting. Most bulimics are near normal weight. An estimated 2–5 % of Americans are bulimic. Onset tends to be slightly later than for AN, and 5–10 % of patients are male. Clinical diagnosis of bulimia is even more difficult. Only if purging, abuse of laxatives, or diuretics are used will dental damage (from stomach acids), hypokalemia, or hypochloremia become apparent.

The **treatment** of both diseases requires multidisciplinary intervention, depending on the degree of severity. Patients must first be hospitalized to stabilize BMI. A BMI <13 is a strong predictor for premature mortality. Beyond that, psychotherapy is the dominant approach. Since many patients have very unrealistic ideas about foods and nutrition, intervention is most promising in combination with nutritional consulting.
As opposed to bulimics, people with **binge eating disorder** do not purge.

┌─ **A. Characteristics** ─────────────────────────────────

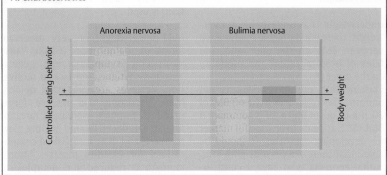

┌─ **B. Anorexia Nervosa** ────────────────────────────────

- Weight ≥15 % below age-appropriate BMI

- Self-induced weight loss through avoidance of high-calorie foods and
  additionally by:
  → Self-induced vomiting
  → Use of laxatives
  → Extreme physical activity
  → Appetite suppressants or diuretics

- Distorted perception of the body weight, size, and shape

- Amenorrhea in women, loss of libido and potency in men

- Delay of normal development at onset of puberty

  According to WHO, ICD 10, F 50.0

┌─ **C. Bulimia Nervosa** ─────────────────────────────────

- Constant preoccupation with food, irresistible cravings for food,
  binge eating

- Avoidance of weight gain through:
  → Self-induced vomiting or
  → Abuse of laxatives or
  → Temporary abstinence from foods
  → Appetite suppressants, diuretics, thyroid hormones

- Abnormal fear of weigh gain

- Preceded by anorexia nervosa

  According to WHO, ICD 10, F 50.2

Underweight

Underweight is as undesirable as overweight; there is a U-shaped relationship between BMI, on the one hand, and rates of hospitalization and mortality on the other (**A**).

Classification of underweight is not uniform. The WHO uses a cut-off BMI of 20, but usage of BMI = 19 is common. A BMI <18.5 appears to be a useful marker for developing countries. It should be noted that there are persons with idiopathic anorexia who have a constitutional BMI below normal range that does not constitute a health risk and who are fully functional. Whereas **prevalence** of underweight is cited as 10–50% in developing countries, it ranges between 3 and 5% in industrialized nations, and it is 2% in the U.S. (women 8%).

The **causes** of underweight in industrialized countries are seldom purely nutritional (**B**). It is usually a symptom of clinical conditions, and in the very old it is usually a symptom of multimorbidity. An exception is the reduced nutrient intake practiced by younger people for the purpose of excessive weight reduction. Malnutrition in the elderly is due mainly to social problems. Approximately 15% of Americans over 65 consume less than 1000 kcal/d. In Americans 75 and older, ~40% of men and 30% of women are ≥10% underweight. If the underweight is caused by insufficient food intakes essential nutrient deficiencies must be expected.

Malnutrition has to be distinguished from underweight. The term **malnutrition** pertains to any kind of inadequate nutritional intake—excess as well as deficiency. For patients with both insufficient energy and protein intakes, the term PEM (protein energy malnutrition) is used.

Mild underweight or very moderate forms of malnutrition usually cause nonspecific symptoms like general weakness, fatigue, and lack of motivation. Reserves are exhausted quickly. More persistent and intense forms manifest through increased rates of infection, reduced wound healing, slow recovery, and increased risk of complications for existing disease. Muscle strength is reduced and neurological and cognitive problems may ensue.

Patients with severe underweight require hospitalization. Feeding occurs either parenterally or enterally/orally. **Treatment** has to primarily address the underlying disease. A nutritional history tends to be a useful tool. If the underweight is mild, a balanced nutrition with minimally processed foods should be offered until positive energy balance is achieved. Nutrient-dense foods like juices, dried fruit, and nuts are suitable. Patients usually like carbohydrate-rich foods. Meals should be tasty, appetizing, and individualized, but small in size. Small amounts of alcohol may help enhance appetite. Hypercaloric dietary foods (>1.25 kcal/ml, available ≤1.6 kcal/ml) are sometimes useful. Light physical activity is recommended. In patients with idiopathic anorexia, weight gain is often not achieved regardless of high caloric intakes.

A. The U-Shaped Relationship Between BMI and Mortality

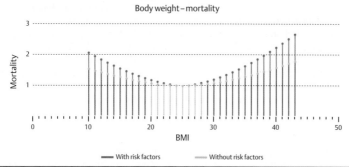

Body weight–mortality

Mortality

BMI

— With risk factors   — Without risk factors

B. Possible Causes of Underweight

1. Inadequate food intake	2. Excessive loss of substrate	3. Increased catabolism
Loss of appetite Anorexia, bulimia Pain syndrome Intoxication Pharmacotherapy Radiation therapy	**Malassimilation syndromes** Maldigestion after gastric resection Cholestasis Crohn disease Malabsorption HIV infection Hereditary enzymopathies (e. g., lactose intolerance) Postoperative malabsorption Parasitoses Radiation therapy Endocrinopathies (hyperthyroidism, diabetic enteropathy) Pharmacotherapy (cytostatic drugs, laxatives, cholestyramine)	**Increased substrate requirement** Chronic consumptive diseases Infection Malignant tumors (cachexia in tumor patients) Catabolism-inducing treatments (immunosuppressive, cytostatic drugs, radiation therapy)
Postaggressive metabolism Postoperative abstention from food Polytraumatic conditions		**Endocrinopathy** Excess of catabolic hormones Hyperthyroidism Lack of anabolic hormones Addison disease Diabetes mellitus Simmonds disease
Head injuries/lesions Cerebral pathologies Trauma, obstruction Chronically inflamed mouth, throat or gums	**Protein deficiency syndrome** Reduced synthesis Liver cirrhosis, liver resection Mushroom poisoning Sepsis Gastroenteropathy Gastric carcinoma, colon adenoma Gastroenteritis, ulcerative colitis Nephropathy	
Gastrointestinal tract obstruction Goiter Esophageal or gastric malignancies Esophageal or pyloric stenosis Pancreatic cancer with duodenal stenosis		
Malnutrition Pathologically altered energy and protein requirements (e. g., in case of malignancies) Inadequate intake during pregnancy Increased energy and protein requirements due to physical activity (e. g., exercise) Socially motivated fasting		

Obesity

Fat accumulation in tissues beyond normal levels is called obesity or adiposity. First, adipocyte (fat cell) volume increases. If caloric intake continues to exceed the requirements, preadipocytes may be transformed into additional adipocytes. Since the triglycerides deposited in these adipocytes undergo constant metabolic transformation, an increase in the levels of all components of lipid metabolism ensues. The resulting hyperlipoproteinemia and hyperinsulinemia may lead to peripheral insulin resistance (see also diabetes mellitus and metabolic syndrome). Visceral fatty tissues have the highest metabolic rates; hence, the android form (apple shape) of obesity tends to have more severe health consequences. Typical diseases associated with obesity are arterial hypertension, type 2 diabetes, coronary artery disease, cardiac insufficiency, breast and colon cancer, as well as orthopedic and psychosocial problems.

For purposes of **evaluating obesity**, BMI tables (see p. 17) are usually used since they correlate well with body fat content. A BMI of ≥25 is considered overweight, ≥30 obese, and ≥40 morbidly obese.

These categories are not suitable for **evaluating the body weight of children**. For children, gender and age specific BMI tables are used (**A**). A BMI above the 90th percentile (P90) is considered overweight, above the 97th percentile (P97) obese.

Figures about the **prevalence of obesity** vary, depending on study design and classification used. In most Western industrialized nations, about a third of the population is considered overweight and 7% obese. In the U.S., the increase in recent years has been, and continues to be, particularly rapid (**B**). In 2002, 31% of the population was obese; figures differ according to race and gender groups. 15% of children and teens 6–19 years of age are overweight (10% of children 2–5) with another 15% at risk (P85–P95).

The **cause of obesity** is always a sustained or repeated positive energy balance. In other terms: energy intake >energy requirements. Both sides of this equation are influenced by exogenous factors. Intake is influenced by taste, upbringing, environment during meals, psychological factors, portion size etc.; requirements depend on physical activity at work and during leisure. Both sides are also subject to hereditary components. Hereditary factors have been shown to affect feeding behavior, hunger and satiation, as well as the efficiency of cellular energy production (see also UCP).

At BMIs >30, the risk of various diseases increases; therefore, **weight reduction** should be attempted. The primary measure is to reduce food intake. If food intake drops below 1500 kcal/d, nutrient deficiencies become likely. Commercial formula diets are based on protein mixtures and are intended to prevent catabolic metabolism. They are enriched with nutrients and contain added carbohydrates and flavors to enhance taste. A disadvantage of formula diets is the fact that they do not modify eating behaviors. Weight reduction programs should be based on the three pillars: diet, behavior modification, and exercise therapy.

A. Evaluation of BMI in Children

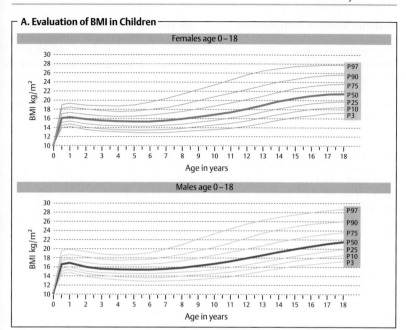

B. Obesity Trends Among U.S. Adults, BRFSS 2002

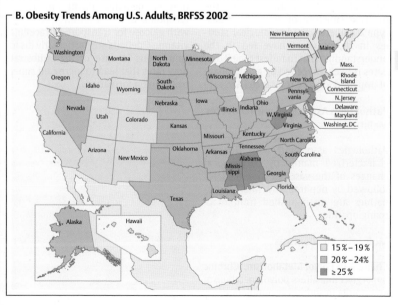

Diabetes Mellitus: Pathogenesis

The name diabetes mellitus (DM) applies to all forms of acute and chronic hyperglycemia with associated aberrations in carbohydrate and fat metabolism. In all forms of diabetes, either the normal feedback loop of the pancreatic beta cells' glucose-dependent insulin secretion or the normal interaction of insulin with its target cells is disturbed. Approximately 95% of DM patients have adult-onset (type 2 or noninsulin-dependent, NIDDM) diabetes with varying degrees of insulin resistance.

Only ~5% of DM patients have juvenile (type 1 or insulin-dependent, IDDM) diabetes, an autoimmune disease, in which the insulin-producing cells are destroyed.

The so-called metabolic syndrome or syndrome X, impaired glucose tolerance, as well as gestational diabetes, should be viewed as different degrees of one and the same primary defect, the most extreme form of which is manifest type 2 diabetes. Epidemiological studies in recent years have led to the understanding that manifest type 2 diabetes is likely preceded by a long phase of impaired glucose tolerance (**A**).

Pathologies Associated with Diabetes Mellitus

Pathologies associated with DM are characterized mainly by pathological changes of the vascular system, later followed by nephropathy. Microangiopathies are distinguished from macroangiopathies.

Molecular Mechanisms

Changes in Polyol Metabolism. Chronic hyperglycemia alters polyol metabolism and results in sorbitol accumulation.

Advanced glycosylation end products (AGE) and activation of protein kinase C (PKC). Formation of AGE and PKC activation due to chronic hyperglycemia (accumulation of diacylglycerol) affects the permeability of the basal membrane and impairs enzyme function and endocytosis of endothelial cells (**B, C**).

Oxidative Stress. Oxidative stress is an important pathogenetic factor for the pathologies associated with DM. Hence, a possible therapeutic approach might be based on strategies to quench reactive oxygen species (ROS) resulting from oxidative stress through supplementation of vitamins or other micronutrients, in particular vitamins C and E (**D**).

Hyperglycemia can cause cellular vitamin C depletion through competitive displacement because absorption of the dehydroascorbic acid form of the vitamin is mediated mainly by GLUT4 receptors, so that vitamin C competes with glucose for transport. Intracellular vitamin C deficits are particularly disadvantageous in case of high substrate flow rates that lead to increased superoxide anion formation.

A. Diabetes Mellitus Type 2

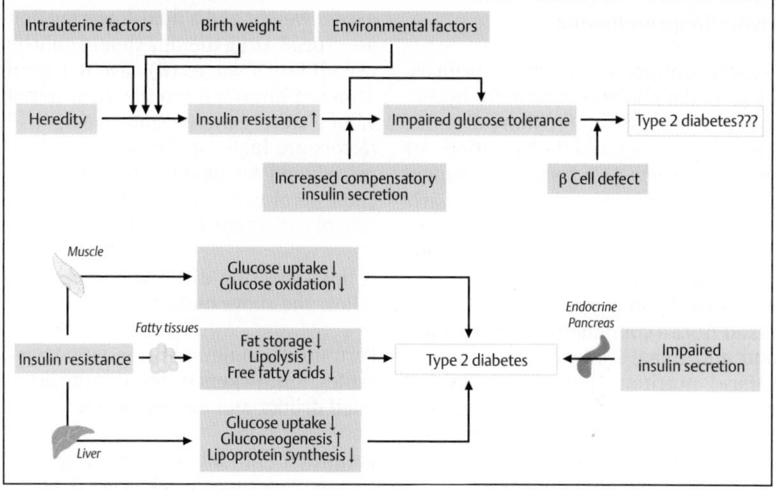

Intrauterine factors | Birth weight | Environmental factors

Heredity → Insulin resistance ↑ → Impaired glucose tolerance → Type 2 diabetes???

Increased compensatory insulin secretion

β Cell defect

Muscle → Glucose uptake ↓ / Glucose oxidation ↓

Fatty tissues → Fat storage ↓ / Lipolysis ↑ / Free fatty acids ↓

Insulin resistance

Liver → Glucose uptake ↓ / Gluconeogenesis ↑ / Lipoprotein synthesis ↓

Type 2 diabetes

Endocrine Pancreas → Impaired insulin secretion

B. Advanced Glycosylation End Products (AGE)

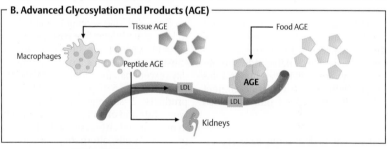

Tissue AGE · Food AGE · Macrophages · Peptide AGE · LDL · LDL · AGE · Kidneys

C. Activation of Protein Kinase C

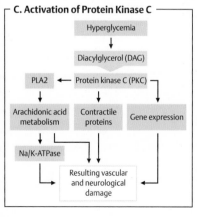

Hyperglycemia

Diacylglycerol (DAG)

PLA2 ← Protein kinase C (PKC)

Arachidonic acid metabolism | Contractile proteins | Gene expression

Na/K-ATPase

Resulting vascular and neurological damage

D. Oxidative Stress

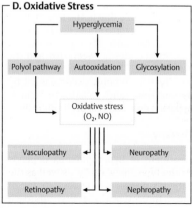

Hyperglycemia

Polyol pathway | Autooxidation | Glycosylation

Oxidative stress (O_2, NO)

Vasculopathy ← → Neuropathy

Retinopathy ← → Nephropathy

Pathologies of Fat Metabolism: Hyperlipoproteinemia

Hyperlipoproteinemia can be primary or secondary. Whereas primary hyperlipoproteinemia is a hereditary disorder and may be caused by a variety of genetic defects (**A**), secondary hyperlipoproteinemia may result from various diseases or from drug side effects, and can usually be corrected by eliminating the cause.

Most cases of hyperlipoproteinemia result from a combination of hereditary and nutritional factors. Besides hypercaloric nutrition with the resulting overweight, the most influential factors are faulty composition of food fats, food cholesterol, as well as improper carbohydrate and low fiber intakes.

Excessive food intake and overweight are the main causes of excessive serum triglyceride levels: the excessive calories increase liver triglyceride synthesis: very low density lipoproteins (VLDL) with high triglyceride content form and are released into the blood stream.

Overweight people often have significantly lower HDL cholesterol levels. This is probably due to the fact that the increase in triglyceride levels stimulates the exchange of cholesterol esters and triglycerides between HDL and triglyceride-rich lipoproteins. Abdominal obesity is commonly accompanied by dyslipidemia and insulin resistance, hypertension, and risk of thrombosis.

Therapy

Treatment of hyperlipidemia depends on the type and severity, as well as the patient's overall risk factors. In any of these three types, the first approach should be nondrug measures. Loss of excess weight and a lipid-lowering diet are crucial. Drug therapy should only be used if target values (**B**) have not been achieved after 3–6 months or if initial values were extreme and overall risk factors are high. Decisions about therapy should be based mainly on LDL-cholesterol values but with consideration of HDL cholesterol values.

A lipid-lowering diet should generally follow the above outline:

Permitted in unlimited amounts: **Vegetables, unthickened soups, unsweetened drinks**, and **mineral water**.

Permitted in moderation: **legumes** ½ cup, 3–4 times/week; **cereal products**, **potatoes** (boiled in skin only) 4–5 servings/day. One serving is equivalent to ½ cup rice or egg-free pasta, one thin slice of whole grain bread, a cup of (unsweetened) cereal. **Fruit** 4 servings/day (except bananas, grapes); **fish, lean meat 100 g** (3.5 oz)/day; **low-fat dairy products** 2 servings/day; 1–2 eggs/week; **fats and oils** 15 g (½ oz)/day, rich in unsaturated fatty acids and vitamin E (e. g., germ oils, alternating with olive oil).

A. Primary Hyperlipidemia

Description	Metabolic defect	Symptoms	Plasma cholesterol	Plasma triglycerides
Polygenic hypercholesterolemia	Multiple gene interactions More than a basic metabolic defect	Arcus corneae, xanthelasma	↑ to ↑↑↑	↑
Familial hypercholesterolemia	LDL receptor defect	Tendinous xanthomas (finger extensors, Achilles tendon), arcus cornea xanthelasma, aortic stenosis	↑↑↑	Normal or ↑
Familial defective Apo B-100	Mutation of Apo B-100, causes reduced LDL receptor activity	Tendinous xanthomas (finger extensors), arcus cornea	↑ to ↑↑↑	Normal or ↑
Familial combined hyperlipidemia	Excessive Apo B production Typical: Intraindividual and interfamilial fluctuation of hyperlipidemia patterns	Arcus cornea, xanthelasma	↑ to ↑↑ or normal	↑ to ↑↑ or normal
Remnant hyperlipidemia	Mutation of Apo E, causes reduced Apo E receptor activity, usually manifests only in combination with other anomalies (diabetes mellitus, adiposity)	Tuberous (elbows) and tendinous xanthomas, palmar xanthomas	↑↑↑	↑↑
Familial lipoprotein lipase deficiency	Lipoprotein lipase or Apo C-III deficiency	Eruptive xanthomas (elbows, buttocks) lipemia retinalis, hepatosplenomegaly, pancreatitis	↑	↑↑↑
Familial hypertriglyceridemia	Unknown	Eruptive xanthomas (elbows, buttocks) lipemia retinalis, hepatosplenomegaly, pancreatitis	↑	↑↑

B. Target Values for Therapeutic Reduction of LDL Cholesterol

Overall risk		Target values for LDL cholesterol
Slightly increased risk	Ex.: pretreatment cholesterol 200 – 300 mg/dl (5.2 – 7.8 nmol/l) Plasma cholesterol (HDL/cholesterol ratio 4 – 5 mg/dl) No additional risk factors	155 – 175 mg/dl (4.0 – 4.5 nmol/l)
Moderately increased risk	Ex.: pretreatment cholesterol 200-300 mg/dl (5.2 – 7.8 nmol/l) plus HDL/cholesterol ratio ≤ 40 mg/dl (≤ 1 nmol/l)	134 – 155 mg/dl (3.5 – 4.0 nmol/l)
High risk	Ex.: coronary or peripheral vascular disease, or familial hypercholesterolemia, or two pronounced risk factors. e.g.: cholesterol 300 mg/dl (7.8 nmol/l) plus 20 cigarettes/d or three or more risk factors	≤ 100 mg/dl (≤ 3 nmol/l)
	Target value for triglycerides: 159 mg/dl (1.7 nmol/l)	

Metabolic Syndrome: Insulin Resistance Syndrome

Obesity plays a central role in **metabolic syndrome**, also called **syndrome X** or **insulin resistance syndrome**. Metabolic syndrome is a combination of **altered lipid metabolism, hypertension, type 2 diabetes mellitus**, and **overweight** (the "deadly four"). The development of metabolic syndrome is gradual, beginning with hyperinsulinemia combined with insulin resistance, moderately altered lipid metabolism, and mild hypertension. With increasing body weight, the metabolic disorder becomes more severe and blood pressure rises. Weight reduction may effectively correct the symptoms of metabolic syndrome at this point. A diagnosis of "metabolic syndrome" requires the presence of at least three symptoms (**A**).

Therapy of metabolic syndrome is based on two pillars: nutrition and exercise. **Nutritionally,** (if overweight) a reduced calorie diet adapted to the insulin resistance (low glycemic index and load) is recommended. Foods or diets with a high glycemic load increase insulin resistance while raising insulin demand. The latter causes exhaustion of the insulin-producing pancreatic β cells, thereby enhancing the onset of type 2 diabetes (**B**). Reduction of postprandial blood glucose peaks may help retard the development of metabolic syndrome (**C**). Intensely processed (carbohydrate-rich) foods like refined flour and refined flour products (breads, pasta, etc.), extensively heated starchy foods (baked potatoes), and instant products like quick rice are poor choices and should, where possible, be replaced by unrefined, whole foods, carefully prepared to maximally maintain integrity (potatoes boiled whole in their skin, brown rice, whole grain pasta) (**D**).

It is not clear at this point, whether reducing carbohydrate in favor of protein intake favorably impacts metabolic syndrome or whether the main measure should be to restrict the glycemic load of individual foods.

Exercise, however, plays an established role in improving clinical symptoms of metabolic syndrome and slows its progression. **Physical activity** reduces insulin resistance by causing breakdown of glycogen and reduces triglyceride levels. There is a negative correlation between physical fitness and systolic blood pressure. Regular exercise reduces plasminogen activator inhibitor (PAI) levels and improves fibrolytic activity. Particularly in combination with a calorie-reduced diet, physical activity reduces abdominal fat. A loss of just 5 kg may, in some cases, normalize one or more symptoms of metabolic syndrome.

A. Diabetes and Insulin Resistance

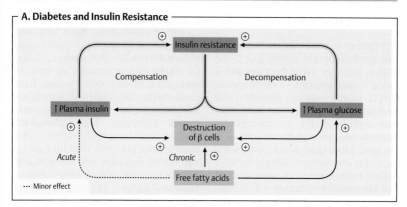

B. Diabetes and Glycemic Load

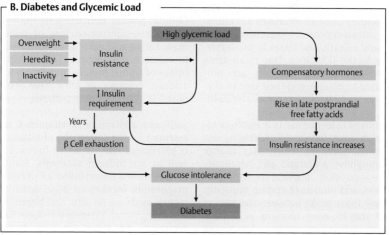

C. Glycemic Load of Foods

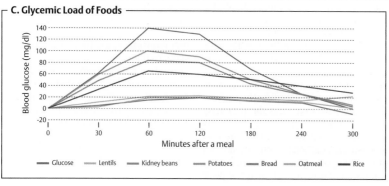

Osteoporosis

A reduction of bone mass to below age and gender-specific norms (–2.5 SD) implies a greater risk of fractures and is called **osteoporosis**. Osteoporosis affects mostly women. However, the significance of estrogens for bone mineralization and for postmenopausal osteoporosis has been overestimated in the past. More than 10 million Americans have osteoporosis, among them ~2 million men. Another 28 million are at risk. Osteoporosis causes 1.5 million new fractures each year. The overall survival rate for hip fractures is 80%. Hip fractures cause an estimated $22 billion in annual expenses, losses through premature death, and losses to productivity, in the U.S. alone. Due to an aging population, their numbers are projected to double, and their cost to skyrocket to $240 billion annually by 2040.

Primary osteoporosis is a multi-factorial disease. Individual underlying risk factors, some of which may change throughout a lifetime are: hereditary predisposition, physical activity patterns, and intakes of certain nutrients. Bone mass peaks between the ages of 20 and 25. After reaching peak bone mass, it first remains on a plateau, and subsequently decreases at a rate of ~1% annually (**A**). Peak bone mass, as well as the rate of decrease in subsequent decades, determine when the fracture risk zone (–2.5 SD) is reached.

The role of many nutrients in sustaining bone integrity is not directly proven. Therefore, the following discussion is based on the basic metabolic functions of the respective nutrient (**B**). The role of **calcium** (Ca) has been researched most extensively. High Ca intake during childhood and youth can increase peak bone mass by 4%. Premenopausal high Ca intake slows down bone loss, and postmenopausal high Ca intake may reduce the risk by ~30%. Hence, optimal Ca intake has preventive as well as therapeutic effects. While various food components may influence Ca metabolism, their impact is minimal on normal mixed nutrition: high phosphate content and complexing agents, like oxalates and phytates, may impede Ca absorption, and table salt, caffeine, and alcohol increase urinary losses. Proper vitamin D status is an essential prerequisite for Ca absorption into bone.

Chronic protein deficiency in the elderly causes increased loss of bone mass. Latent acidosis is also considered to enhance osteoporosis. That a high intake of animal protein contributes to acidosis, however, as some have proposed, is a speculative hypothesis.

Sufficient availability of **vitamin C** is essential for the conversion of vitamin D precursors into its active forms, as well as for collagen synthesis. Some studies show a strong influence of high **magnesium intakes** on bone density, related evidence for **zinc** and **boron** is less unequivocal. **Vitamin K** reduces Ca excretion and stimulates new bone growth. Osteocalcin and matrix GLA protein are vitamin K-dependent proteins that have a function in bone metabolism. Epidemiological studies show that low levels of vitamin K correlate with higher bone loss. The results of clinical studies indicate that vitamin K has great importance for osteoporosis prevention—particularly through its interactions with vitamin D.

A. Bone Mass

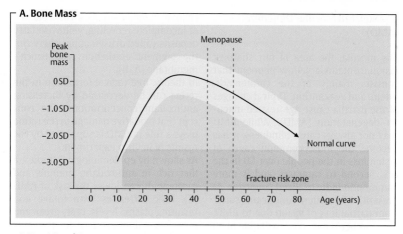

B. Nutritional Factors

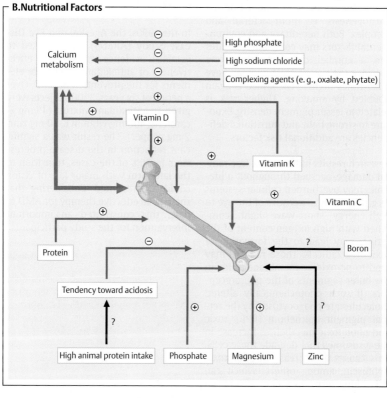

Age-Related Macular Degeneration (AMD)

The macula, the area of our sharpest vision, contains a yellow pigment that consists mainly of the carotenoids, lutein, and zeaxanthin. Typical changes of the macula cause age-related macular degeneration (AMD). While AMD may not always cause blindness, it has become the most common cause of vision loss in the people over 60 in the U.S., second to cataracts, and is more common in industrialized countries. At present, 1.7 million Americans suffer from partial loss of vision due to AMD. The number is expected to double in 30 years, due to an aging population. Its **pathogenesis** is multi-factorial and complex. Both hereditary and environmental factors may contribute. Besides age, a number of other risk factors enhance the risk of AMD: women have a 2.5 times higher risk, which is again doubled by smoking. Higher risk is related to lesser pigment density. Exposure to strong light and nutritional deficiencies are additional risk factors.

Research results indicate that free radical damage, accrued throughout a lifetime, may overburden cellular systems (e.g., pigments). Exposure of the eye to high-energy short-wave light, combined with high oxygen content of the retina, may lead to the formation of toxic free radicals. Those radicals may tend to peroxidize membrane lipids in the outer segments of the photoreceptors. If such photochemically altered molecules are phagocytosed by the retinal pigment epithelium (RPE), toxic and phototoxic metabolites increase in the lysosomes that degrade those cells. This causes an increase in phototoxic lipofuscin, among others, which can have long-term negative effects on cellular metabolism. As a consequence of incomplete recycling, yellowish fatty deposits called drusen appear between the pigment epithelium and Bruch's membrane (**A, B**).

In theory, free radical formation in the retina can be decreased by increasing antioxidant concentrations. The concept that oxidative damage to the retina plays a role in AMD is supported by the results of in vitro experiments.

As shown by epidemiological studies, a diet rich in antioxidant vitamins and carotenoids can lower the risk of AMD (**C**). Risk correlates with intake and resulting plasma levels. Leafy green and other vegetables are best for this purpose (**D**).

In the 1990s, the **Age-Related Eye Disease Study** (**AREDS**) was initiated to establish evidence regarding the effectiveness of antioxidants and trace elements for the prevention of AMD. Over a period of six years, 3500 subjects were given an antioxidant mixture (15 mg β-carotene, 400 mg vitamin E, 80 mg zinc, 2 mg copper). The result was a significant reduction in the disease progression. In 25% of the cases, transition to the late form with major loss of vision could be prevented. Considering that there is no effective therapy for AMD to date, this constituted an important intervention for the study participants.

A. Demographic Risk Factors

The risk of blindness increases drastically with age

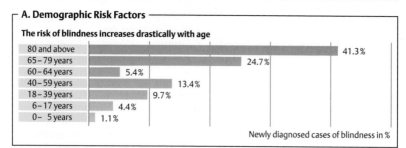

Age	Newly diagnosed cases of blindness in %
80 and above	41.3%
65–79 years	24.7%
60–64 years	5.4%
40–59 years	13.4%
18–39 years	9.7%
6–17 years	4.4%
0–5 years	1.1%

B. Lipid Peroxidation, Drusen Formation, and Neovascularization

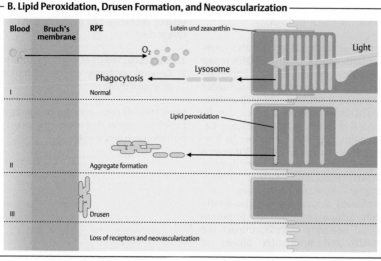

Blood | Bruch's membrane | RPE

Lutein und zeaxanthin

Light

O_2

Lysosome

Phagocytosis

I   Normal

Lipid peroxidation

II   Aggregate formation

III   Drusen

Loss of receptors and neovascularization

C. Serum Carotenoids and AMD Risk

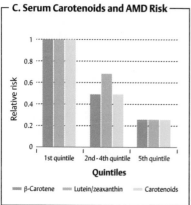

Relative risk

Quintiles: 1st quintile | 2nd–4th quintile | 5th quintile

■ β-Carotene   ■ Lutein/zeaxanthin   ■ Carotenoids

D. Sources of Lutein and Zeaxanthin

Amount of vegetables required to obtain 1 mg lutein and zeaxanthin

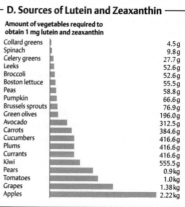

Collard greens	4.5 g
Spinach	9.8 g
Celery greens	27.7 g
Leeks	52.6 g
Broccoli	52.6 g
Boston lettuce	55.5 g
Peas	58.8 g
Pumpkin	66.6 g
Brussels sprouts	76.9 g
Green olives	196.0 g
Avocado	312.5 g
Carrots	384.6 g
Cucumbers	416.6 g
Plums	416.6 g
Currants	416.6 g
Kiwi	555.5 g
Pears	0.9 kg
Tomatoes	1.0 kg
Grapes	1.38 kg
Apples	2.22 kg

Cancer

Nutrients can influence carcinogenesis in many ways during tumorigenesis:

Vitamin C and other **antioxidants**, for instance, are able to block the conversion of nitrite into carcinogenic N-nitrosamine in the stomach. Antioxidants are often able to directly block the carcinogen, which is commonly a free radical, neutralize it, or prevent adduct formation by methylating DNA.

Carcinogenic chemicals can also interfere with genetic control of DNA repair (possibly an extremely important mechanism). Micronutrients influence activation of oncogenes as well as deletion of tumor suppressor genes, thereby impacting cell differentiation. **Carotenoids** may stabilize tissues by having effects via gap junctions. **Vitamin A** impacts cell differentiation directly. Growth-stimulating factors (energy supply, growth hormones, and cytokines), as well as **ω-3 and ω-6 fatty acids**, which modulate the immunological behavior of cells, impact the growth and promotion phases of tumors.

Primary Prevention: The causality of many of the correlations shown in the table (**A**) is poorly established. Therefore, the general guidelines for cancer prevention have to remain very general:
- Avoid overweight, normalize body weight
- Reduce fat intake to <30% of caloric intake. Use monounsaturated oils with high antioxidant content preferentially
- Consume sufficient vitamins, minerals and trace elements; more fruit and vegetables, less meat, more fish, and calcium-rich foods
- Use fiber-rich foods preferentially
- Reduce salt intake
- Consume alcoholic beverages in moderation or avoid them

Nutrition and Nutritional Therapy for Cancer Patients: In ~50 percent of patients with malignancies, disturbances in food intake, nutrient processing, or metabolism can be diagnosed with varying frequencies, depending on the type of tumor. These nutrition-related problems can be divided in two categories:

1. Effects caused directly by the tumor
2. General, systemic effects of tumor and treatment

Especially during anticancer therapy, problems appear that require particular nutritional attention (**B**).

A. Associations Observed During Epidemiological Studies

Cancer site	Fat	Body weight, energy intake	Fiber	Fruit, vegetables	Alcohol	Smoked, cured foods
Lung				●	●	
Breast	●	●		●	●	
Colon	●	●	●	●		
Prostate	●	●		●		
Bladder	●			●		
Rectum	●				●	
Endometrium		●				
Mouth				●	●	
Stomach					●	●
Kidneys		●				
Cervix		●		●		
Thyroid		●				
Esophagus					●	●

● Positive correlation, risk factor   ● Negative correlation, protective factor

B. Nutritional Recommendations for Cancer Patients

Symptoms	Nutritional recommendations for cancer patients during chemo- and cancer therapy
Difficulty swallowing	– No solid foods – High-caloric, liquid food supplements – Drink small amounts frequently (mint tea)
Inflammation of the upper digestive tract	– Avoid hot spices – Avoid salty foods – Avoid acidic foods (vinegar, fruit, rhubarb, tomatoes) – Don't consume foods too hot – Avoid carbonated drinks – Vitamin, mineral, and trace mineral supplements may be necessary
Diarrhea, vomiting	– No fresh fruit – No gas-producing vegetables and salads – Lots of fluids (2.5 – 3 l) – Supplement minerals and trace minerals
Altered sense of taste	– Taste threshold for bitter taste lowered – Taste threshold for sweet taste raised – Dislike of meat and sausages: switch to milk, dairy products, eggs, and fish
Loss of appetite	– Eat when there is appetite – Avoid strong food odors – Small portions – Arrange meals to be appetizing and attractive – Appetite-enhancing drinks

Chronic Inflammatory Bowel Disease (CIBD)

Nutritional factors. There are huge differences in the incidence of Crohn disease (Morbus Crohn) and ulcerative colitis among developing and industrialized countries. This provides a basis for the assumption that low fiber and high sugar intake are causative factors in the development of these diseases.

Fiber provides a substrate for the growth of healthy microbial flora and is converted to short-chain fatty acids (butyrate) in the colon. Butyrate is an essential nutrient for the colonocytes. ω-3 fatty acids are precursors of the anti-inflammatory leukotrienes 3 and 5, whereas ω-6 fatty acids favor the formation of the proinflammatory leukotrienes 4 and 6. Exogenous antioxidants like carotenoids and also vitamin C and E protect colonocytes from free radical damage (**A/1**). Low antioxidant and fiber intakes and an unfavorable ratio of ω-3 to ω-6 fatty acids are major causative factors in the pathogenesis of Crohn disease and perhaps ulcerative colitis as well (**A/2**).

However, there is no proof to date of a direct causative link between nutritional factors and the onset of ulcerative colitis.

Vitamin and trace mineral deficiencies. In-patients, as well as ambulatory patients with chronic inflammatory bowel disease (CIBD), often exhibit signs of general malnutrition, more commonly patients with Crohn disease, especially if large areas of the small intestine are affected (**B**). Trace elements, which are important cofactors of enzymes, are commonly deficient (**C**).

The following conditions contribute to malnutrition: lack of appetite, one-sided nutrition, food sensitivities, vomiting, enteric fistulas, reduced absorptive surface, bacterial overgrowth of the small intestine, lack of bile acids, exudative enteropathy, drug side effects, increased energy needs after operations, and during sepsis. In children and teenagers, the resulting catabolism causes reduced growth rates and delayed puberty. Signs of general malnutrition (underweight, negative nitrogen balance, decreased serum albumin) can usually be quickly reversed through artificial, enteral, or parenteral feeding. If possible, nutrients should be introduced through the intestinal tract. Because of their greater tendency to hemorrhage, patients with ulcerative colitis more commonly suffer from iron deficiency anemia than Crohn disease patients.

There are no confirmed data on successful treatment of ulcerative colitis patients with chemically defined formula diets during acute attacks. For milder cases, a light whole food diet is sufficient in addition to adequately dosed steroids.

A. Nutritional Factors

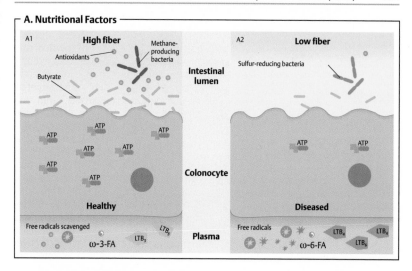

B. Micronutrient Deficiencies (% of patients)

	Crohn disease	Ulcerative colitis
Iron	25–50 %	80 %
Folic acid	50–60 %	30–40 %
B$_{12}$	50 %	10 %
Vitamin A$_1$	10–50 %	>90 %
Vitamin A$_2$	25–75 %	35 %
Vitamin A$_3$	?	40 %
Zinc	40 %	?

C. Trace Element Deficiencies in CIBD Patients

Micronutrient deficiencies	Effect	
Copper	SOD ↓	
Selenium	GPX ↓	
Zinc	Immune system ↓	
Chromium	Glucose tolerance ↓	
Manganese	SOD ↓	
Molybdenum	Thiol/disulfide ↑↓	

Appendix

Table of Measures

Weight

Metric		English (U.S.)
1 milligram (mg)	=	0.002 grain (0.000035 oz)
1 gram (g)	=	0.04 oz. (1/28 of an oz)
1 kilogram (kg)	=	35.27 oz, 2.20 lb
1 metric ton (1000kg)	=	1.10 tons

English (U.S.)		Metric
1 grain	=	64.80 mg
1 ounce (oz)	=	28.35 g
1 pound (lb)	=	453.60 g, 0.45 kg
1 ton (short – 2000 lb)	=	0.91 metric ton (907 kg)

Volume

Metric		English (U.S.)
1 milliliter (ml)	=	0.03 oz
1 liter (l)	=	2.12 pt
1 liter	=	1.06 qt
1 liter	=	0.27 gal

English (U.S.)		Metric
1 ounce	=	0.03 liter (30 ml)
1 pint (pt)	=	0.47 liter
1 quart (qt)	=	0.95 liter
1 gallon (gal)	=	3.79 liters

Additional Metric and Other Units Commonly Used in Nutrition

Unit / Abbreviation		Other Equivalent Measure
1 milligram/mg	=	1/1000 of a gram
1 microgram/µg	=	1/1,000,000 of a gram
1 deciliter/dl	=	1/10 of a liter (about 1/2 cup)
1 milliliter/ml	=	1/1000 of a liter (5 ml is about 1 tsp)

General References

Biesalski HK, Köhrle J, Schümann K (eds.). Vitamine, Spurenelemente und Mineralstoffe. Prävention und Therapie mit Mikronährstoffen. 2nd ed. Stuttgart: Thieme; 2002.

Biesalski HK et al. Ernährungsmedizin. 3rd ed. Stuttgart: Thieme; 2004.

Despopoulos A, Silbernagl S. Color Atlas of Physiology. 5th ed. Stuttgart–New York: Thieme; 2003.

Eastwood M, Stewart AT. Principles of Human Nutrition. 2nd ed. Oxford: Blackwell Publishers; 2003.

Gibney M. Introduction to Human Nutrition. Iowa: Iowa State Press; 2002.

Hidgon J. An Evidence–Based Approach to Vitamins and Minerals. Health Benefits and Intake Recommendations. Stuttgart–New York: Thieme; 2003.

Kastner J. Chinese Nutrition Therapy. Dietetics in Traditional Chinese Medicine. Stuttgart–New York: Thieme; 2004.

Koolman J, Röhm KH. Color Atlas of Biochemistry. Stuttgart–New York: Thieme; 2005.

Mann J. Essentials of Human Nutrition. Oxford: Oxford University Press; 2002.

Quick Access: Professional Guide to Conditions, Herbs, and Supplements. Stuttgart–New York: Thieme; 2000.

Quick Access: Professional Access 2.0 CD–ROM. Stuttgart–New York: Thieme; 2000.

Silbernagel S, Lang F. Color Atlas of Pathophysiology. Stuttgart–New York: Thieme; 2000.

Stipanuk MH. Biochemical and Physiological Aspects of Human Nutrition. Philadelphia: WB Saunders Co.; 2004.

Theml H, Diem H, Haferlach T. Color Atlas of Hematology. Stuttgart–New York: Thieme; 2004.

Whitney EN, Rolfes SR. Understanding Nutrition. 10th ed. Belmont, CA: Wadsworth/Thompson Learning; 2005

Zimmermann M. Pocket Guide to Micronutrients in Health and Disease. Stuttgart–New York: Thieme; 2001.

Zimmermann M. Burgerstein's Handbook of Nutrition. Micronutrients in the Prevention and Therapy of Disease. Stuttgart–New York: Thieme; 2002.

Selected Websites

American Dietetic Association (ADA): http://www.eatright.org/Public/

American Nutriceutical Association (ANA): http://www.americanutra.com/

American Society for Clinical Nutrition (ASCN): http://www.ascn.org/

Food Processor and Genesis R&D; NutritionCalc Plus+, von ESHA Research, Salem, OR/USA: http://www.esha.com/

Orthomolocular Medicine Online: http://www.orthomed.org/

International Society for Orthomolecular Medicine (ISOM): http://www.orthomed.org/isom/isom.htm

Linus Pauling Institute: http://lpi.oregonstate.edu/

Medline: http://www.ncbi.nlm.nih.gov/entrez/query.fcgi

Natural Standard Online Database @ www.thieme.com/cam

Nutritional Therapy Association (NTA): http://www.nutritionaltherapy.com/

Nutrition Data: http://www.nutritiondata.com

Vitamins and Nutrition Center: http://www.vitamins–nutrition.org/

Figure Sources

Biesalski, H.K.: Ernährungsmedizin. Georg Thieme Verlag, Stuttgart, New York, 1995. [469]

Biesalski, H.K.: Vitamine. Georg Thieme Verlag, Stuttgart, New York, 1997.
[234, Fig. 87 a, b
color plate 2, Fig. 2a
color plate 3, Fig. 6, 8
color plate 6, Fig. 15a, 16
color plate 7, Fig. 18, 22]

Faller, A., M. Schünke: Der Körper des Menschen. Georg Thieme Verlag, Stuttgart, New York, 1995. [220, Fig. 6.8] = 59 B

Gerlach, U., et al.: Innere Medizin für Pflegeberufe. Georg Thieme Verlag, Stuttgart, New York, 2000.
[15, Fig. 1.5
78, Fig. 2.6a, 2.6b
79, Fig. 2.7b]

Reichl, F.-X.: Taschenatlas der Toxikologie. Georg Thieme Verlag, Stuttgart, New York, 1997. [267]

Riede, U.-N., M. Werner: Color Atlas of Pathology. Georg Thieme Verlag, Stuttgart, New York, 2004. [399, Fig. B]

Sohn, C.: Ultraschall in Gynäkologie und Geburtshilfe. Georg Thieme Verlag, Stuttgart, New York, 1995. [151, Fig. 6.1–57]

Theml, H., H. Diem, T. Haferlach: Color Atlas of Hematology. Georg Thieme Verlag, Stuttgart, New York, 2004. [33, Fig. 9e; 133, Fig. 45b]

Washington Department of Fish and Wildlife. wdfw.wa.gov/wlm/cwd/ [333 B]

Index

A

AA *see* amino acids
AAS *see* amino acid score
absorption 42–5, 52–3
    carbohydrates 58–9
    medication 326–7
absorptive phase 60–1
ACAT *see* acyl–CoA cholesterol acyl–trans-
    ferase
Acceptable Macronutrient Distribution Range
    (AMDR) 8–9, 82, 114
acesulfame K 282–3
acetaldehyde 273
acetate 273
acetoacetate 102, 165
acetoacetyl–CoA 102, 105
acetolactate synthase 169
acetone phosphates 70–1
acetyl carboxylase 185
acetyl salicylic acid 280, 326
acetyl–CoA
    biotin 185
    carboxylase 98, 102–3, 184
    cholesterol biosynthesis 104–5
    citrate cycle 169
    energy transfer 24–5
    fasting 32–3
    fatty acid metabolism 102–3
    glycolysis 70–1, 73
    pantothenic acid 181
acetyl–LDL receptor 94
acetylcholine 128–9, 208
acid secretion 50–1
acidic amino acids 118–19
acidosis 126–7
acne 238
acrodermatitis enterohepatica 248
acyl transferases 139
acyl–CoA 102–3
    cholesterol acyl transferase (ACAT) 94,
        107
    acyl–CoA–retinol acyl transferase
        (ARAT) 138
acyl–SCoA 90–1
acylation 111
acylglycerols 84–5, 91, 103, 209
additives 280–1
adenosine diphosphate (ADP) 34–5, 128
adenosine monophosphate (AMP) 256
adenosine triphosphate (ATP) 26–7, 34–5,
    70–1, 102–3
    athletes 322
    ATPase 41

hydrolysis 27
synthetase 39
S-adenosyl-homocysteine 201
S-adenosyl-methionine 201
adenylate cyclase 102–3
Adequate Intake (AI) 8–9, 82, 114
ADH *see* alcohol dehydrogenase; antidiuretic
    hormone
adhesion factors 204
adipocytes 98, 103, 260, 340
ADP *see* adenosine diphosphate
adrenaline 165
    -adrenergic receptor 103
advanced glycosylation end products
    (AGE) 342–3
Adverse Reaction Monitoring System (ARAS)
    280
aerobic metabolism 24–5
afferent control 36–7
age
    body mass index 16–17
    YOPIs 300
age-related eye disease study (AREDS) 350
age-related macular degeneration (AMD)
    350–1
aglycones 268
Agrobacterium tumefaciens 296
AHEI *see* Harvard School of Public Health
    Alternative Healthy Eating Index
AI *see* Adequate Intake; average intakes
Airola 327
alanine (A; Ala) 62–3, 120–1, 180
albumin 98, 172, 247, 251, 255
alcohol 84–5, 272–7
    abuse 170, 276
    consumption 277
    dehydrogenase (ADH) 272
    fetal alcohol effects (FAE) 276
    fetal alcohol syndrome (FAS) 276
    reductase 73
    sugar 72–5
aldehyde
    dehydrogenase (ALDH) 272
    oxidase 256–7
    reductase 73
aldehydes 77
aldol reductase activity 72–3
aldolase 73
aldose reductase 71, 73
aldosterone 225–6, 304–5
α cells 67
alitame 282–3
alkaline phosphatase 212
alkoxy radical 203

all-trans-retinoic acid 142–3
all-trans-retinol 141
all-trans-retinylpalmitate 141
allergies 122, 262–3
allicin 222, 278
allosteric regulation 62–3
Amadori reactions 76
AMD *see* age-related macular degeneration
AMDR *see* Acceptable Macronutrient Distribution Range
amino acid score (AAS) 132
amino acids (AA) 95, 118–19
    basic 118–19
    branched (BCCA) 324–5
    essential 120–1
    glucogenic 62–3
    long-chain neutral (LNAA) 130–1
    polar 118–19
    pools 124
    proteinogenic 120–1
    proteins 122–3, 126–7
amino-oligopeptidases 123
aminobenzoic acid 196
aminoglycans 71, 100, 223
aminolevulinate synthase 231
aminopeptidases 122–3
ammonia 126–7
AMP *see* adenosine monophosphate
amphetamines 316
amylopectin 57
amylose 56–7
AN *see* anorexia nervosa
anaerobic metabolism 24–5, 62–3
anemia 234
    hypochromic 190, 232
    iron deficiency 233
    megaloblastic 198
    megoblastic 195
    pernicious 194
ANF *see* atrial natriuretic factor
angina pectoris 128
angiotensin 225
    converting enzyme 225
angiotensinogen 225
animals
    cells 20–1
    husbandry 287
anorexia nervosa (AN) 336–7
antagonists 220
anthocyanidins 268–9
anthocyanins 268–71
anthropometrics 10, 16–17
antibiotics 286–7, 296, 326–7
antidepressants 302, 305
antidiuretic hormone (ADH) 214
antioxidants 205, 278, 352
    -carotene 148

carotenoids 354
    endogenous 250
    phytochemicals 270
    site-specific 246
    vitamin E 158
aortic stenosis 335
apoenzymes 185
apolipoproteins 98–9
apoproteins 90–1, 100
    A 92–3, 96–7
    B 101
    B_{48} 92–3
    B_{100} 92–3, 335
    receptor 94
    C 92–3, 97
    CII 92–3, 100–1
    E 92–3, 97, 101, 106–7, 345
    receptor 92–4, 99, 157
apotransferrin 229
appetite 36–9, 178
arabitol 75
arachidic acid 87
arachidonic acid 87, 110–12, 114–15, 343
ARAT *see* acyl-CoA-retinol acyl transferase
arcus cornea 345
AREDS *see* age–related eye disease study
arginase 254
arginine (R; Arg) 120–1, 129, 325
arsenic (As) 266–7
    trioxide (As_2O_3) 266
arterial hypertension 340
arteriosclerosis 128, 198
ascites 275
ascorbic acid 164–7, 206–7
    alcohol 277
    chromium 259
    dehydroascorbic acid 164–5, 207
    lactation 316–17
    osteoporosis 348–9
    recommended intakes 166–7
    semidehydro-L-ascorbic acid 164
    seniors 320–1
    tumors 271, 352
ascorbic acid-2-sulfate 223
asialoglycoproteins 76–7
asparagine (N; Asn) 120–1
aspartame 282–3
aspartic acid (D; Asp) 120–1, 321
aspirin (acetyl salicylic acid) 280, 326
asthma 222, 262
atherosclerosis 94, 100, 200
athletes 322–23
Atkins, Dr. R.C. 4
ATP *see* adenosine triphosphate
atrial natriuretic factor (ANF) 224–5
autoimmune diseases 122
autoprothrombin 161

Average Intakes (AI) 8–9
azoospermia 277

B

B *see* boron
bacteria
    colon 46–7
    GM foods 297
    nitrogen fixation 116
Bacteroides 46–7, 162
basal membranes 43, 91
basic amino acids 118–19
basic metabolic rate (BMR) 28–31, 312, 320
BCCA *see* amino acids, branched
beef tallow 115
behenic acid 87
benzopyrene 287
beriberi 170–1
β cells 67
BIA *see* bioelectrical impedance
Bifidobacteria 288–9
Bifidus 46–7
bile 88–9, 147
    acids 48–9, 88–9, 98–9, 164–5, 222–3
    cholesterol 105
    salts 91, 104–5
bilirubin 48–9, 229
biliverdin 231
binge eating disorder 336
bioelectrical impedance (BIA) 18–19
bioflavonoids 21, 209, 211
biological value (BV) 132–3
biotin 184–7
Bircher-Benner diet 313
Bitot spot 145
blindness 256, 350
blood
    coagulation 160–1, 277
    copper 250
    glucose 66–9
    lipids 98–9, 101
    pressure 113
    supply 204
blood-brain barrier, proteins 130–1
BMR *see* basic metabolic rate
BN *see* bulimia nervosa
body composition 12–23
Body Mass Index (BMI) 16–17, 340–1, 346–7
body weight *see* weight
bomb calorimetry 26
bombesin 51, 164
bones 152
    boron 264
    deformities 150
    density 214
    loss 218
    mass 349
    mineralization 218
borage oil 113
boric acid 264
boron (B) 264–5, 348–9
bovine spongiform encephalopathy (BSE) 330–1
bowel disease, chronic inflammatory (CIBD) 354–5
bradykinin 128–9
brain 32–3, 128
Broca 16
Bruch's membrane 350–1
brush borders 91, 122–3
BSE *see* bovine spongiform encephalopathy
buccal cavity 52–3
Buchinger diet 313
bulimia nervosa (BN) 336–7
burning feet syndrome 182
butyrate 169, 354
butyric acid 37, 87
BV *see* biological value

C

Ca *see* calcium
CaBP *see* calcium-binding protein
CAD *see* coronary artery disease
cadmium 287
caffeine 324–5
calcidiol 25-(OH)-D *see* 25-hydroxychole-calciferol
calciol *see* vitamin D₃
calcitonin 214–15
calcitriol 1, 25-(OH)2-D *see* 1, 25-dihydroxy-cholecalciferol
calcium (Ca) 212–17
    calmodulin 128
    chondroitin sulfate 213
    citrate 213
    homeostasis 152–3
    lactation 316–17
    magnesium absorption 220
    osteoporosis 348
    phosphate 213, 218
    seniors 317
    transport 152–3, 214
    zinc absorption 246
calcium-binding protein (CaBP) 152, 212
calmodulin 128–9, 212–13
calories 26–9, 326
Campylobacter jejuni 298
cancer 307
Candida albicans 248
capric acid 87
caproic acid 87

caprylic acid 87
capsaicin 278
carrageenan 79
carboanhydrase 41
carbohydrates 2–3, 52–3
  absorption 58–9
  athletes 322
  digestion 58–9
  distribution 60–1
  fiber 78–81
  foods 83
  fructose *see* fructose
  galactose *see* galactose
  glucose *see* glucose
  glycoproteins 76–7
  intake 82–3
  metabolism 64–7
  requirements 82–3
  structure 56–7
  sugar alcohols 72–5
carbon dioxide 103
  blood-brain barrier 130–1
carbon monoxide 231
carboxylases 184
  -glutamyl 160
  proprionyl–CoA 184
  pyruvate 184–5, 254
  -carboxylation 161
carboxylesterase 88–9
carboxylic acids 86–7
carboxypeptidases 122–3, 196
carcinogens 270–1, 352
carcinomas 274–5, 353
cardiomyopathy 244
cardiovascular disease 267, 270, 274
carnitine 102, 164–5, 181, 211
  L-carnitine 324–5
  synthesis 230
  palmitoyl transferase 102
  transporter 103
carnosol 278
carnosolic acid 278
carotenoids 146–9, 206, 268–71
  age-related macular degeneration 350–1
  alcohol abuse 277
  -carotene 136, 146–9
  chronic inflammatory bowel disease
    (CIBD) 354
  tumors 352
carpoptosis 267
catabolism 277
catalase 204–5, 251
cataracts 277
catecholamines 102–3, 164–5, 256–7
  LPL regulation 92–3
CCK *see* cholecystokinin
CCO *see* cytochrome C oxidase

CE *see* cholesterol esters
cells 20–1, 67
  chief 40–1
  enteroendocrine 43
  fatty foam 200
  goblet 43
  intercellular 43, 90–1
  lipoproteins 93, 95, 97, 101
  membrane fluidity 112
  mucosa 40–1, 58–9, 91, 98–9, 138
  NK 246
  nutrient uptake 44–5
  paracellular diffusion 42–3
  Pareth's granular 43
  parietal 40–1
  Schwann 72
  stem 43
cellular retinal-binding protein (CRALBP)
  140–1
cellular retinol-binding protein (CRBP) 138–
  40
celluloses 78–9
central nervous conduction 36–7
cephalic phase 40–1
ceramides 84–5
cereal 83
cerebrosides 84–5, 222
ceruloplasmin (Cp) 250, 252, 322
CETP *see* cholesterol ester transfer protein
CH_3-Pte *see* methyltetrahydrofolic acid
cheilosis 175, 187
chelatases 230–1
chief cells 40–1
children 252, 318–19
chili peppers 278
chitin 79
cholecalciferols 150, 218
  see also vitamin D_3
cholecystokinin (CCK) 36–7, 50–1
cholesterol
  7-dehydrocholesterol 150–1
  24(S),25-epoxycholesterol 105
  absorption 91
  biosynthesis 99, 104–5
  cellular 106
  ester transfer protein (CETP) 93, 96–7
  esterase 88–9, 91
  esterification 98–9
  esters (CE) 88–91, 93, 95–7, 101, 106–7
  exogenous 106–7
  free (FC) 91, 93–5, 101, 106
  genetic factors 106
  homeostasis 106–7
  lipoproteins 95
  macrophages 107
  membranes 106, 108–9
  reduction 270

synthesis 260
uptake 96–7
cholesterol-7-hydroxylase 165
cholesterol-7-hydroxylase 105
cholesterolemia 252, 345
choline 84–5, 208–9
chromium (Cr) 258–9, 351
chronic inflammatory bowel disease (CIBD) 350–1
chronic protein deficiency 348
chronic wasting disease (CWD) 332–1
chylomicrons (CM) 45, 96–9, 138–9, 147
prechylomicrons 90–1
remnants (REM) 92–3, 98–9
chyme 45–6, 88–9
chymotrypsin 122
CIBD *see* chronic inflammatory bowel disease
cirrhosis 120
Indian childhood 252
liver 120, 274–5
citrate 255
cycle
biotin 185
energy transfer 24–5, 34–5
fasting 32–3
pantothenic acid 181
sorbitol 73
thiamin 169
isocitrate 169
methyl 185
citrate-malate shuttle 102–3
L-citrulline 129
CJD *see* Creutzfeldt-Jakob disease
clathrin 94–5
Clostridium 284, 288–9
CM *see* chylomicrons
CoA *see* coenzyme A
cobalamin 192–5, 264
cobalt (Co) 192, 264–5
cobamides 265
cocaine 316
cocoa butter 115
coenzymes
A (CoA) 180–2
see also individual CoA compounds
biotin 184
cobalamin 192
niacin 176
pyridoxine 188
Q 211
Q$_{10}$ 206, 210, 324–5
riboflavin function 172
thiamin 169
cofactors 128–9
apolipoprotein CII 100
ascorbic acid 164
magnesium 220

vitamin K 160
colic 267
colipase 89, 100
collagen 165
colon 46–7
absorption 44–5
cancer 277
colonocytes 354
coma 256
contaminants 284–7
copper (Cu) 172, 246, 248, 250–3, 355
toxicosis 252
copper-superoxide dismutase (Cu-SOD) 250–1
Cori cycle 62–3
corn 294
oil 115
syrup, high fructose (HFCS) 57
coronary artery disease (CAD) 112, 158, 274
corrinoids 192
corticoids 39
receptors 338–9
corticosteroids 225
corticotropin releasing factor (CRF) 36–7
cortisol 237, 338–9
cortisone 338–9
coumestans 268
Cp *see* ceruloplasmin
Cr *see* chromium
CRALBP *see* cellular retinal-binding protein
CRBP *see* cellular retinol-binding protein
creatine 172, 324–5
phosphate 325–6
creatinine 324
cretinism 236–7
Creutzfeldt-Jakob disease (CJD) 330–5
CRF *see* corticotropin releasing factor
CRIP *see* cysteine–rich intestinal protein
Crohn disease 256, 355
crotonyl-CoA 185–6
crotonyl-glycine 185
cryptoxanthine 147
crypts 42–3
Cu *see* copper
Cu-SOD *see* copper-superoxide dismutase
Curcuma longa 278
CWD *see* chronic wasting disease
cyanide 270
cyclamate 282–3
cyclases 128–9
cyclic AMP 102–3
cyclic AMP-dependent protein kinase 103
cystathionine 201
synthase 200–1
cysteine (C; Cys) 120–1, 201, 222–3, 258
pantothenyl 181
cysteine-rich intestinal protein (CRIP) 246

cystic fibrosis 158
cytochrome C 230, 257
    oxidase (CCO) 250–1, 253
cytochrome P$_{450}$ 164–5, 272
    oxidases 203
cytoplasm 91

D

deamination 203
decarboxylases 169
dehydroascorbic acid 164–5, 207
7-dehydrocholesterol 150–1
dehydrogenases
    11-hydroxysteroid dehydrogenase 307
    -ketodehydrogenase 168–9
    L-iditol 72
    lipoamide 207
    pyruvate 168–9
    retinol 140–1
    sorbitol 72–3
    succinate (SuccDH) 172–3
3-dehydroretinol 137
1,25-dehydroxycholecalciferol 150
delirium tremens (DT) 274
δ cells 67
dementia 178
demosterol 105
dental fluorosis 240
dermatitis 178, 190
-6-desaturase 112
desaturation 111
dextrin 57
DFE see dietary folate equivalents
diabetes mellitus (DM) 72–4, 305, 342–3,
    346–7
    lipolysis 102
diacylglycerol 91, 103, 343
diarrhea 166, 178, 248
diclofenac 307
dietary folate equivalents (DFE)
Dietary Reference Intakes (DRI) 8–9, 14
dietary requirements
    carbohydrates 82–3
    fatty acids 114
    fluids 14–15
    lipids 114–15
    protein 134–5
    see also individual chemicals
diets 310, 312–13
digestion 50–3, 58–9
diglycerides 102
dihomo-linoleic acid 111, 113
dihydrolipoic acid 207
dihydroxyacetone phosphate 70–1
1,25-dihydroxycholecalciferol 218
dihydroxymandelic acid 257

diiodotyrosine 235
dimethyltocol see tocopherols
dioxin 286
dioxygenases 230–1
dipeptidases 122–3
dipeptidyl-aminopeptidase 123
direct calorimetry 28–9
disaccharides 56–7, 59
DM see diabetes mellitus
DNA
    free radical 203
    GM foods 296–7
L–dopa 230
dopamine 237
dopamine-hydroxylase 251, 253
dopamine-monooxygenase 164–5
DRI see dietary reference intakes
DRP see vitamin D-binding protein
DT see delirium tremens
dulcitol 73, 75
duodenum 42–3, 88–9, 122

E

EAR see Estimated Average Requirements
eating disorders 336–7
eczema 262–3
EDRF see endothelium–derived relaxing fac-
    tor
EER see estimated energy requirement
efferent control 36–7
eicosanoids 84–5, 110–13
eicosapentaenoic acid 112
eicosatrienoic acid 114
elastase 122
electrocardiograms 191
electromechanical coupling 212
electron transport chain 230
ellagic acid 268
embryos 141, 276
emulsification 90–1
encephalins 51
encephalopathy 267, 330–1
endergonic processes 34–5
endiol 77
endocrine system 274
endocytosis 92–5
    receptor-mediated (RME) 94–5, 98–9
endogenous antioxidant system 250
endogenous defense system 204
endopeptidases 122–3
endoplasmic reticulum (ER) 90–1, 95, 102,
    273
    cholesterol 104, 106
endosomes 95
endothelium 128–9

endothelium-derived relaxing factor (EDRF) 128
energy
    athletes 322
    charge 34
    consumption 28
    metabolism 32–5
    requirements 28–31
    transfer 24–5
    use of 26–7
Enterococcus 46–7, 289
enterocytes 43, 229
enteroendocrine cells 43
enteroglucagon 51
enterohepatocytes 48–9, 196
enteropeptidase 122
enzymes 44–5, 52–3
    see also individual enzymes
epimerases 71
epinephrine 164
epithelium 143
epoxidases 104–5
2,3-epoxide 160
24(S),25-epoxycholesterol 105
5,6-epoxyretinol 137
ER see endoplasmic reticulum
ergogenic agents 324–5
erucic acid 87
erythritol 75
erythrocyte carboanhydrase 246
erythrocytes 189, 231, 256
    alcohol 276
erythropoiesis 230–1
erythrose-4-phosphate 169
Escherichia coli 46–7, 162, 300
essential amino acids 120–1
essential fatty acids 86–7
esterification 90–1, 96–7
Estimated Average Requirements (EAR) 8–9
Estimated Energy Requirement (EER) 9
estrogens 268–71, 287
ethanol 272–3
etheric oils 268, 279
ethyl maltol 282
Eubacteria 288–9
evening primrose oil 113
Evers diet 312–13
excitatory phase 40–1
excretion 212–13, 250
exergonic processes 34–5
exocytosis 90–1
exotic ungulate encephalopathy 331

F

F see fluorine
F⁻ see fluoride

FA see fatty acids
FABP see fatty acid binding protein
factor X see autoprothrombin
FAD see flavin adenine dinucleotide
FAE see fetal alcohol effects
farnesyl diphosphate 104–5
    synthase 105
FAS see fetal alcohol syndrome
fasting 32–3, 60–3, 100, 102, 312–13
fat 52–3
    particles 88–92
    pig 115
    saturated 115
    storage 98–9
fat-soluble vitamins 84–5
    see also individual vitamins
fatty acid binding protein (FABP) 90–1
fatty acid synthase 98, 102
fatty acids (FA) 32–3, 95, 99, 113, 352
    absorption 90–1
    athletes 323
    digestion 88–9
    eicosanoids 110–13
    elongation 185
    essential 86–7
    food effects 112–13
    free (FFA) 66–7, 86–7, 93, 102–3
    hepatocytes 103
    membranes 108–9
    metabolism 102–3
    monounsaturated (MUFA) 86–7, 115
    nomenclature 86
    polyunsaturated (PUFA) 86–7, 115, 202, 292
    regulation 112–13
    requirements 114–15
    structure 84–7
    synthesis 185
    tissue-specific uptake 100–1
fatty foam cells 200
fatty liver 274–5
fatty tissues 32–3, 98
FBPase 35
FC see free cholesterol
Fe see iron
feces 48–9, 80–1, 93
Federal Food, Drug and Cosmetic (FD&C) 280
feline spongiform encephalopathy 331
Fenton reaction 202
ferritin 228–9, 231, 261
ferrochelatase 230–1
ferrotransferrin 229
fetal alcohol effects (FAE) 276
fetal alcohol syndrome (FAS) 276
FFA see free fatty acids
fiber 78–81, 246
fibrin 161

fibrinogen 161
fish oils 112–13
flavanoids, isoflavanoids 268
flavin adenine dinucleotide (FAD) 128–9, 172–3, 257
flavin mononucleotide (FMN) 128–9, 172–3
   oxidase 189
flavokinase 172
flavones 269
flavonoids 268–71
flavonoles 269
flax seed oil 113
flour 83
fluid requirements 14–15
fluid-mosaic model 108–9
fluoride (F⁻) 240, 261
fluorine (F) 240–1
FMN see flavin mononucleotide
folic acid 196–9, 201, 317, 355
   deficiency 194, 277
food
   allergies 122
   carbohydrate 83
   genetic modification 296–7
   groups 306–7
   intake 10–11, 36–9
   lipid distribution 98–9
   and medication 328–29
   organic 292
   processing 298
   quality 292–301
   safety 328–31
   storage 298–9
   vitamin A 145
   water content 14–15
free cholesterol (FC) 91, 93–5, 101, 106
free fatty acids (FFA) 66–7, 86–7, 93, 102–3
free radicals 148, 158, 202–3
fructokinase 73
fructose 56-7, 59, 70–3
fructose-1,6-bisphosphate 73
fructose-1-phosphate 70–1, 73
fructose-5-phosphate 169
fructose-6-phosphate 35, 73
fructose-bisphosphate 35
fumarate 165, 169
funicular myelosis 194
futile cycles 34–5

G

G-protein 103
G6P see glucose-6-phosphate
GABA 37
GAGs see glycosaminoglycans
galactitol 70–3, 75
galactokinase 71

galactose (Gal) 56–7, 59, 70–1, 84–5
galactose-1-phosphate 70–1
galactose-1-phosphaturidyl–transferase 71
galactose-4-sulfate 79
galactosemia 70
   -galactosidase 71
galacturonic acid 79
gall bladder 49, 88–9, 93, 97, 104
gangliosides 84–5
garlic 278
gastrectomy 194
gastric acid reflux disease (GERD) 274
gastric lipase 88–9
gastric pylorus 88–9
gastrin 50–1, 164
gastrocolic reflex 46
gastrointestinal 274
   disorders 267
   hormones 50–1
   inhibitory peptide 51
   peptides 50–1
Generally Recognized As Safe (GRAS) 280, 296
genes
   genetic factors 36–71, 106
   genetic modification (GM) 296–7
   genetic variability 2
   obesity 38
geranyl diphosphate 105
GI see glycemic index
GL see glycemic load
GLC see glucose
GlcNAc see N-acetyl-glucosamine
Gln see glutamine
globulins 118–19, 234–5
GLU see glucuronic acid; glutamate
glucagon 37, 64–7, 105
glucagon-like peptide 1 (GLP-1) 37–9, 51
glucocorticoids 39
glucocorticosteroids 225
glucogenic amino acids 62–3
glucokinase see hexokinase
glucomutases 71
gluconeogenesis 32–3, 66–7, 102, 254
glucuronic acid (GLU) 209
glucose (GLC)
   biotin metabolism 185
   blood 66–9
   blood-brain barrier 131
   brain 32
   carbohydrates 56–9
   carriers 58–9
   fasting 32–3
   glycolipids 84–5
   glycolytic pathway 70–1
   homeostasis 64–7
   inositol 209

levels 68–9
loading test 68–9
storage 62–3
sugar alcohols 72–3
syrup 57
tolerance 332, 351
    factor (GTF) 258–9
UDP 70–1
glucose-1-phosphate 62–3, 71
glucose-6-phosphatase 71
glucose-6-phosphate (G6P) 32–3, 62–3, 70–1, 73
    dehydrogenase (G6PDH) 250–1
glucosinolates 268–9, 270–1
glucuronides 48–9
glutaconyl-CoA 185
glutamates 196–7
glutamic acid (GLU) 196–7, 258
glutamine (Q; Gln) 120–1, 126–7, 176–7
glutaminic acid (E; Glu) 120–1
-glutamyl carboxylase 160
-glutamyl carboxypeptidases 196
glutamyl transpeptidase 123
glutathione 204–5
    oxidized (GSSG) 250–1
        translocase 205
    peroxidase (GSH–Px) 204–5, 242–3, 250–1
    reduced (GSH) 250
    reductase (GR) 204–5, 250–1
    translocase 205
glutathione-S-transferase (GST) 250
Gly see glycine
glycemia
    hyperglycemia 73, 258, 342–3
    hypoglycemia 130–1, 312
glycemic index (GI) 68–9, 306
glycemic load (GL) 68–9, 335
glyceraldehyde 70–1, 73
glyceraldehyde–3–phosphate 73, 169
glycerides
    diglycerides 102
    monoglycerides 90–1, 100, 102
    triglycerides see triglycerides
glycerin 84–5
aldehyde-5-phosphate 169
glycerols 73, 91, 103
    -glycerophosphate 91, 99
glycerophospholipids 84–5
glycine (G; Gly) 120–1, 258, 325
    peptidase 123
glycosaminoglycans 222
glycogen 32–5, 56–7, 60–1, 70–1
    athletes 322–23
    liver 63
    muscle 62–3
    phosphorylase 34–5

glycogenolysis 66–7
glycolipids 71, 84–5
    membranes 108–9
glycolysis 24–5, 71, 73, 102
    anaerobic 62–3
glycoproteins 71, 76–7
glycosaminoglycans (GAGs) 71, 100, 223
glycosidic bonds 56–7
glycosylamines 76
glycosylation 90–1
glycyrrhetic acid 308–9
Glycyrrhiza glabra 308
glycyrrhizic acid 308–9
glycyrrhizin 282, 308
GM see genes, genetic modification
goblet cells 43
goiter 238
Golgi bodies 90–1, 95, 106
GR see glutathione reductase
grain 20–1
granulocytes 195
grapefruit juice 304
GRAS see Generally Recognized As Safe
Graves disease 238
griseofulvin 302–3
growth 314–15
    hormones 286–7
    vitamin D 152
GSH see glutathione, reduced
GSH-Px see glutathione peroxidase
GSSG see glutathione, oxidized
GST see glutathione-S-transferase
GTF see glucose tolerance factor
guanidinoacetic acids 325
guanosine monophosphate (GMP) 129, 256
guanosine triphosphate (GTP) 103, 129
guanylate cyclase 128–9
guar gum 326
Guillain-Barre syndrome 300
L-gulonolactone oxidase 164
gynoide adipocytes 102–3

H

H_2S see hydrogen sulfide
H_3C–PteGLU see 5-methyl-tetrahydrofolic acid
H_4-PteGLU see tetrahydrofolic acid
hallucinations 254
haptocorrins 192
Harvard Food Pyramid 6–7
Harvard School of Public Health Alternative Healthy Eating Index (AHEI) 8–9, 306–7
Hay diet 310–11
Hb see hemoglobin
HCA see hydroxy citrate

HDL 92–3, 96–9, 157, 209, 345
  nascent (n–HDL) 96
  receptor 107
headaches 256
heart disease 305
heavy metals 286
HEI *see* USDA Healthy Eating Index
helices 118–19
Heliobacter pylori 274
hematology 267
heme 231
hemicelluloses 78–9
hemoglobin (Hb) 231
  methemoglobin 284
hemoglobulin 230–1
hemoglobulinemia 222
hemolytic uremic syndrome (HUS) 300
hemorrhages 160, 162–3, 167
hemoxygenase 229, 231
Henle, loop of 220
heparan sulfate 92–3, 100–1
heparin 222
  lipoprotein lipase-heparin complex 100
  LPL complex 100
hepatitis, alcoholic 274
hepatocytes 92, 96
  cholesterol 104
  enterohepatocytes 48–9, 196
  fatty acid metabolism 103
hepatosplenomegaly 345
herbs 278–9
hereditary factors *see* genes genetic factors
heroin 316
heterodimerization 142–3
hexokinase 73
hexose 4-epimerase 71
high fructose corn syrup (HFCS) 57
high-density lipoprotein *see* HDL
histamine 128
histidine (H; His) 120–1
HMB *see* hydroxymethyl butyrate
HMG-CoA 94, 99
  reductase 104–7
    inhibitors 302
  synthase 104–5
holo-RBP-transthyretin complex 140–1
homeostasis 22–3
homo-linoleic acid 112
homocysteine 198, 200–1
  methyl transferase 201
  vegetarians 308–9
homocysteinemia 200
homocysteinuria 120
hormones 102–3, 165, 306
5HT *see* 5-hydroxytryptamine
human growth hormone, recombinant
  (rBGH; rBST) 286

hunger *see* appetite
HUS *see* hemolytic uremic syndrome
3-hydoxy-3-methyl-glutaryl-CoA 104–5
hydrochloric acid 41
hydrogen peroxide 251
hydrogen sulfide (H_2S) 222
hydrolases 139, 141
hydrolysis 90–3, 98–101
hydroperoxide 203
hydroxy citrate (HCA) 325
3-hydroxy isovalerianic acid 185
3-hydroxy-2-methyl–pyridine *see* vitamin
  B_6
hydroxyaldehyde 77
25-hydroxycholecalciferol 150
hydroxycinnamonic acids 269
hydroxyl
  apatite 213, 218
  radical 203
hydroxylases 165, 219
hydroxymethylbutyrate (HMB) 324–5
hydroxymethylglutaryl *see* HMG
4-hydroxyphenylpyruvate dioxygenase 165
3-hydroxyproprionic acid 185
11-hydroxysteroid dehydrogenase (11-
  OHSD) 305
5-hydroxytryptamine (5HT) 130–1
  receptor 131
  see also serotonin
hygiene 300–1
hypercalcemia 216
hypercholesterolemia 94, 252, 345
hyperglycemia 73, 258, 342–3
hyperinsulinemia 340
hyperkalemia 226–7
hyperlipidemia 344–5
hyperlipoproteinemia 340, 344–5
hyperparathyroidism 218
hypertension 274, 340
hyperthyroidism 236, 238
hypertriglyceridemia 345
hypervitaminosis 144, 166
hypochromic anemia 190, 232
hypoglycemia 130–1, 312
hypokalemia 226
hypothalamus 37–9, 237
hypothyroidism 236
hypoxanthine 257

I

I *see* iodine
ICAM 204
IDDM *see* insulin-dependent diabetes melli-
  tus
L-iditol dehydrogenase 72

IDL 92–3, 98–9
IF *see* intrinsic factor
ileum 42–3
iminopeptidase 123
immune system 246, 355
  vitamin D 152–3
  YOPIs 298
Indian childhood cirrhosis 252
indirect calorimetry 28–9
inflammation 112–13, 260, 270
inhibitory phase 40–1
inolates, glucosinolates 268–71
inorganic phosphates 71
inositol 208–9
  phosphate (IP) 209
inositol-1, 4, 5-triphosphate (IP_3) 208
insulin 36–7, 39, 66–7, 246, 259
  blood-brain barrier 130–1
  LPL regulation 92
  receptor 64–5
  resistance 340, 346–7
  secretion 64–5
  thyroxine 105
  vitamin D 152
insulin-dependent diabetes mellitus (IDDM) 342–3
insulinemia 340
intercellular communication 43
intercellular space 90–1
interleukin-2 246
intermediate-density lipoproteins *see* IDL
interphotoreceptor retinol-binding protein (IRBP) 140
intestines 88–9, 93, 97
  see also gastrointestinal; small intestines
intrinsic factor (IF) 192–3
invert sugar 57
iodide 235
iodine (I) 234–9, 316–17
Iododerma tuberosum 238
iodothyronines 234–5
iodotyrosines 235
IP *see* inositol phosphate
IPP *see* isopentenyl disphosphate
IRBP *see* interphotoreceptor retinol-binding protein
iron (Fe) 172, 228–33, 246, 251, 313, 351
  deficiency anemia 233
  and nickel 262
  sulfide (FeS) 257
  vegetarians 308–9
iron-transferrin 228
IRS *see* insulin receptor substrate
ischemia 204–5
islets of Langerhans 64–5, 67, 72–3
isocitrate 169

isoflavanoids 268
isoflavones 269
isoleucine (I; Ile) 120–1
isomaltitol 75
isomerases 141
isopentenyl diphosphate (IPP; isoprene) 84–5, 104–5
isopentenyladenine 105
isoprenoids 104–5
isothiocyanates 268
isotope dilution methods 18–19
isovaleryl-CoA 185

jaundice 48–9, 194
jejunum 42–3, 168
juniper berries 278–9

K *see* potassium
kalemia 226–7
Kellog diet 313
Keshan disease 244
2-keto isocapronic acid 185
ketoaldehyde 77
ketoaminomethylol 77
  -ketobutyrate 201
  -ketodehydrogenase 207
ketogenesis 102–3
  -ketoglutarate 169
    dehydrogenase 168–9
ketolases 169
ketone bodies (acetacetate) 32–3, 102
ketones 103
4-ketoretinol 137
ketosis 66–7, 82, 312
kidneys 120, 126–7, 216
  ascorbic acid 164
  renal tubules 214, 225
  stones 166, 216
  vitamin A 139
kinases
  hexokinase 73
  phosphofructokinase (PFK) 34–5, 73
  protein kinase C (PKC) 206, 342–3
Kushi/Ohsawa diet 313

L-dopa 230
lactase 59
lactate 35, 70–1, 185, 322

lactation
  niacin 178
  and nutrition 316–17
lactitol 75
Lactobacillus 288–9
lactose 56–7, 59
  intolerance 212
  synthetase 71
laetrile 21
lanosterol 105
lanosterol-14-demethylase 105
lauric acid 87
LCAT *see* lecithin cholesterol acyl-transferase
LDL 98–9, 147, 209, 344
  oxidized 128–9
  particles 92–3
  receptor 94–5, 100, 107, 157
    endocytosis 92–3
lead (Pb) 266–7, 286–7
leaky gut syndrome 122
lecithin 84, 98–9, 208
  cholesterol acyl-transferase (LCAT) 96–9
lecithin-retinol-acyl-transferase 139
lectins 77
leptin 37–9
leucine (L; Leu) 120–1, 185
leukocytes 110, 128
  polymorphonuclear (PMN) 204
leukotrienes 84, 110–12, 354
Li *see* lithium
licorice 226, 308–9
life style 30–1
light 203
lignans 268
lignin 79
lignocellulose 79
D-limonene 269
lingual lipase 88–9
linoleic acid 86–7, 110–11, 114–15
  dihomo-linoleic acid 111, 113
  -linoleic acid 86–7, 115
  -linoleic acid 111–13
lipases 88–9, 139
  hormone-sensitive 102–3
  lingual 88–9
  phospholipases 88–9
lipemia retinalis 345
lipidemia 344–5
lipids 2–3, 20–1
  absorption 90–1
  bilayers 108–9
  classification 84–5
  digestion 88–9
  distribution 98–9
  early absorption phase 98
  fatty acids *see* fatty acids
  glycolipids 71, 84–5, 108–9

lipoproteins *see* lipoproteins
  membranes 108–9
  peroxidation 148
  peroxide 158
  phospholipids *see* phospholipids
  structure 84–5
  transport 92–3
lipoamide dehydrogenase 207
lipogenesis 73, 102–3
lipoic acid
  dihydrolipoic acid 207
  -lipoic acid 206–7, 211
  -lipoid acid 325
lipolysis 100–1, 103
lipoprotein lipase (LPL) 92–3, 98–101, 157
  deficiency 335
lipoproteinemia 334–5, 342
lipoproteins 90–3, 101, 105
  see also individual lipoproteins
lipoxygenase 112
Listeria monocytogenes 300
lithium (Li) 264–5
liver 32–3, 98
  amino acid homeostasis 126–7
  cirrhosis 120, 274–5
  fatty 274–5
  fructose 70
  glycogen 63
  HDLs 97
  hepatosplenomegaly 345
  lipoproteins 90–2
  portal circulation 48–9
  portal hypertension 274
  vitamin A 139
long-chain neutral amino acids (LNAA)
  130–1
  -loop structure 118–19
low-density lipoproteins *see* LDL
LPL *see* lipoprotein lipase
lutein 147, 346–7
lycopene 147
lymph 90–1, 98
lysine (K; Lys) 120–1
lysosomes 95, 97, 106–7, 229
lysyl oxidase 252

M

macrobiotics 312
macrocytosis 276–7
2-macroglobulin 255
macrophages 97, 107, 128
macular degeneration, age-related (AMD)
  346–7
magnesium 317, 324, 348–9
malate 98, 169

malitols 75
malnutrition 338–9
malonyl-CoA 102–3, 185
maltase 59
maltol 282
maltose 56–7, 59
maltotetraitol 75
maltotriitol 75
mandelic acids 257
manganese (Mn) 172, 254–5, 355
manganese–superoxide dismutase (Mn–SOD) 250–1, 254
D-mannitol 75
MAO see monoamine oxidases
marijuana 316
matrix GLA proteins (MGP) 160, 348
meat production 286
medication 306–7
Mediterranean Diet, The 4–5
megaloblastic anemia 198
membranes
  arsenic 267
  basal 43, 91
  cholesterol 106, 108–9
  fatty acids 108–9
  fluidity 108–9, 112
  glycolipids 108–9
  mucous 267
  phospholipids 108–9
  plasma 90–1, 95, 102
men 30–1
menadion see vitamin K$_3$
menaquinone see vitamin K$_2$
menopause 216
MEOS see microsomal ethanol oxidation system
mercapturic acids 251
mercury 287
metabolic rate, basic (BMR) 28–31, 312, 320
metabolic syndrome 342, 346–7
metabolism 24–7, 64–5, 90–1, 124–5
metallothionein 247, 251
metals 286
methemoglobin 284
methionine (M; Met) 120–1, 201, 222
  sulfonium chloride 211
methyl citrate 185
3-methyl crotonyl–CoA 185
  carboxylase 184
3-methyl crotonyl-glycine 185
3-methyl glutaconyl-CoA 185
D-methyl malonyl-CoA 185
methyl methionine sulfonium chloride 211
methyl transferase 200
methyl-butyrates 324–5
methyl-tetrahydrofolate (H$_3$C-PteGLU) 196–7

5-methyl-tetrahydrofolic acid (5-methyl–THF; H$_3$C-PteGLU) 196, 200–1
5,10-methylene-tetrahydrofolic acid 201
8-methyltocol see -tocopherol
mevalonate 104–5
  kinase 104–5
MGP see matrix GLA-proteins
micelles 45, 147
  absorption 90–1
  mixed 88–9, 91
microsomal ethanol oxidation system (MEOS) 272–3
middle chain triglycerides (MCT) 98
mineral corticoid receptors 304–5
minerals 2–3, 20–1
mineralization 212, 218
mitochondria 102–3, 273
Mn see manganese
MnSOD see manganese-superoxide dismutase
molybdate (MoO$_4^{2-}$) 256
molybdenum (Mo) 172, 223, 256–7, 355
molybdopterin 256
monoacylglycerol 91, 103
  lipase 103
monoamine oxidase (MAO) 172–3
  inhibitors 328–9
monocytes 97
monoglycerides 90–1, 100, 102
monoiodotyrosine 235
monooxygenases 230–1
monosaccharides 56–7
monoterpenes 268–71
monounsaturated fatty acids (MUFA) 86–7, 115
motilin 51
mucins 77
mucosa 99
  cells 40–1, 58–9, 91, 98–9, 138
mucous membranes 267
muscle 32–3
  amino acid homeostasis 126
  athletes 322–3
  glycogen 62–3
  ocular 274
  smooth cell 128
myelosis, funicular 194
myoglobin 231
myoglobulin 230
myristic acid 87
myrosine 268

N

N-acetyl neuraminic acid 84–5
N-acetyl-galactosamine (GalNac) 79

N-acetyl-glucosamine (GlcNAc) 79
N-HDL *see* HDL, nascent
NA *see* nicotinic acid
NAD+ 34–5, 70–1, 73, 177, 272
NAD 176
NADH 34–5, 70–1, 73, 207, 251
NADP+ 73, 251, 273
NADP 176
NADPH 73, 128–9, 207, 273
1,4-naphtoquinone *see* vitamin K
2-methyl-1,4-naphtoquinone *see* vitamin K$_3$
nascent high-density lipoproteins *see* HDL,
    nascent (N-HDL)
NE *see* nicotinamide
neogenesis 32–3, 66–7, 102, 254
neohesperidine 282–3
neotame 282–3
nervonic acid 87
nervous system 36–7, 274, 277
net protein utilization (NPU) 132
neurodermatitis 113
neuroendocrine hormones 164–5
neuromedin K 51
neuromuscular disturbances 220
neuropathy 274
neuropeptide Y (NPY) 38–9
neurotensin 37, 51
neurotransmitters 130
NFκB 206
NH^{4+} *see* ammonia
niacin 176–9
niacinamide 178
nickel (Ni) 262–3
nicotinamide (NE) 176–7
    adenine nucleotide *see* NAD+
    adenine nucleotide phosphate *see* NADP
    see also niacin
nicotinic acid (NA) 176–7, 258
    amide 177
    mononucleotide (NMN) 176–7
    see also niacin
NIDDM *see* non-insulin dependent diabetes
    mellitus
night blindness 256, 277
nitrite 284–5
nitro-vasodilators 128
nitrogen
    amino acid homeostasis 126–7
    balance 124
    fixation 116–17
    protein biosynthesis 116–17
nitrogen monoxide (NO) 120
    endothelium 128–9
    synthase (NOS) 128–9
nitroglycerin 128
nitrosamines 165, 284–5
S-nitrosocysteine (NO-R) 128

NK cells 246
NMN *see* nicotinic acid mononucleotide
NO *see* nitrogen monoxide
NO-R *see* S-nitrosocysteine
non–insulin dependent diabetes mellitus
    (NIDDM) 332–3
noradrenaline 103, 165
norepinephrine 164
NOS *see* nitrogen monoxide synthase
NPU *see* net protein utilization
NPY *see* neuropeptide Y
nucleus 95
Nutrient RDA 8–9
nutrients 20–3, 40–53
    lactation 316–17
    pregnancy 314–15
nutrition 4–7
    assessments 10–11
    athletes 322–5
    children 318–19
    diets 312–3
    and growth 318–19
    and health 304–7
    and illness 304–5
    and lactation 316–17
    and medication 326–9
    and pregnancy 314–15
    seniors 320–1
    separation 310–11
    vegetarians 248, 308, 309, 316
    vegetarianism 308–9

O

O-bound sugar chains 95
obesity 17, 18, 38–9, 130, 340–1, 344, 346–7
    ob gene 38
11-OHSD *see* 11-hydroxysteroid dehydro-
    genase
oils 112–13, 115
OLAN *see* 24(S), 25-oxidolanosterol
oleic acid 87, 114
olive oil 115
OP *see* organophosphate
Oral Reference Dose (RfD) 284
organophosphate (OP) 292
ornithine 325
orotic acid 210–11
osteoblasts 152, 212–13
osteocalcin 160, 348
osteoclasts 152, 212–14
osteomalacia 154–5, 277
osteoporosis 216, 277, 348–9
oxalic acid 212–13, 259
oxaloacetate 169, 185

oxidases
    L-gulonolactone 164
    lysyl 252
    monoamine (MAO) 172–3
        inhibitors 328–9
oxidation
    microsomal ethanol system 27–273
    -oxidation 102–3, 111
oxidative deamination 203
oxidative phosphorylation 24–5
oxidative stress 342–3
oxidocyclases 105
24(S),25-oxidolanosterol (OLAN) 105
oxidoreductases 172, 230–1
oxygen 128
    blood–brain barrier 130–1
    radicals 129
    singlet 148
oxygenases
    4-hydroxyphenylpyruvate dioxygenase
        165
    dioxygenases 230–1
    hemoxygenase 229, 231
    monooxygenases 230–1

P

P see phosphate
PAF see platelet activation factor
PAH see phenylalanine hydroxylase; polycy-
    clic aromatic hydrocarbons
PAI see plasminogen activator inhibitor
PAL see physical activity level
palatinite 75
palmitic acid 87, 102–3
pancreas 51, 88–9, 152
pancreatic amylase 58–9
pancreatic lipase 89
pancreatitis 345
pangamic acid 211
pantetheine 181
D-panthenol 180
pantoic acid 180
pantothenic acid 180–3
pantothenyl cysteine 181
paprika 278
para-aminobenzoic acid 196
paracellular diffusion 42–3
paracetamol 326–7
parathormone 214
parathyroid hormone 219
Pareth's granular cells 43
parietal cells 40–1
Parkinson's disease 254
Pb see lead
PDCAAS see protein digestibility-corrected
    amino acid scores

peanut oil 115
pectins 78–9
    amylopectin 57
pellagra 178–9
    preventative (PP) vitamin see niacin
PEM see protein energy malnutrition
penicillamine 326–7
pentose phosphate shunt (PPS) 72–3, 98, 209
pepsinogens 40–1, 50–1, 122
pepsins 40–1, 122–3
peptidases 122–3, 196
peptides 117–19, 122–3
peristalsis 40–1
pernicious anemia 194
peroxidase 235
peroxides 128, 203
peroxy radical 203
pesticides 292
PFK see phosphofructokinase
PG see polygalacturonase
phagocytosis 231
Phe see phenylalanine
phenolic acids 268–71
phenols 268
phenylalanine (F; Phe) 120–1, 280
    hydroxylase (PAH) 120
phenylketonuria (PKU) 120
phenylketonuronics 280
phenylpropane 79
phosphatase 261
phosphate (P) 218, 246, 255
    homeostasis 152–3
    inorganic 71
phosphatidates 85
phosphatidyl 84
    inositol (PI) 209
phosphatidylcholine see lecithin
phosphatidylethanolamine 84
phosphatidylserine 84
3′-phosphoadenosine-5-phosphate 223
phosphofructokinase (PFK) 34–5, 73
phosphoglucomutase 71
phosphoketolase 169
phospholipases 88–9
phospholipid transfer protein (PTP)
    96–7
phospholipids (PL)
    absorption 91, 98–9
    digestion 88–9
    glycerophospholipids 84–5
    LDL receptor 95
    lipoproteins 91, 100–1
    membranes 108–9
    resynthesis 90–1
    structure 84–5
    transfer 96–7
4–phosphopantetheine 181

5-phosphoribosyl-1-diphosphate (PRPP) 176
phosphorus 218–21
phosphorylation 24–5
phylloquinone *see* vitamin K$_1$
physical activity 28–9, 346
   level (PAL) 30–1
phytate 213, 255
phytic acid 212, 246, 270–1
phytoestrogens 268–71
phytosterins 268–71
phytosterols 268
PI *see* phosphatidyl inositol
pig fat 115
pigments 203
pituitary 36–7, 237
PKC *see* protein kinase C
PKU *see* phenylketonuria
PL *see* phospholipids; pyridoxal
plants
   breeding 295
   cells 20–1
plasma membranes 90–1, 95, 101
plasmalogens 85
platelet activation factor (PAF) 204
pleated sheets 118–19
plexus choroideus 39
PM *see* pyridoxamine
PMN *see* polymorphonuclear leukocytes
polar amino acids 118–19
polycyclic aromatic hydrocarbons
   (PAH) 286–7
polyglutamates 196–7
polymorphonuclear leukocytes (PMN) 204
polyneuropathy 274
polyphenols 268
polyprenyls 84–5
polysaccharides 56–7, 59
polyunsaturated fatty acids (PUFA) 86–7, 115,
   202, 292
porphyrin 230
potassium (K) 226–7, 321
PP *see* pellagra preventive
PPS *see* pentose phosphate shunt
prebiotics 288–9
prechylomicrons 90–1
pregnancy
   folic acid 198
   iron 232
   niacin 178
   and nutrition 314–5
   vitamin A 144
   YOPIs 300
prenyls 84–5
preservation 294–5
prions 330–33
probiotics 288–9
processing 298–9

prolactin 37
proline (P; Pro) 120–1
   dipeptidases 123
propionyl-CoA 185
   carboxylase 184–5
propionic acid 185
prostaglandins 84, 110
protease inhibitors 270–1
protein kinase C (PKC) 206, 342–3
protein-digestibility-corrected amino acid
   scores (PDCAAS) 132–3
proteinogenic amino acids 120–1
proteins 2–3, 20–1, 32–3, 52–3
   amino acids 120–3, 126–7
   blood-brain barrier 130–1
   chronic deficiency 348
   efficiency ratio (PER) 132
   endothelial function 128–9
   energy malnutrition (PEM) 124
   evaluation 132
   food content 135
   free radicals 204
   globular 118–19
   glycoproteins 71, 76–7
   metabolism 124–5
   nitrogen 116–17
   peptides 122–3
   prions 330–1
   quality 132–3
   recommended intakes 134–5
   requirements 134–5
   selenoproteins 242
   seniors 321
   steady state 124–5
   structure 118–19
   transfer 96–7
   vegetarians 248, 308–9, 316
proteoglycans 100–1
prothrombin 161
proton pump 40–1
protoporphyrin IX 231
provitamins 138
   A 148
   D$_3$ 150
PRPP *see* 5-phosphoribosyl-1-diphosphate
pteridine (Pte) 196
pteroyl
   glutamate *see* folic acid
   monoglutamate 197
   polyglutamate 197
PTP *see* phospholipid transfer protein
PUFA *see* polyunsaturated fatty acids
pyridoxal (PL) 188–9
   phosphate 200
pyridoxal-5-phosphate 189
pyridoxamine (PM) 188–9
pyridoxamine-5-phosphate 189

pyridoxine 188–91
pyridoxine-5-phosphate 189
pyridoxol *see* pyridoxine
pyruvate 102, 169, 185, 223, 325
    carboxylase 184–5, 254
    decarboxylase 169
    dehydrogenase 168–9

| Q |

quintiles 350–1

| R |

R *see* retinol
R-groups 118
RA *see* retinoic acid
radiation 203
radicals
    free 148, 158, 202–3
    peroxy 203
rapeseed oil 115
RAR *see* retinoic acid receptor
rBGH *see* human growth hormone, recombinant
RBP *see* retinol-binding protein
rBST *see* human growth hormone, recombinant
RE *see* esterified retinol; retinol equivalents; retinyl ester
reactive oxygen species (ROS) 202
rearrangement, posttranslational 118
receptor-independent pathways 94
receptor-mediated endocytosis (RME) 94–5, 98–9, 193
Recommended Daily Amounts (RDA) 8–9
recommended daily intakes (RDI) 9
Recommended Dietary Allowances (RDA) 8–9
redox systems 202
reduced glutathione (GH) 250
reductants 204
reductases 172, 230–1
Reference Nutrition Intake (RNI) 9
REM *see* chylomicron remnants; remnants
remnants (REM) 98, 138
renin 225
renin-angiotensin system 128
renin-angiotensin-aldosterone system 224
reperfusion 203, 205
respiration
    respiratory chain 24–5, 35
    respiratory tract 260
retinal 137, 140, 147
    pigment epithelium (RPE) 350

11-cis-retinal 140–1
    aldehyde 137
    dehydrogenase 140–1
retinic acid 137
retinoic acid (RA) 136, 138, 140, 142
    receptors (RAR) 143
    9-cis-retinoic acid 142
retinoids 136
retinol (R) 22–3, 136–40, 147
    3-dehydroretinol 137
    5,6-epoxyretinol 137
    dehydrogenase 140–1
    equivalents (RE) 136
    esterified (RE)
    isomerase 141
retinol-glucuronide 137
retinol-binding protein (RBP) 138
    interphotoreceptor (IRBP) 140
    RBP-transthyretin complex 140–1
retinyl
    acetate 136
    ester (RE) 138–9, 144, 147
        hydrolase 141
    palmitate 137, 141
retinyl-acyl-transferase 141
retinyl-palmitate-hydrolase 139
reversible modification 34
RFBPs *see* riboflavin-binding proteins
RfD *see* Oral Reference Dose
rheumatic disease 113
rhodopsin 140–1
riboflavin 172–5, 277
    kinase 172
riboflavin-binding proteins (RFBPs) 172
ribose 79
ribose-5-phosphate 169
ribosomes 95
ribotol 75
rickets 154–5
RME *see* receptor-mediated endocytosis
RNI *see* reference nutrient intake (UK)
rods 141
ROS *see* reactive oxygen species
rosemary 278
roughage 292
royal jelly 182
RPE *see* retinal pigment epithelium

| S |

saccharides 56–7, 59
saccharin 280, 282–3
saccharose *see* sucrose
SAD *see* seasonal affective disorder
saliva 50–1
salivary amylase 58–9

Salmonella 300
salt 224
saponins 268–71
satiety 36–8
saturated fats 115
scavenger receptor 94, 107
Schwann cells 72
scrapie 330
scurvy 166, 277
Se *see* selenium
seasonal affective disorder (SAD) 130
second messengers 212
secretin 37, 50–1
sedoheptulose-7-phosphate 169
selenate (SeO$_4^{2-}$) 242–3
selenite (SeO$_3^{2-}$) 243
selenium (Se) 242–5, 251, 355
selenocysteine 242
selenomethionine 242
selenoproteins 242
semidehydro-L-ascorbic acid 164
seniors 320–21
separation diet 310–11
serine (S; Ser) 120–1, 201
serotonin 36–7, 128
   see also 5-hydroxytryptamine
sialoglycoproteins 76–7
sickle-cell crisis 166
signal transduction 64–5
silicate (SiO$_4^{4-}$) 266
silicic acid 266
silicon (Si) 266
   oxide (SiO$_2$) 266
singlet oxygen 148
skeleton 214–15
skin
   arsenic 267
   -carotene 149
   lesions 249, 260
   vitamin D 152
sleep 178
slow waves 40
small intestines 42–3, 52–3, 94
   absorption 44–5
Sn *see* tin
SO$_3^{2-}$ *see* sulfite
SO$_4^{2-}$ *see* sulfate
SOD *see* superoxide dismutase
sodium 58–9
   chloride 224–5
somatostatin 37, 51, 67
sorbitol 72–3, 75
   dehydrogenase 72–3
soy 296
   oil 115
spasms 260
specified risk materials (SRM) 330, 332

sphingolipids 84–5
sphingomyelin 84–5
sphingophospholipids 84–5
sphingosine 84–5
spices 278–9
spina bifida 199
spleen 94
sports 322–3
squalene 104–5
SRM *see* specified risk materials
Staphylococcus 289
starch 56–7
starvation 32–3
   lipolysis 102
   LPL activity 100
stearic acid 87
steatorrhea 213
Steiner diet 313
stem cells 43
sterins 268–71
steroids 84–5
   cholesterol
   hormones 104–5
sterols 268
stevioside 282–3
stilbenes 287
stomach 40–1, 50–3, 88–9
   absorption 44–5, 122–3
   digestion 122–3
   gastric acid reflux disease (GERD) 274
   gastric pylorus 88–9
   gastrocolic reflex 46
stomatitis 190
storage 296–7
Streptococcus 289
stress, oxidative 342–3
strokes 274, 305
substance P 51, 128
succinate 169, 207
   dehydrogenase (SuccDH) 172–3
succinyl-CoA 169, 185
sucralose 282–3
sucrase 59
sucrose (saccharose) 56–7, 59
sugar 83
   alcohols 72–5
   chains 95
   invert 57
sulfatases 222–3
sulfate (SO$_4^{2-}$) 222
sulfhemoglobinemia 222
sulfides 268–71
sulfite (SO$_3^{2-}$) 222
   oxidase 222, 256–7
sulfiteoxidase 223
sulfonyl pyruvate 222
sulfur 222–3

superoxide 203
  dismutase (SOD) 204–5, 250–1, 253–4,
    351
sweeteners 282–3
  see also sugar
syndrome X 342, 346–7
synthases 105

T

T lymphocytes 246
tachycardia 256
tannin 213
taurine 222, 324–5
TBG see thyroxine-binding globulin
TDP see thiamin diphosphate
terpenes 84–5, 268
  menthol 84
  monoterpenes 268–71
  triterpenes 269
tetany 220
tetrahydrofolate (THFA) 196–7
tetrahydrofolic acid (H₄-PteGLU) 196–7,
    200–1
tetraiodothyronine 234–5
TfR see transferrin receptors
TG see triacyl glycerols; triglycerides
thaumatin 282–3
thiamin 168–71
  diphosphate (TDP) 168
thiocyanate 234–5
thionein 247
thrombosis 270
threonine (T; Thr) 120–1
thrombin 161
thrombocytes 112–13, 128
thrombosis 162
thromboxanes 84, 110
thymocytes 246
thymulin 246
thyreocytes 234
thyreostatika 237
thyretins 139–41
thyroglobulin 234–5
thyroid 234–5
  hormones 219, 236–7
  hyperthyroidism 218
  hypothyroidism 236
thyroxine–binding globulin (TBG) 234
tin (Sn) 262–3
tissues, fatty 32–3, 98
tocopherol esters 156
tocopherols 104, 156–7, 206–7
  –tocotrienol 207
Tolerable Upper Intake Levels (UL) 8–9, 14
tomatoes 296

toxicosis 222, 252
trace elements 2–3, 20–1
transcellular transport 42–3
transcobalamin II 192–3
transcuprein 251
transfer proteins 96–7
transferases 141
transferrin 228–9, 231, 258–9, 261
  ferrotransferrin 229
  receptors (TfR) 228–9
transketolase 169
translocases 205
transmissible mink encephalopathy 331
transmissible spongiform encephalopathies
  (TSEs) 330–1
transpeptidases 123
transport 42–3
transthyretin (TTR) 139
  RBP–transthyretin complex 140–1
tranylcypromine 329
triacylglycerols (TG) 84–5, 91, 103, 209
triglyceridemia 345
triglycerides (TG)
  digestion 88
  energy 32–3
  fatty acid metabolism 102, 344
  hydrolysis 101
  lipid transport 92–3, 95, 99
  medium-chain (MCT)
    transport 96
triiodothyronine 234–5
5,7,8-trimethyltocol see tocopherols
triterpenes 269
troponin C 212
trypsin 122
trypsinogen 122
tryptophan (W; Trp) 120–1, 177–8
  blood brain barrier 130–1
  PDCAAS 133
  5-OH-tryptophan 230
TSEs see transmissible spongiform encephalopathies
TTR see trans-thyretin
tumors 271, 352–3
turmeric 278
tyramine 328–9
tyrosine (Tyr) 120–1, 164, 235, 329
tyrosyl 234
  kinase 261

U

ubiquinol 207
ubiquinone 206–7, 211, 230
UCP see uncoupling protein
UDP-galactose 70–1
UDP-glucose 70–1

UDP-glucose-pyrophosphorylase 71
UDP-hexose 4-epimerase 71
UL *see* Tolerable Upper Intake Levels
ulcers 326
uncoupling proteins 38–9
underweight 338–9
urea cycle 254
uric acid 257
uridine phosphate *see* UDP
urine 126–7, 255, 261
urobilinogen 48–9
urobilirubin 49
USDA Food Pyramid 7, 306–7
USDA Healthy Eating Index (HEI) 9
UWL *see* water, unstirred water layer

V

V *see* vanadium
valerianic acid 87, 184
    3-hydroxy isovalerianic acid 185
valine (V; Val) 120–1
vanadate (VO_4^{3-}) 260
vanadium (V) 161, 260–1
vanadyl (VO^{2+}) 260
vascular tone regeneration 128
vasoactive intestinal peptide 51
vasodilators 128
vegetarians 308–9
very low density lipoproteins *see* VLDL
villi 42–5
vision
    alcohol 274
    pantothenic acid 182–3
vitamin A 136, 140–1
vitamin A 22–3, 136–45, 313, 352, 355
    and -carotene 147
    cirrhosis 276–7
    deficiency 143–4
    food content 145
    pregnancy 144
    recommended intakes 145
    requirements 145
    seniors 321
    vision 136, 140–1
vitamin B 200–1, 276, 321
    B_1 168–9, 276–7, 317
        see also thiamin
    B_2 *see* riboflavin
    B_3 *see* niacin
    B_6 188, 190, 201, 276–7, 317
        see also pyridoxine
    B_{12} 194–5
        alcohol abuse 277
        chronic inflammatory bowel disease
        355

homocysteine metabolism 200–1
    lactation 312–13
    vegetarians 308–9
    see also corrinoids
    B_{13} *see* orotic acid
    B_{15} *see* pangamic acid
    B_{17} *see* laetrile
    BT *see* carnitine
vitamin C *see* ascorbic acid, L-ascorbic acid
vitamin D 150–5, 276–7, 309, 317, 321
    D_3 150–1, 215
vitamin E 156–9, 206–7, 271, 277, 354
vitamin F 210
vitamin H *see* biotin
vitamin K 46, 160–3, 277, 348–9
vitamin P *see* bioflavonoids
vitamin PP *see* niacin
vitamin U *see* methyl methionine sulfonium
    chloride
vitamins 2–3, 20–1
    defense mechanisms 204–7
    food processing 296–7
    free radicals 202–3
    hypervitaminosis 144, 166
    nonvitamins 210–11
    see also individual vitamins
VLDL 92–3, 96–9, 147, 209, 344
-VLDL 107
VO^{2+} *see* vandyl
VO_4^{3-} *see* vanadate

W

W *see* tryptophan
waist-to-hip ratio 16–17
water 2–3, 14–15
    blood-brain barrier 130–1
    unstirred water layer (UWL) 90–1
waxes 84–5
weight 28–9, 38–9
    loss 178, 258, 312–13, 340
    obesity 340–1
    pregnancy 314–15
    underwater weighing 18–19
    underweight 338–9
Wernicke-Korsakoff syndrome 170, 274, 277
Wilson's disease 248, 252
women 30–1

X

X5P *see* xylulose-5-phosphate
xanthelasma 345
xanthine 257
    oxidase (XO) 256–7

xanthomas 335
xanthophylls 146
xerophthalmia 144–5
xylitol 72–3, 75
xylulose 72
  reductase 72
xylulose-5-phosphate (X5P) 72, 169, 209

 Y

Y *see* tyrosine
YOPIs (young, old, pregnant, and
  immunocompromised) 300

 Z

zeaxanthin 147, 346–7
zinc (Zn) 118, 246–9, 317, 348–9, 355